PRAISE FOR

LIFE, LIBERTY, AND THE PURSUIT OF FOOD RIGHTS

"It seems far-fetched to think that 'police' in black suits would make an assault on what we-the-people have forever assumed was our right to eat what we want to eat. Based on an extraordinary journalistic investigation, David Gumpert makes a compelling case that we are witnessing a concerted national program to shut down the buying and selling of pure, wholesome, unadulterated food — farm by farm and state by state. These assaults, being carried out on farmers in the name of 'food safety,' are jeopardizing our basic liberties, which must include access to foods that keep us healthy. There is no bigger story, and Gumpert has told it in a compelling, highly readable fashion."

— **ABBY ROCKEFELLER**, president of The ReSource Institute for Low Entropy Systems and author of the scientific paper "Civilization and Sludge"

"The 18th century was the century of political rights; the 19th century was the century of women's rights; the 20th century was the century of civil rights. The challenge of the 21st century will be the struggle for food and farming rights. Thanks to the work of David Gumpert in chronicling this ongoing battle, we have a roadmap for establishing the right to access the foods of our choice. *Life, Liberty, and the Pursuit of Food Rights* is highly recommended for anyone interested in family farms and nutrient-dense food."

— **SALLY FALLON MORELL**, president of The Weston A. Price Foundation

"A wakeup call for anyone who eats, *Life, Liberty, and the Pursuit of Food Rights* is an exposé on the American government's calculated attack and sinister use of brute force on family farmers and consumers involved in the local food movement. Through harrowing tales of government spying and raids, David Gumpert demonstrates how complacency has allowed corporations to manipulate federal agencies and gain complete control of our entire food supply. If you care about what your family eats, read this book."

— **LINDA FAILLACE**, author of *Mad Sheep: The True Story of the USDA's War on a Family Farm*

"An issue this important should have its own revolutionary flag. The image would show a farmer and a neighbor exchanging food above the classic motto 'Don't tread on me.' This is a revolution that needs to happen. What could be more important to all of us than control over the quality of food we put in our bodies?"

— ELIOT COLEMAN, author of *The Winter Harvest Handbook,*
Four-Season Harvest, and *The New Organic Grower*

"With incredible clarity and masterful storytelling, David Gumpert leads us on a journey into the trenches of America's battle over food rights. No one knows this terrain and understands the implications as thoroughly as Gumpert, and the result is a book that will by turns enrage and inspire you. The battle for the right to nourish our bodies with real food must be won, and this book is an essential part of making that happen."

— BEN HEWITT, author of *The Town That Food Saved:*
How One Community Found Vitality in Local Food

"This book will get you fired up! David Gumpert makes an eloquent case for the importance of food rights and documents the actions of government regulators against small farms and buyers clubs. These infuriating stories are woven together and contextualized by Gumpert's insightful legal and political analysis. For anyone interested in reclaiming food, this book shows you that you are part of a larger political struggle."

— SANDOR ELLIX KATZ, author of *The Art of Fermentation,*
The Revolution Will Not Be Microwaved, and *Wild Fermentation*

"David Gumpert plucks out some of the most salient battles in this current food war and brings them to our awareness with the storytelling genius of a spy novel. The intrigue, the angst, the heartache, and the heroism are all displayed."

— JOEL SALATIN, from the Foreword

LIFE, LIBERTY
AND THE PURSUIT
OF FOOD RIGHTS

THE ESCALATING BATTLE OVER WHO
DECIDES *WHAT WE EAT*

DAVID E. GUMPERT
FOREWORD BY JOEL SALATIN

CHELSEA GREEN PUBLISHING
WHITE RIVER JUNCTION, VERMONT

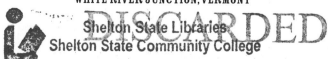

Project Manager: Hillary Gregory
Developmental Editor: Brianne Goodspeed
Copy Editor: Eric Raetz
Proofreader: Nancy Ringer
Indexer: Shana Milkie
Designer: Melissa Jacobson

Printed in the United States of America.
First printing May, 2013
10 9 8 7 6 5 4 3 2 1   13 14 15 16

green press
INITIATIVE

Chelsea Green Publishing is committed to preserving
ancient forests and natural resources. We elected to print
this title on 30-percent postconsumer recycled paper,
processed chlorine-free. As a result, for this printing, we
have saved:

18 Trees (40' tall and 6-8" diameter)
8 Million BTUs of Total Energy
1,550 Pounds of Greenhouse Gases
8,406 Gallons of Wastewater
563 Pounds of Solid Waste

Chelsea Green Publishing made this paper choice because
we and our printer, Thomson-Shore, Inc., are members
of the Green Press Initiative, a nonprofit program dedicated to supporting authors, publishers, and suppliers
in their efforts to reduce their use of fiber obtained
from endangered forests. For more information, visit:
www.greenpressinitiative.org.

Environmental impact estimates were made using the Environmental Defense Paper Calculator.
For more information visit: www.papercalculator.org.

Our Commitment to Green Publishing

Chelsea Green sees publishing as a tool for cultural change and ecological stewardship. We strive to align our book
manufacturing practices with our editorial mission and to reduce the impact of our business enterprise in the environment. We print our books and catalogs on chlorine-free recycled paper, using vegetable-based inks whenever possible.
This book may cost slightly more because it was printed on paper that contains recycled fiber, and we hope you'll
agree that it's worth it. Chelsea Green is a member of the Green Press Initiative (www.greenpressinitiative.org), a
nonprofit coalition of publishers, manufacturers, and authors working to protect the world's endangered forests and
conserve natural resources. Life, Liberty, and the Pursuit of Food Rights was printed on FSC®-certified paper supplied by
Thomson-Shore that contains at least 30% postconsumer recycled fiber.

Library of Congress Cataloging-in-Publication Data
Gumpert, David E.
 Life, liberty, and the pursuit of food rights : the escalating battle over who decides what we eat / David
E. Gumpert ; foreword by Joel Salatin.
    pages cm
 Includes bibliographical references and index.
 ISBN 978-1-60358-404-3 (pbk.) — ISBN 978-1-60358-405-0 (ebook)
 1. Food industry and trade — United States. 2. Local foods — United States. 3. Farmers' markets — United
States. 4. Food supply — Government policy — United States. 5. Food — Biotechnology — Government
policy — United States. I. Title.

 HD9005.G86 2013
 338.1'90973 — dc23
                          2013008071

Chelsea Green Publishing
85 North Main Street, Suite 120
White River Junction, VT 05001
(802) 295-6300
www.chelseagreen.com

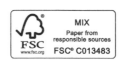

MIX
Paper from
responsible sources
FSC
www.fsc.org   FSC® C013483

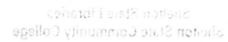

To the brave men and women,
some of whom are described in the pages that follow,
who are risking their personal security and livelihoods
so that many others may have access
to fresh and wholesome food.

CONTENTS

Foreword   ix

Abbreviations   xiv

The Players   xv

Introduction   1

1: A Daughter's Resolution   11

2: Is There Such a Thing as Private Food?   19

3: The Hundred-Year War against Raw Milk   37

4: "We Have Just Been . . . Handed a Fantastic Case!"   59

5: Local Food and Second Chances   81

6: The Violent Birth of the Food Rights Movement   99

7: Since When Are We Afraid of Food?   121

8: Food Rights and the Buzz Saw of Law Enforcement   147

9: The Flickering Promise of Food Sovereignty   179

10: The Search for a Rosa Parks Moment   199

    Epilogue   229

    Acknowledgments   233

    Appendix: Declaration of Food Independence   237

    Notes   238

    Index   252

FOREWORD

G rowing up in a middle-class, white, southern, Protestant home in the 1960s, I literally did not know about the abuses incurred daily by African Americans in our community. If any family was not prejudiced, it was ours. After all, my mom and dad had spent a decade in Venezuela buying land and starting a farm, only to have it expropriated in a coup when I was four years old.

Fleeing the back door as guerillas entered the front, we spent a few desperate weeks in Caracas trying to get protection for our property. The highest-level government ministers offered nothing but excuses. Unable to stay there, our family returned to the United States and found the cheapest, most worn-out piece of land in a three-state area.

We started over in Virginia's Shenandoah Valley, breadbasket of the Confederacy. Although our family was politically savvy, I don't remember any discussions about racial discrimination. The fifteen-minute drive from town (Staunton) to our farm took us by the county's black high school. After desegregation, which occurred in my preteen years, our integrated schools exposed me to numerous black kids and I became good friends with many of them.

At least once, our family visited the largest African American church in the area during a special participatory performance of "Negro spirituals." We were the only white family there. I still remember how slow they sang "Swing Low, Sweet Chariot." In our white circles, we always sang it upbeat, but the African Americans sang it in a drawn-out, contemplative, yearning attitude. It was extremely moving, and with more mature retrospect, I can only imagine why slaves would not sing it in a joyous, upbeat demeanor.

In my white circles, as a teen, I don't remember discussing racial prejudice or being exposed to anything about abuses against African Americans. For several years our little independent church group met Sundays in a black Seventh-Day Adventist Church, which, to my child's eyes, offered numerous fleeting interactions with the owners. They were always clean, courteous, and professional.

At today's mid-fifties juncture of my life and awareness, I'm discomfited by my ignorance about what was happening in our culture at the time. It rattles my spirit. It scares me. What am I allowing myself to be apathetic and ignorant about today? Will my grandchildren think me myopic, cowardly, or even complicit in some terrible injustice of our day? I can imagine them trying to figure out why Grandpa never apprised them of this wrong, this abuse. Allowed to persist, perhaps, and enslaving them in the natural extensions of unchecked abuse, would these injustices make them resentful toward my inaction, my disinterest?

In today's world, injustice exists on many fronts. We could argue whether it's worse than ever, but certainly our exposure via electronic communication saturates our lives with its sordid details in unprecedented volume. The problem with injustice is that it generally starts benevolently.

Prohibition started as a backlash against alcoholism. The War on Terror started as vengeance for 9/11. Affirmative action started as remuneration for racial discrimination and slavery. The Food Safety and Inspection Service started as a solution to the abuses in mega processing plants exposed by Upton Sinclair's *The Jungle*.

Oh, you were with me just fine until that last one, I'll bet. Up until 1908, food enjoyed unregulated commerce. The fact that neither the Declaration of Independence nor the U.S. Constitution ever mentions the word *food* indicates that it was such a ubiquitous and common part of human experience that the framers of our country couldn't imagine its restriction. Like air for breathing or sunshine for growing plants.

But today, the U.S. government denies perhaps the most fundamental right: freedom of food choice. After all, what good is it to possess the right to own guns, assemble, speak, or worship if we can't choose good fuel for our bodies to propel us to shoot, pray, or preach? Is not food even more basic than religion? What religion can you practice without food?

In America, this great land of plenty, why would I even mention access to food? Isn't every supermarket full of food? What's the problem? After all, we have all sorts of choice. We can get milk from any number of suppliers, right? Wrong. What if it's raw milk?

Look at the meat case. It's full of choices. But what if you want chicken untouched by chlorine? That's a different story. What if I'd rather buy chicken from my neighbor, who dresses a few hundred in her backyard every year?

In the name of food safety and fueled by a veritable paranoia toward food, the U.S. government has declared war on people who would dare to exercise their most fundamental human right to choose their food. Ultimately, this ideological clash is over who owns me as an individual.

Who owns me? God? My neighbor? Society? If I am simply a societal asset, like copper fittings on an assembly line, then certainly society has a justified vested interest in keeping me from engaging in risky behavior that may land me in the hospital or an insane asylum. It has an interest in keeping me out of churches that may make me an unproductive societal asset.

But what if society does not own me? What if I am free to practice my own beliefs and actions, even if someone considers them risky? Generally, personal rights extend as far as my neighbor's nose. I can be noisy unless the noise infringes on my neighbor's property. I can move my cow around wherever I want to, but not on my neighbor's property. I can make a compost pile on my property, but it can't spill over on my neighbor's. And I can cut a tree on my property, but I can't cut my neighbor's.

How much personal liberty can society tolerate? The founders of America decided it should be quite a lot, actually. Perhaps more than in any other civilization in history. But in the name of protection and security, our leaders are taking away these rights to free exercise, essentially criminalizing whatever fringe activity dares question governmental orthodoxy.

This assault on food is simply another permutation of Prohibition and the war on drugs. To demonize and criminalize something as fundamental to self-actualization and personal liberty as drinking and eating, to subject this most basic human function to the strong arm of the government, is an abusive overreach that our founders would find intolerable. The most tragic part of this injustice is that most people don't have a clue it's happening — and most don't even care.

An entire alternative scientific and personal belief system exists in our day. It disagrees vehemently with such audacious agencies as the U.S. Centers for Disease Control, the U.S. Food and Drug Administration, the U.S. Department of Agriculture, and the Food Safety and Inspection Service.

What does a culture do with its fringe folks? Does it arrest them and stand them before the inquisitors, pulling them apart on the regulators' rack?

The Romans had an axiom that you could tell a lot about the strength of a society by the number of laws it has. The stronger a society, the more it can abide differing opinions and lifestyles. The more fragile and weak a society, the more laws it needs to keep freethinkers from questioning orthodoxy.

David Gumpert is a quintessential journalist. Impeccable to a fault, he plucks out some of the most salient battles in this current food war and brings them to our awareness with the storytelling genius of a spy novel. The intrigue, the angst, the heartache, and the heroism are all displayed to bring the personal element to something perversely impersonal . . . at least to those he calls our nation's food police.

My growing awareness of how our culture treated Native Americans and African Americans causes deep remorse. That is good, healing, cleansing. I would like to think that had I been living in those critical days of the most egregious injustice, I would have tried to stop it. Indeed, would I have gone along with Pizarro and the conquistadors as they slaughtered the Incas in Peru?

You see, the very freedom to feed my child foods that I think will nourish her brain development and keep her away from hospitals is at stake. The very freedom to acquire for my own body the health-giving foods I believe it demands no longer exists. To equate this to these terribly unjust cultural clashes between native and immigrant or slave and free is a fair assessment of the current food struggle.

If we as a culture do not become concerned, aware, and participatory in this great clash over life, liberty, and the pursuit of food rights, will our children's children forgive us for standing by while the government-corporate-industrial food complex destroyed their freedom to choose raw over pasteurized, homemade over processed, living over dead? As you read this book, realize that for every story Gumpert publicizes, countless threatening letters, sick children, and food farmers with destroyed integrity remain anonymous.

May this book awaken in each of us a righteous anger toward government injustice and a burning desire to encourage with words and patronage these heroes who dare to defy the powers of our day. These are my heroes. It's one thing to fight when the culture is backing you. It's quite another to fight your culture when it's wrong. You will join the ranks of those who know about this desperate struggle. It's more important than gun rights, tax rights, retirement rights, or education rights.

Thank you, David Gumpert, for giving all of us the information we need to bolster our resolve in this historic struggle. May we devote ourselves afresh to being food freedom allies.

— JOEL SALATIN

ABBREVIATIONS

CDC: U.S. Centers for Disease Control and Prevention

CDFA: California Department of Food and Agriculture

CFSAN: Center for Food Safety and Applied Nutrition (part of the FDA)

CSA: community supported agriculture

CSO: Consumer Safety Officer (for the FDA)

DATCP: Wisconsin Department of Agriculture, Trade, and Consumer Protection

FDA: U.S. Food and Drug Administration

FTCLDF: Farm-to-Consumer Legal Defense Fund

GDA: Georgia Department of Agriculture

IMGC: International Milk Genomics Consortium

LLC: limited liability company

MDA: Minnesota Department of Agriculture

ODA: Ohio Department of Agriculture

RTCHF: Right to Choose Healthy Food

USDA: U.S. Department of Agriculture

THE PLAYERS

DANIEL ALLGYER: A lanky, soft-spoken Amish farmer from Lancaster County, Pennsylvania, who provided food to a budding food club in Maryland as a way to escape the impersonal commodity food system.

VICTORIA BLOCH: A Los Angeles graphic designer who spent her weekends manning farmer Sharon Palmer's booth at several farmers markets.

KARINE BOUIS-TOWE: A young mother and one-time U.S. Labor Department employee. Bouis-Towe formed the Washington DC–area food club Grassfed on the Hill and recruited Amish farmer Daniel Allgyer to be its supplier.

KARL DAHLSTROM: The founder of ProAdvocate, a legal advisory organization. Dahlstrom took over legal oversight of several food clubs and Amish farmers from Aajonus Vonderplanitz's Right to Choose Healthy Food.

DENISE DIXON: A raw milk cheese aficionado and articulate mother of twelve. Dixon started as an unpaid intern at Morningland Dairy and eventually became one of its owners.

MICHELLE DOFFING-BAYNES: The Minneapolis assistant city attorney charged with prosecuting Minnesota farmer and food club organizer Alvin Schlangen.

DON FALLS: A veteran inspector with the Missouri Milk Board who oversaw the state's investigation of Morningland Dairy.

ROSS GOLDSTEIN: A U.S. Justice Department lawyer who oversaw a federal investigation into Amish farmer David Hochstetler of Indiana.

NATHAN HANSEN: The defense lawyer for Minnesota farmer Alvin Schlangen who argued his case before a Minneapolis jury.

VERNON HERSHBERGER: A Wisconsin dairy farmer who left an Amish community as an adult. Hershberger became a target of Wisconsin regulators who sought to shut down his tiny farm store serving 200 local food club members.

MARY HETHERINGTON: A young mom in the midst of building a new home north of Los Angeles who was attracted to invest in Sharon Palmer's effort to launch a new farm in Ventura County.

DAVID HOCHSTETLER: A tall, full-bearded Amish farmer from Indiana who provides food clubs in the Midwest with raw milk.

DONALD HOENIG: The Maine state veterinarian who oversaw a state investigation into raw dairy farms over a possible connection with illnesses from a parasite.

KATHRYN NIFLIS JOHNSON: A holistic health counselor who had trained as a registered nurse and was a member of two Minneapolis-area food clubs. She became a key court witness in a case involving one club.

MAX KANE: A Wisconsin food club organizer who became an activist after the Wisconsin attorney general sought to force him to disclose names of farmers who supplied his food club.

WILLIAM MARLER: A dead ringer for Newt Gingrich, in both voice and appearance, Marler nearly single-handedly elevated food safety into a high-priority legal and policy issue.

AMOS MILLER: An upbeat entrepreneurial Amish owner of a farm just a few miles from Daniel Allgyer's farm in Pennsylvania's Lancaster County.

LARRY OTTING: A successful Venice Beach real estate investor who used his good credit to help Sharon Palmer buy her Ventura County farm.

SHARON PALMER: Fresh off felony convictions and jail time for defrauding elderly victims in a mortgage scam, this single mother of three was trying to begin life anew as a Southern California chicken and dairy farmer.

LIZ REITZIG: A passionate advocate of raw milk who helped organize a national food rights group that committed itself to engaging in civil disobedience to challenge the U.S. Food and Drug Administration's actions against raw dairy farmers.

HEATHER RETBERG: The owner of a small Maine dairy and chicken farm who became an activist on behalf of food sovereignty by local towns in the state.

BRAD ROGERS: An Indiana sheriff who became involved in trying to head off FDA enforcement efforts against Amish farmer David Hochstetler.

RAE LYNN SANDVIG: A homeschooling suburban Minneapolis mother of four whose home was raided by local public health and police officials seeking evidence she was reselling food from a local farmer after she made her driveway and garage available as a neighborhood food drop site.

ALVIN SCHLANGEN: This Minnesota egg farmer became a target of state regulators and prosecutors when he formed a food club. Schlangen was abandoned by several members of his family as a result.

JOHN SHEEHAN: Director of the FDA's dairy division and the government's most ardent opponent of raw milk.

JAMES STEWART: He helped resuscitate raw milk in California at the turn of the century and formed the Rawesome food club, which became a target of numerous local, state, and federal agencies.

SCARLETT TREVISO: A veteran senior investigator with the California Department of Food and Agriculture (CDFA) who initiated and led the investigation of Sharon Palmer and the Rawesome food club.

AAJONUS VONDERPLANITZ: An evangelist for raw milk and other raw foods, he originated an animal-leasing arrangement between food clubs and small farms that became a target of food police around the country.

KEN WARD: A senior investigator with the Los Angeles district attorney, he became a key player in the undercover investigation of the Rawesome food club.

INTRODUCTION

Sometime late in the evening of Sunday, June 17, 2012, enforcement agents at a northern Florida weigh station operated by the state's department of agriculture pulled over a large refrigerated truck barreling down I-95. It had just crossed from Georgia into Florida, carrying a substantial load of goods, including about $45,000 worth of food from two Pennsylvania farms destined for several hundred members of three private food clubs in the Miami–Fort Lauderdale area. The agents asked the driver for his bills of lading, which are the legal documents between the shippers and trucker detailing what is being delivered and to whom.

The enforcement agents didn't like what they saw — apparently they considered the bills of lading too terse — so the agents told the driver they needed to look inside. As one agent began opening boxes, he noticed some bottles containing brown liquid, labeled KOMBUCHA. He called for agents from the Florida Department of Alcohol, Tobacco, and Firearms.

"Moonshine," said an agent.

"That can't be moonshine," said the driver.

"Shut up!" the agent told the driver, slapping handcuffs on the man.

Next into the truck were agents from the Florida Department of Agriculture and Consumer Services Food Safety Division. They opened more boxes and didn't like what they saw either. Boxes of beef, chicken, and pork — all missing United States Department of Agriculture (USDA) stamps, indicating they came from custom slaughterhouses and not facilities regularly monitored by the USDA. Fermented vegetables and cheeses labeled in black magic marker with the most basic descriptions — SAUERKRAUT and GOAT CHEESE.

The driver was thrown into a Jacksonville-area jail, charged with a third-degree felony for illegally shipping alcoholic beverages into the state. The cargo, the hundreds of pounds of farm-fresh food, was ordered taken to a landfill. Under Florida law, food that is confiscated because of concerns about its origins and safety is usually set aside pending a court hearing. But if the inspectors judge it to be "poisonous," it can be dumped immediately. And so that Monday morning, within hours of being seized, hundreds of pounds of fresh meat, dairy products, eggs, fermented vegetables, and other foods were trucked over to a local landfill, dumped, and buried. The farmers who shipped the food, and the members of the food club receiving it, didn't have insurance covering it, so together they were out the $45,000. In addition, the trucking company was assessed a dumping fee of nearly $2,000, which was charged to the farmers.

That wasn't the end of the incident. Before the week was out, Pennsylvania state police were visiting the trucking company, inquiring into the circumstances of the shipment. An agent from the USDA was visiting with the managers of one of the Florida food clubs, warning them that it was against the law to ship meat not inspected by the USDA across state lines. One of the Pennsylvania farmers whose food was on the truck was noticing strange cars cruising back and forth and parking outside his farm.

I heard about the incident a few days after it occurred, via an e-mail from a friend of one of the farmers whose food was on the truck. "Breaking News!" was the subject line of his e-mail. He figured I'd want to broadcast on my blog this troubling incident of government authorities interfering in people's access to food.

He was partially correct. As a journalist, my first instinct was to confirm what happened, and then publish an account of this seemingly outrageous incident exclusively on my blog, The Complete Patient (www.thecomplete patient.com). But my second instinct, as an advocate journalist — one who has covered for five years the emergence of the food rights movement and sympathizes with its concerns about attempts to limit access to certain food — was to hesitate while mulling over some questions.

Was this food seizure and disposal a setup, possibly arranged by the U.S. Food and Drug Administration (FDA) and/or the USDA, to ensnare the farmers in a legal morass aimed at shutting them down? There had been any number of "stings" and undercover investigations of small farms around the country over the previous five years. If it was a setup, how much did the authorities know? For example, did they know about only one farmer, or both?

If it was an isolated incident, then publicizing it might give the federal authorities information that they didn't have and encourage them to go after the farmers. My particular fear was of the FDA, since it had become especially aggressive in enforcing food laws — especially concerning the distribution of raw milk — against farmers. I didn't know for sure if raw milk was even on the truck, though I assumed it was. In any event, I didn't want to be responsible via my blog for putting one or another farmer in danger of a protracted and expensive legal tangle with the FDA.

If it was a setup, a sting operation of some kind, then I would want to report on it — but only after I felt comfortable about what the authorities knew and didn't know. I had long made it a professional rule to try my best to avoid endangering farmers and food clubs by releasing information that could become intelligence for the food police.

Over the next few weeks, it became increasingly apparent that the seizure was an isolated incident. A local prosecutor decided not to file charges against the driver. The strange cars stopped cruising by one of the farms. There were no official actions against the farmers or the Florida food clubs whose members had ordered the food. The main hassle, aside from the financial loss on the confiscated food, appeared to be that the farmers had to shift to a different trucker, since the original one decided it didn't want to risk any more such problems.

Still, the event stayed with me long after it had seemingly blown over (and I felt enough time had elapsed to discuss it here, without naming names). For one thing, I couldn't easily get over the fact that the Florida officials had so quickly condemned, and then disposed of, so much perfectly good food. Couldn't they have checked a little further to find out who was getting the food? If there was a violation of labeling requirements, couldn't there have been a warning — or even a fine — and a commitment to straightening out the labeling problem in the future? I spoke with officials in the Florida agencies, and they basically said the decision was made by the agents on the scene, and that they had followed "policy."

Had our national concerns about food safety become so obsessive that agriculture agents would, within hours, send to a landfill $45,000 worth of food that they could tell was fresh and wholesome from a simple taste and smell? If they had concerns about pathogens, couldn't they have quickly tested samples?

I was bothered as well by the fact that the farmers and food club members I consulted about the situation felt reluctant to complain about what had happened. There had been many other similarly sad and upsetting events concerning the distribution of fresh-from-the-farm food, especially dairy and meat; everyone felt intimidated about making a fuss, and possibly bringing down even greater penalties than the confiscation and disposal of $45,000 worth of good food. The attitude didn't seem that far removed from that of women who are sexually harassed on the job or in the military and feel intimidated about complaining, knowing there could be reprisals.

I was also unnerved personally that I had felt compelled to compromise my journalistic instincts and recommend to the farmers and food club members that we pull back from reporting on a questionable exercise of authority. Questionable on so many levels — to dispose of so much good food during a time when people are going hungry, to dump that food in a landfill when we are all needing to rethink the amount of waste we produce on a finite planet, and to confiscate a significant amount of private property from people without even a hint of due process of law.

Complicating my own concerns about my journalistic instincts was the knowledge that, outrageous as the incident seemed to me, it likely wouldn't seem that way to other journalists. They would be inclined to accept the explanation of Florida authorities that the food had been judged unsafe, and thus required immediate disposal — if they were even interested in the event at all. In my experience covering this sort of story over the previous five years, more often than not few or no members of the media question regulatory judgment about food safety, whether at the state or federal level. What the Centers for Disease Control and Prevention (CDC), FDA, and state public health and agriculture authorities determine is "safe" or "dangerous" is typically accepted; the few individuals like me who question them are seen as reckless and unconcerned about public health.

Finally, I was unnerved by a larger issue: the huge and expanding amount of authority we have entrusted to geographically remote and seemingly arbitrary government officials to regulate our food. This applied not just to the mass-produced food sold in supermarkets, big box stores, convenience stores, and other retail outlets, but increasingly to food exchanges that have traditionally been out of their view and authority — church suppers, bake sales, neighborhood lemonade stands, and agreements between farmers and their neighbors for the sale of food direct from a farm.

This extension of regulation has happened to coincide with the growing popularity among Americans to obtain more and more of their foods directly from farmers and other producers, including some people who go to extraordinary lengths to access food they consider healthy and wholesome. The result is a tension between regulators attempting to impose the rules of the marketplace and individuals who consider themselves to be operating privately, outside of the marketplace and beyond the purview of government.

The fear and powerlessness underlying the Florida food confiscation was representative as well of a Wild West atmosphere that now prevails around the issue of "private food," so that it's not always clear who the enemy is. To Americans determined to choose what foods to put into their bodies without the government getting in the way, the regulators and agents who are interfering with those choices have taken on the role of the Wild West's outlaws and renegades. Yet to the regulators and agents, these farmers and consumers are the outlaws and renegades.

The struggle has been cast by regulators as one in which food safety must take precedence over "food rights." For those targeted by the authorities, the struggle is more fundamental; it's about expanding government control into ever more areas of our lives versus individual freedoms promised by the American Revolution and the U.S. Constitution that grew out of it.

This struggle over private food rights appears to be unique to America (and its cousin to the north, Canada, on a smaller scale). In no other countries that I am aware of is such a struggle — pitting government authorities against groups of ordinary citizens trying to access farm-fresh food — presently going on, aside from countries like North Korea and Cuba where control of the food supply is part of the totalitarian effort to control the population.

All of which raises some fundamental questions: When did we lose our right to buy whatever food we want directly from farmers and assorted food producers, outside of the regulatory system of permits and inspections? Or stated more fundamentally, when did the custom of people exchanging food — a natural and essential part of community-based life and commerce since nearly the beginning of humankind — become transformed into such an intense source of conflict that it now is being cast as a "right"?

Was it in 1788 when the U.S. Constitution was ratified without making a single mention of the word "food"?

Was it in 1906 when Congress enacted the Pure Food and Drug Act, and the first regulators were hired to watch over our food system?

Was it immediately after World War II, when the memories of the Great Depression and rationing caused by wartime shortages were still fresh in people's minds, and we committed to modernizing and improving our agriculture sector's productivity?

Was it in the 1950s and 1960s, when many states outlawed unpasteurized milk, and in the process outlawed the sale of raw dairy products or confined such sales to farms that obtained special permits?

Was it in the 1970s, when Secretary of Agriculture Earl Butz repeatedly urged farmers to "get big or get out"?

Was it in 1987, when the FDA, in response to a federal court order, enacted a regulation outlawing the interstate shipment of unpasteurized dairy products?

Was it in 1995, when a Seattle product liability lawyer earned $15.6 million in a settlement of a food-borne illness case caused by a fast-food chain's tainted hamburgers, the largest settlement at that time for damages associated with such illness?

Was it in the aftermath of the 9/11 terrorist attacks on the United States, when food security and bioterrorism became big concerns?

Was it in spring 2011, when public health inspectors issued cease-and-desist orders to shut down ForageSF, an underground food market in San Francisco that gathered monthly for producers of everything from kimchi to chocolate cupcakes, selling to members who paid $5 to join each event? A few months later when San Francisco public health officials shut down a nursery school bake sale? Or the Friday night a couple months after that when a Nevada public health inspector tried to halt a farm's private fork-to-plate event just as dozens of guests were preparing to sit down to an elegant dinner of lamb meatballs and fresh vegetables?

Or was it in September 2011, when a judge in Wisconsin, the nation's "Dairy State," in ruling on a case involving the distribution of raw milk by two farmers there, declared that they "do not have a fundamental right to own and use a dairy cow" and "do not have a fundamental right to consume the milk from their own cow"?[1]

Surely it wasn't any single event, but by the end of the first decade of the twenty-first century, the quickening pace of legal and enforcement challenges demonstrated that the once universally accepted custom of farmers, friends, and neighbors exchanging food without regulatory oversight had been so reduced in consciousness that it was actually under official attack — and that the right to privately obtain the foods of one's choice was in jeopardy across the United States and Canada. In the process of simultaneously promoting cheap food and fomenting fear around the dangers of pathogens in food, something strange has occurred. Traditional avenues of private food acquisition have gradually disappeared.

I can remember seemingly endless farm stands as I traveled across the United States in the 1950s and 1960s. I can also recall various produce trucks with vegetables, meats, and eggs that traversed our neighborhood in Chicago during that time. Even after I became a homeowner in suburban Boston in the late 1970s, we had a milk man and a chicken-egg man who came around with farm-fresh food.

Over the last few years, with the growing interest in fresh locally grown food and fears about commercially available food and the presence of genetically modified organisms (GMOs) and processed ingredients, more people have begun trying to re-create these traditional sources of privately obtained food via members-only food clubs and communal ownership of cows and goats. Many of these efforts were originally begun to secure sources of the increasingly popular unpasteurized milk and then expanded to include beef, chicken, eggs, honey, fermented vegetables, and other so-called nutrient-dense foods.

Unfortunately, when groups of ordinary people began organizing themselves to obtain food directly from farms on a private basis, they ran into trouble. Such foods weren't properly labeled, they were told. Such foods weren't safe. The producers required retail licenses. Such foods needed to be inspected by public health and agriculture regulators. The stories of the farmers and organizers entangled in the enforcement crackdown are the basis of this book.

In the big picture of history, the conflict is sadly ironic, since these battles aren't happening in a time of food scarcity or widespread outbreaks of animal or human illness, but rather during a period of seeming abundance and plenty.

Throughout history, food has often had a political tinge. Food shortages fomented the French Revolution and a number of riots in nineteenth-century America. As recently as the 1930s and 1940s, food availability was a major problem for members of my family. My aunt, Inge Joseph, spent her teen years hiding from the Nazis in the French countryside with one hundred other children; sometimes they had to make do eating plants and herbs scavenged from the woods. My mother, who was lucky enough to escape the Holocaust by being sent to the United States in the years just before World War II, often went to bed hungry while living with foster families in Chicago, who themselves were so financially strapped by the difficulties associated with the Great Depression and World War II that they couldn't afford enough food for a growing teenager.

Food shortages have been nearly unknown to members of the baby boomer generation that began sprouting in the years after World War II. In those years of readjustment, America's political and industrial leaders came up with a uniquely modern capitalist solution to chronic worries about food supplies and prices: use the principles of automation and economies of scale learned from manufacturing automobiles, radios, textiles, and shoes to mass-produce food. The key mass-production tools would be newly developed fertilizers, powerful pesticides, and huge tractors, combines, and balers. The results would be the same as with manufactured goods — we'd lower unit costs and increase production, creating such vast quantities that there would be abundant cheap food. Politicians wouldn't have to worry about the populace having empty stomachs and could focus instead on getting people to spend all the money saved on food for other things, like homes, cars, furniture, and televisions — thereby growing the economy.

The strategy seemed to work in important ways. It reduced the burden of food as a component of living expenses for all Americans. Since World War II, the percentage of income the average American family spends on food has declined by nearly half, from 22 percent in 1951[2] to 15 percent in 1980, and from there to 12 percent in 2008.[3] Macro-economically it seemed to work as well, in the sense that the American economy exploded after World War II, and other countries around the world have adopted at least some of our cheap-food technologies to grow their economies as well. Thus, even though baby boomers like me have lived through five wars since the end of World War II (Korea, Vietnam, Iraq I, Afghanistan, Iraq II), not one of them has led to even a hint of food shortages.

Unfortunately, the industrialization of food has had a number of serious consequences: environmental pollution (from all the manure the mass-produced pigs, cattle, and chickens generate); poisoning of our food with pesticides; excessive processing and reliance on sugar, which may play a role in exploding obesity and diabetes rates; the overuse of antibiotics, which has likely encouraged the development of antibiotic-resistant bacteria; and the introduction of previously unknown pathogens into our food. But while the pollution, poisoning, and processing have likely led to huge increases in chronic disease, it's the pathogens that our public health establishment has identified as the most serious public health risk at hand. Indeed, it has used a few highly publicized outbreaks of illness to convince legislators, judges, and consumers that we have been lax in protecting the public from food-borne illness, and that we must do more to stamp out pathogens. Even though the CDC counts only 13,000 to 27,000 cases of food-borne illness each year, the agency argues (using complex and, frankly, convoluted mathematical modeling) that the real number is nearly 50 million, since it assumes huge numbers of cases aren't reported.

From a business perspective, there is almost no way food quality couldn't suffer from industrialization. The overriding incentive for producers under the "get-big-or-get-out" philosophy is to continually lower costs so as to increase profit margins. That means (without some kind of technological magic of the sort that has lowered the cost of computers and other digital technologies) lowering the quality of food inputs — cheaper animal feed, more crowding of farm animals, greater use of antibiotics to counter disease threats from the crowding, reliance on hormones or other artificial agents to speed animal growth, and adding cheap fillers and flavorings.

It's one thing to cheapen the inputs on furniture and refrigerators (we all know those things generally don't last like they used to), but quite another to cheapen stuff we are putting into our bodies. Gradually we have learned some of the effects. For example, much of the meat sold in American super-markets and other retail outlets like Wal-Mart contains residues of antibi-otics, which may be contributing to the expansion of antibiotic-resistant bacterial illnesses, and possibly three-fourths or more of chicken contains the pathogens campylobacter or salmonella.[4]

Corporate food producers, of course, don't want to tell customers that the quality of mass-produced food has been declining. So they have fostered the notion, backed up by the public health and medical communities, that all food is the same nutritionally, whether conventional or organic, CAFO (confined animal feeding operations) beef or beef raised on a small local farm, mass-produced eggs or eggs produced from chickens that spend time on pasture and searching out bugs. This is despite research suggesting that eggs, for instance, can differ in the amount of nutrients and cholesterol they contain depending on what the chickens are fed, or that unpasteurized milk helps counter asthma and allergies in children. Most of the emphasis from the medical and public health communities is on steering clear of disease by avoiding "bad" foods like excessive fats and sugar, as opposed to ingesting naturally produced nutrient-dense foods like fermented and locally produced vegetables or even acknowledging that there are "good" animal fats.

The cheap-food push fosters the perception that price is the prime differentiator among foods — cheaper is better, and cheapest is best. I know any number of health-conscious people who diligently exercise and eat low-fat, low-sugar foods and yet seek out the cheapest supermarket chicken, eggs, and milk — paying no heed to the likelihood that the animals that produced the food were raised in dirty and unbelievably crowded conditions, and that their products likely contain antibiotic residues to counter disease from the filth. They try not to think about the possibility that they could join the rapidly growing number of, for example, women experiencing chronic urinary tract infections that antibiotics can't help. These same people will turn away from chickens raised on small farms and pasture that cost two dollars a pound more as "too expensive."

Finally, the focus on safety has led to confusion between "bacteria" and "pathogens." Bacteria, of course, come in both friendly and unfriendly forms, and there is growing appreciation that the friendly forms are ever more essential to building up our immune systems. But our growing obsession with "safety" has led regulators to push ever harder to sanitize our food system by enforcing standards and processes that eliminate all bacteria.

What happens when a lot of people begin to demand food devoid of the problems that industrialization has fostered? When they begin demanding real food, raised the old-fashioned way? For starters, we begin to see new forms of "community" take shape as people organize privately to obtain food they think will be more healthful — for example, uncommon alliances among suburban soccer moms and Amish farmers, involved arrangements between urban professionals and small farms miles outside the city to coordinate food purchases and group deliveries, and efforts by city folks to pool their funds to launch community-based farms.

All of which means there is a second question that needs to be asked in addition to the one I posed about when we lost the right to obtain the foods of our choice directly from farmers and other producers: How do we get that right back? That is the focus of this book.

CHAPTER 1

A DAUGHTER'S RESOLUTION

There's never a good time to lose your mother. It's made sadder when you feel your mother suffered because she didn't care properly for her physical health. I had that experience when my mother died in 2007. While she lived to the seemingly ripe age of eighty-five, she spent the last dozen or so years of her life dealing with a series of ever-worsening health problems — hip pain, exacerbated by excess weight, that made walking torturous; a recurrence of breast cancer; edema that created terrible swelling in her legs (probably a sign of heart failure). And those were just the worst problems.

During that time, I tried to encourage my mother to exercise — even hiring a physical trainer to work with her for several months in hopes she would latch on to a customized routine — and to eat healthy foods. But she wouldn't latch on to either the exercise or the diet. Food was especially problematic. She had a sweet tooth and loved carb-heavy meals with pasta or potatoes and a rich dessert, often topped off by a Swiss chocolate bar. I even bought her a juicer and tried making her fresh vegetable smoothies, as a way to steer her toward healthy foods. She would sip the smoothies and smile kindly at my suggestions that she incorporate such foods into her meals, but she made clear in her failure to adopt new eating habits that she never truly believed good food could make a difference in her health. She had more faith in the doctors, with their surgical solutions and their prescription pills. When my mother finally died in her sleep, it was almost a relief — an end to the ever-increasing suffering she was going through while confined to a wheelchair and living in a nursing home.

So when I met Karine Bouis-Towe in 2011 — a mother of two young children in Washington DC — and asked what got her interested in devoting herself to making healthy food more available in her community, I could relate to the story of her journey being precipitated by her mother's death in 2004. Her mother's circumstances were more dramatic than mine, if only because she was struck down at age fifty-five by ovarian cancer. Bouis-Towe's response to the tragedy was more dramatic than mine as well; she took the traumatic event as a challenge. She was used to challenges — at the time, she was an overachieving professional helping manage a huge database for the U.S. Department of Labor. "I was determined not to feel helpless regarding my fears of cancer — my mother's death made me question everything. I wanted to feel more secure about living a long, productive life. My mother was wise but she grew up during the era of 'doctors know best' and she followed their advice in ways that I question now that she has passed on. My mother was a good cook but natural ingredients and nutrient density were not an emphasis in her cooking."

In the interests of making a full commitment to learning about and searching out a healthier way of eating, Bouis-Towe decided to give up her high-intensity career path. "It required way too much responsibility outside of normal business hours," especially given that she had just become a mom: "I decided I would be different; I would find a diet that was in line with my heritage — making food from scratch, obtaining the raw ingredients from local farms, and minimizing my visits to the grocery store. I was already vegetable gardening and eating food mostly without chemical additives. My goal was to use food as my medicine, along with minimizing unnecessary stress and staying active both mentally and physically."

Bouis-Towe's search led her way beyond organic and into an exploration of "traditional diets of healthy cultures." That led her, first, to "fresh, unheated milk" — better known as raw milk.

It had nearly disappeared from the American food scene following World War II — the result of the nearly universal conclusion by America's public health and agriculture professionals, following large-scale disease outbreaks in the late 1800s and early 1900s, that raw milk constituted a serious health risk from an assortment of pathogens potentially passed on by cows and their manure. By the 1980s and 1990s, raw milk was consumed mainly by small clusters of health advocates, many of them in California. But with the closure there in the late 1990s of the largest raw dairy in the country (which had shipped widely out of state), raw milk became ever less accessible — except from reclusive Amish farmers scattered in small eastern and Midwestern communities, mainly in Pennsylvania, Ohio, Indiana, and Minnesota.

The Amish are mysterious to most of us, mysterious because they keep to themselves. They place a premium on family, community, religious observance, and tradition. The tradition part is so powerful that they have persisted with the old-time ways of living — forgoing modern technology like cars and computers as well as living off the electric grid. The women dress in bonnets and plain cotton dresses and shawls, and the men in white or blue cotton collared shirts and black trousers (without zippers) held up by suspenders. The children play on scooters and metal tricycles. Thousands of tourists visit the largest enclave of Amish, in Pennsylvania's Lancaster County, each year to experience and observe a long-past era. The Amish oblige the tourists by selling them trinkets, jams, relishes, and even horse-and-buggy rides.

Beyond cultural tourism, however, Amish traditions have become important to a growing number of Americans — ordinary Americans who have become worried about the hormones, antibiotics, and other drugs that are used in raising most farm animals, and the effects of processing and chemical additives on other staples like milk and cereals. The Amish have a rich agricultural tradition. Most avoid the fertilizers, hormones, and antibiotics commonly used by American farmers. Equally significant, most avoid monoculture — raising just one or two crops. Their tendency toward agricultural diversity means they rotate crops and raise various animals like dairy cows, pigs, and chickens. The farms tend to be run sustainably, which means the cows eat grass and live alongside chickens and pigs, with the manure from all the animals helping replenish the soil for new grass as well as vegetables and grains. The calves stay with their mothers and nurse for some weeks, instead of being immediately separated and fed formula. And the cattle and pigs are slaughtered right on the farm — with a bullet from a revolver to the brain. A local Mennonite butcher cuts up the carcasses and ages the meat.

There are some Amish who have adopted the more "modern" agricultural techniques, confining animals in close quarters or relying on pesticides, often for the same reasons as other farmers — to increase production, and earnings, by selling into the conventional food system. But by and large, there's no need for energy-intensive tractors and tillers and artificial fertilizers, no need for proprietary Monsanto seeds, no need for feeds filled in with genetically modified (GM) soy or laced with antibiotics, no necessity to purchase hormones to help the animals grow faster and fatter, no need to shop for cattle semen to breed the cows, and no need to ship cattle and pigs on expensive rides to far-off slaughterhouses.

For much of the last half of the twentieth century, the Amish and their old ways of growing food were a curiosity at best — a relic of a nearly forgotten past, of little interest to DC professionals, FDA scientists, and U.S. Justice Department lawyers. Indeed, in a number of places like Pennsylvania and New York, the Amish have been squeezed off their land as prices have risen while their markets for agricultural products have failed to grow — or declined. Some Amish have migrated from Pennsylvania to Indiana, Kentucky, Wisconsin, and other spots in the Midwest to seek out cheaper land.

But a shift in attitudes about food during the early and middle years of this century's first decade meant changes for the Amish. Suddenly, the old-fashioned and seemingly outdated ways of the Amish became cool, or maybe I should say hot, to people like Karine Bouis-Towe. When she began her search for healthy food in 2005, the Amish didn't have a huge market for unpasteurized milk outside their own communities. Typical of the Amish dairy farmers was Daniel Allgyer, whose thirty-cow dairy was representative of what you find in Lancaster County, between Philadelphia and Harrisburg.

Like many of his neighbors, Allgyer sold into the huge wholesale dairy market. Every few days a tanker truck would come creeping down his long farm driveway and cart off all the milk his cows produced. Some weeks later, he'd receive a check for an amount dependent upon how much butterfat the milk contained and how much of various types of naturally occurring bacteria it included. The more the butterfat and the lower the bacteria counts, the higher the price he received. Generally, it worked out to between $2 and $2.50 a gallon.

But by 2005, there were more and more consumers like Bouis-Towe researching food and health and concluding that the brief intense heat from pasteurizing milk kills off important good bacteria and alters enzymes and proteins — all essential for building a healthy immune system. These people wanted their milk straight from the cow as an important component of a nutrient-dense diet.

But living in Washington DC, Bouis-Towe couldn't easily access raw milk. As she extended her research and asked around, she found that nearby

Virginia farmers could make raw milk available under private "herdshare" arrangements, but they weren't willing to risk being accused of violating a regulation the FDA had added to existing federal rules in 1987, which prohibited sales of raw milk across state lines. "The next closest option was Maryland and all raw milk sales there were illegal and the dairy industry was declining rapidly," she recalls.

She then began looking in Pennsylvania and found Allgyer's Rainbow Acres Farm listed on a nutrition website. She telephoned him and instantly liked what she heard from the soft-spoken farmer. While the Amish are known for maintaining older traditions of dress and living, most of the farmers have telephones out in the barn to handle business matters (and some use diesel-powered generators to power coolers and freezers in order to store their meat and dairy products).

"Our philosophies were in line," Bouis-Towe recalls. "Pastured animals feeding on fresh grass with hay in the winter, traditional dairy cows, and holistic health and breeding practices. In addition, I spoke with him from the beginning about not pricing consumers out of the market. I explained to him that fresh milk was critical to many, including those on special diets that recommend raw milk, kefir, and other probiotic foods, as well as families with young children, those with lactose intolerance, those recovering from illness, and those who just want to consume the best food they can. Dan understood this and felt the same way."

Next, she took the two-hour car trip to his farm. "Dan and his family were welcoming to my family and we were all enthusiastic about starting the deliveries."

For Allgyer, a tall lanky man of about forty, the appearance of Bouis-Towe was a welcome development. He liked the idea of selling directly to consumers who appreciated his traditional foods as opposed to a corporation. He also liked the idea that he'd receive about $4.50 a gallon for his milk, which was about double what the dairy processing corporation paid. (Over time, his price would rise to $6.50 a gallon.) Moreover, he'd now have a regular market for some other foods he produced (like yogurt, butter, and cheeses), which weren't in demand by the big dairy companies because they made their own, as well as for other foods like eggs, lard, whey, and fermented vegetables. Bouis-Towe was sold on Allgyer, except for one problem: there was no way she could travel four hours round-trip each week to pick up groceries, no matter how healthy and tasty they were. To make an arrangement with Allgyer workable, she'd need to convince other people to share in transporting the food.

She had some friends who shared her interest in nutrient-dense food. "We determined that to start off we would need twenty families and each family would take a turn picking up directly from the farm every two weeks until demand increased enough to cover the cost of a driver. Like any new endeavor, the beginning was rough as we worked on growing the customer base and keeping the orders up during the holiday season." Among her friends, and friends of friends, a tiny buying club gradually took shape. "The group started to gain momentum in the spring of 2006," remembers Bouis-Towe. "Word was spreading about the good products from Rainbow Acres."

One of the people who got the word was Liz Reitzig, a longtime raw milk drinker and mom who had lost her supplier to a crackdown by Maryland public health and agriculture officials. Home to FDA headquarters, Maryland was completely intolerant of raw milk. While most states that prohibited the sale of raw milk allowed private herdshare arrangements, Maryland's legislature passed a law banning herdshares — and the law was upheld by the state's supreme court in a challenge by food rights advocates that included Reitzig. In the process of fighting the Maryland raw milk battle, Reitzig had become a fiery and outspoken defender of food rights, doing television and newspaper interviews about state and federal hostility toward raw milk and its producers. "They were turning ordinary people into criminals," she complained.

Once Reitzig teamed up with Bouis-Towe, the group "grew exponentially," according to the founder. The online ordering system the moms had helped develop "could handle infinite growth, provided the community would support more drop locations." By 2007, two hundred households participated in the group; by 2009 it grew to one thousand households — mostly DC-area professionals such as lawyers, congressional aides, consultants, and officials of nonprofits and nongovernmental organizations (NGOs). With input from others, Bouis-Towe and Reitzig named the club Grassfed on the Hill to honor its commitment to grass-fed dairy, meat, and other healthy foods.

But in point of fact, there was a limit to the number of locations that could be established. When the locations became so widely scattered that delivering to all of them became a major transportation challenge, would-be members who couldn't easily be served by Grassfed on the Hill formed entirely new food clubs to serve additional locales around Maryland and Virginia.

Grassfed on the Hill gave rise to at least seven more food clubs in Maryland and Virginia as word spread, and people in various far-flung locales used the model Bouis-Towe and Reitzig had pioneered. Sometimes they purchased Allgyer's food, and sometimes the new clubs contracted with other Amish farmers. Three other clubs in the region sprouted independently of the spin-offs Bouis-Towe and Reitzig were responsible for. Thousands more consumers were buying Amish food.

Even as the number of participants expanded sharply, Bouis-Towe and Reitzig tried hard to keep the club focused on its founding ideals, a big part of which had to do with the club's relationship with its supplying farmer, Daniel Allgyer. They encouraged members to visit his farm when they were in Pennsylvania and, in particular, to partake of the annual "Customer Appreciation Day" the farmer and his wife hosted each August at the farm.

The event was really an old-fashioned family-style picnic. The Allgyers served a buffet-style lunch of pulled pork, roast chicken, coleslaw, beans, and such, topped off with wonderful raw milk ice cream. It was a great scene, with Allgyer's Amish friends and neighbors mixing it up with dozens of DC professionals who drove out with their children and, perhaps, some chocolate chip cookies or a salad to add to the feast. After lunch, the city kids would take rides in a kid-size horse-drawn wagon, climb the high bales of hay stacked in Allgyer's huge barn, and chase each other around. The adults would sit around and talk about food and farming before the DC contingent would get back into their cars in the late afternoon and head back to the city. It was a nice relaxed time.

The growing popularity of the DC-area food clubs would have been cause for public celebration except for the fact that they operated in a legal no-man's-land. There was that pesky federal prohibition on shipping raw milk for interstate commerce. Was a private club, which didn't operate to earn a profit, engaged in interstate commerce when it transported milk ordered and paid for by individual members from Pennsylvania to Maryland? The courts hadn't provided any clear rulings since the federal prohibition on interstate sales of raw milk went on the books back in 1987.

Allgyer wasn't concerned. He felt that the sale of his products to the members of Grassfed on the Hill was a private matter, not "interstate commerce." After all, the Amish led much of their lives outside the purview not only of interstate commerce but of public education, fashion, entertainment, and communication.

Bouis-Towe and Reitzig tried to warn all new members to keep their neat food arrangement confidential. In their online information package for members, they had a section entitled "Sharing Information about This Group." Its assessment and advice consisted of the following: "Most government officials and all government agencies are highly skeptical of the benefits of raw milk or at least state this publicly. Government agencies are quick to point fingers at raw milk as the cause for illness, typically due to their lack of education on properly raised dairy cows (grassfed only), living in healthy conditions, and proper handling of raw milk. Keep this in mind when you go to the doctor or share information with people you don't know very well. We ask that you do not share information about our group and certainly not about our farmer with individuals that you can't fully trust."[1]

One issue they didn't discuss in any detail with Allgyer was how they would all handle a government challenge to their arrangement. The Amish adhere to a tradition of pacifism; they don't fight in wars. And they avoid fighting in court, as well, steering clear of the American judicial system's reliance on combative lawyers and seemingly endless hearings, delays, technicalities, and costs.

In retrospect, it was nearly impossible to keep the information about Grassfed on the Hill and its supplier confidential given how quickly the buying club was growing — especially given its membership including professionals in the Washington DC area such as government workers and congressional aides. Someone could easily have bragged about the wonderful fresh wholesome food they were buying from the Amish. How the chickens, when roasted, were so much tastier than anything from the grocery store; how the butter was an eye-catching yellow instead of the off-white color of store butter; and how the eggs had thick shells with yolks that were a bright orange, compared with the thin-shelled ovals that held the pale yellow yolks of factory eggs.

It's possible that someone who heard the bragging about Grassfed on the Hill, rather than being impressed, became upset to learn that parents were feeding raw milk, unwashed eggs, and uninspected (by the government) meats to their children. That person may have had a friend at the FDA.

CHAPTER 2

IS THERE SUCH A THING AS PRIVATE FOOD?

At 9:40 on the morning of February 4, 2010, two FDA agents in an SUV pulled up the long driveway of Daniel Allgyer's farm in Kinzers, Pennsylvania. The agents, Joshua Schafer and Deborah Haney, were from the FDA's Delaware office to do an inspection, they told Allgyer.

Allgyer objected. "This is a private farm. I do not sell anything to the public."

One of the agents replied, "You sell milk to the public, therefore we have jurisdiction." When Allgyer said he wasn't going to cooperate, the agents said he would be reported to their superiors for his "refusal to have an investigation," as Allgyer recalls it.[1]

Less than three months later, the agents followed through on their threat. At 5:00 a.m. on April 20th, two FDA agents showed up again — this time accompanied by two U.S. Marshals and a Pennsylvania state trooper. As if to justify the accompanying armed officers, one of the FDA agents took a photo of the signs on several farm building doors: WARNING: NO TRESPASSING . . . ATTN: GOVERNMENT EMPLOYEES, INSPECTORS, AND OTHERS: THIS IS A PRIVATE AREA, NOT A PUBLIC AREA. WARNING TO ALL STATE AND FEDERAL OFFICIALS AND INFORMANTS: YOU MUST HAVE AN APPOINTMENT AND PERMISSION FROM THE OWNER TO ENTER THIS LAND/FARM/PROPERTY OR BUILDING.

As Allgyer recalled the situation: "They drove past my two PRIVATE PROPERTY signs, up to where my coolers were, with their headlights shining right on them. They all got out of their vehicles — five men altogether — with big bright flashlights they were shining all around. My wife and family were still asleep. When they couldn't find anybody, they prepared to knock on the door of my darkened house. Just before they got to the house I stepped out of the barn and hollered at them, then they came up to me and introduced themselves. Two were from the FDA, agent Joshua C. Schafer who had been there in February, and another [David Pearce]. They showed me identification, but I was too flustered to ask for their cards. I remember being told that two were deputy U.S. Marshals and one a state trooper.

"They started asking me questions right away. They handed me a paper and I didn't realize what it was. Agent Joshua C. Schafer told me they were there to do a 'routine inspection.' At 5:00 in the morning, I wondered to myself. 'Do you have a warrant?' I asked, and one of them, a marshal or the state policeman, said, 'You've got it in your hand, buddy.'

"I asked, 'What is the warrant about?' Schafer responded, 'We have credible evidence that you are involved in interstate commerce.'

"They wanted me to answer some questions, my name, middle initial, last name, wanted to know how many cows we have on the farm. I answered those questions and some more. Finally, I got over my initial shock and said I would not be answering any more questions. They said OK, we'll get on with the 'inspection.'"[2]

The FDA's report of the inspection, written by investigator Schafer, pretty much jibes with Allgyer's. "After answering questions stating that the firm is a sole proprietorship, he has owned the farm for two years, and he has 31 dairy cows that are milked two times per day, Mr. Allgyer wanted to know why we were asking these questions. I told Mr. Allgyer these questions are part of a routine inspection. Mr. Allgyer then stated that he will not answer any more questions." The Schafer inspection report says that during the inspection "Mr. Allgyer alternated between going into his dairy barn and standing in the driveway watching us perform our inspection."[3]

One of the inspection's primary goals, based on twenty-eight pages of photos that accompanied the written inspection report, appeared to be to confirm the bare-bones labeling of food products. One photo showing half-gallon and gallon containers of milk was labeled: "Products resembling milk. Photo 1 is of unlabeled containers and photo 2 is of containers labeled GOAT."[4]

The farmer's objection and the federal agents' highlighting of his minimal labeling illustrate differing perceptions of what constitutes "private food." Allgyer was supplying individual members of the food club with products produced on his farm. There were no wholesale distributors and supermarkets or mass-market retailers like Wal-Mart involved between him and the end consumers. He packaged each member's food separately and sent the packages directly from his farm to the individual buyers.

In both his view and that of Grassfed on the Hill members, there was no need for oversight from the USDA, the FDA, or state and local public health and agriculture departments. These regulators, under the authority of federal food and drug legislation first signed into law a century earlier (and added to in subsequent years), enforce regulations governing food's processing and labeling: pasteurization of milk, inspection of meat slaughtering and butchering, refrigeration and washing of eggs, the aging of cheese. But this official oversight is intended for commercially available products, not — in the view of food club members and farmers — foods that individuals produce and sell or trade to friends, neighbors, and acquaintances.

The plastic and glass jugs of yogurt, kefir, cream cheese, goat milk, sauerkraut, and cultured butter that Daniel Allgyer's farm supplied to members of Grassfed on the Hill were hand-labeled in black marker: KEFIR, CREAM CHEESE, YOGURT, CULTURED BUTTER, SAUERKRAUT, GOAT (for the goat milk), and so forth. After all, there were no wholesalers or distributors who needed to know the exact source of the food. The food never came close to any retail store's shelves. The food club members didn't need or want ingredient labels beyond the handwritten identification given that there were no thickeners, sweeteners, preservatives, or artificial colors added to any of it. In the event Allgyer needed to supplement his farm's products with milk or butter from a neighboring Amish farm, he alerted Karine Bouis-Towe and Liz Reitzig, the administrators of the club, and they included a note in e-mails to members that a particular product came from a neighbor of Allgyer.

What was it about privately distributed food, direct from an Amish farm, that aroused so much attention from federal regulators that they thought it necessary to conduct an investigation and recruit armed escorts for the investigators? After all, we weren't that far removed from a time when most food in the United States was distributed the way Daniel Allgyer was doing it, direct from farms to the individuals who ate it.

For much of human history, well into the nineteenth century, food was a private matter. People raised their own food and traded for what they didn't produce themselves. In the United States, as the country became more urbanized, people purchased more of their food, often from farm stores and stands on the outskirts of towns and cities or from small specialty shops — butchers, fish stores, bakeries, fruit and vegetable sellers — who obtained it directly from producers. In suburban areas in the 1940s and 1950s, even into the 1970s in some areas, farmers would deliver. Peddlers came around with meat and eggs. And there was the ever-present milkman.

The advent of huge supermarkets in the 1950s and 1960s, with convenient locations and vast selections of foods, began to supplant the butchers, fish stores, and peddlers. It also heralded the formalization of a regulated "public" commercial system of food distribution. This new system of clean and modern food outlets presented consumers with bins of glistening vegetables and fruits, neatly cut meat and fish in wrapped plastic trays, and milk in plastic or waxed cardboard containers. The public system has continued to expand — chains of 7-Elevens, huge Wal-Marts on highways outside towns large and small, and fast-food franchises crowding strip malls across the country.

In the public system's expansion, farming has become increasingly removed from the output process of the nation's food. More and more of the nation's farms have become essentially subcontractors to huge corporations that dictate the feed, breed, housing, and life span for chickens, pigs, and cattle. The corporations pay fixed prices that often allow the farmer little or no profit. These contractor-farmers have ever less negotiating leeway since the Big Ag corporations behind the contracts have consolidated into only a few producers. These corporations have effectively taken control of the meat business in this country.

According to an analysis in *Forbes* by two academics from the University of Kansas and Northern Michigan University, "Just four companies provide us with 79 percent of our beef, 65 percent of our pork, and 57 percent of our poultry. So, no matter what kind of meat we have for dinner, most likely it comes from the same handful of companies: Tyson Foods, JBS, Cargill, Smithfield Foods. You can never decide which bacon to bring home? Armour, Eckrich, Farmland, Gwaltney, John Morrell, Smithfield — all owned by Smithfield Foods.

"Virtually all the chickens sold in the United States are grown under production contracts to a handful of companies, who own the birds from egg to supermarket. Tyson Foods, the largest U.S. poultry company, contracts with about 6,000 of what it calls family farmers to raise its chickens. They are expected to grow birds to slaughter weight under strict company guidelines as quickly and as cheaply as possible. If Tyson is not satisfied, it may cancel their contracts with little notice and even less recourse, leaving them under a mountain of debt for their otherwise useless chicken houses."[5]

Countering these trends, some private means of distribution have continued to survive, and even thrive — church suppers, bake sales, block parties, lemonade stands. More recently, field-to-fork farm dinners, urban farmers markets, community-supported agriculture (CSA), and small cooperatives and food clubs like Grassfed on the Hill have become popular. Traditional or new systems, they all involve either farmers or other producers selling food directly to consumers or an organization distributing food directly to participants of a particular community, like members of a church or parents of a school's students. They are also decidedly noncommercial and generally avoid advertising beyond the particular confines of the community — in other words, they aren't presented to the general public.

But something happened, beginning in this century, to change the seeming independence of the private food sector and foretell the targeting of Daniel Allgyer. Both before and since the inspection of his farm, other small private food endeavors have also come under regulatory scrutiny and enforcement procedures.

One case notable for its force and threat of violence involved the Manna Storehouse food club in Ohio. The family-run club, organized as a private outlet, had been providing grass-fed beef, lamb, turkey, eggs, flour, and other items from local farms to dozens of neighbors and friends who were members beginning in 2000. On December 1, 2008, officers from the Lorain County Sheriff's Office, dressed in full tactical armor, arrived at the home of the club's owners in LaGrange (outside Cleveland) with Lorain County Health Department and Ohio Department of Agriculture inspectors. With weapons drawn and trained on one owner, Jacqueline Stowers, her in-laws, and eight small children Stowers was homeschooling, the officers herded the family into a home living room and kept them under armed guard for about seven hours. The agriculture and health inspectors executed a search warrant, taking cell phones, three computers, business records, and a year's worth of frozen meat — mostly lamb from the Stowerses' own herd. Jacqueline's husband, John Stowers, was out running errands when the raiding party arrived.

The food club's offense? Failure to obtain a retail license. Jacqueline Stowers told me that at the time she had received notification a year earlier that she needed a license, and when she wrote back to question it based on Manna Storehouse being a private membership organization, she didn't receive a response — until the raiding party showed up.

The search warrant used by the armed officers was similar to that used for drug dealers, giving the agents permission to confiscate anything on the premises.[6] The affidavit authorizing the warrant cited the Stowerses for operating a retail food establishment without a license, according to the Farm-to-Consumer Legal Defense Fund. It filed suit against Ohio officials on behalf of the Stowerses, arguing that the search and seizure had been unlawful and the Stowerses denied due process and equal protection. After a number of hearings, a county judge in early 2010 rejected the arguments, ruling that Manna Storehouse was subject to the state's retail licensing rules because it was a profit-making operation; an appeals court in 2011 upheld the ruling.[7]

Another incident occurred in July 2011, when San Francisco regulators shut down the Underground Market, which was launched in 2009 as a private market by an organization known as ForageSF, with vendors peddling foods ranging from foraged seaweed to Belgian waffles. Iso Rabins, the founder, explained the market's rationale and growth in a statement to supporters: "I started the Underground Market in 2009 as a reaction to the high bar of entry that has been created to start a food business, something that I experienced personally. Starting in a house in the Mission with seven vendors and 150 eaters, the market has grown to feed over 50,000 people and help over 400 vendors get their start."

That ended on July 11, 2011, when the city's health department "served us a cease and desist letter, stating they no longer considered the market a private event." Rabins said the private organization was actually *launched* at the suggestion of local health department officials, who were trying to help organizers circumnavigate the regulations and presumably figured it would stay small. "Everyone who walks through the door is a member who knows they are eating un-certified food, so technically the health department doesn't have to be involved. They have decided (apparently with pressure from the state level) that the market is no longer a private event, and can therefore not continue as it has."[8] (The market did open for a "final" market December 22, 2012.)

Within three months of the San Francisco market's 2011 shutdown, Quail Hollow Farm in Nevada came under public health scrutiny on the evening it was serving its first-ever farm-to-fork dinner to dozens of area customers. In a letter to the Farm-to-Consumer Legal Defense Fund, farm owner Laura Bledsoe described how her carefully planned evening was nearly ruined: "The evening was everything I had dreamed and hoped it would be. The weather was perfect, the farm was filled with friends and guests roaming around talking about organic, sustainable farming practices. . . . Our guests were excited to spend an evening together. The food was prepared exquisitely. The long dinner table, under the direction of dear friends, was absolutely stunningly beautiful. The music was superb. The stars were bright and life was really good.

"And then, . . . for a few moments, it felt like the rug was pulled out from underneath us and my wonderful world came crashing down. As guests were mingling, finishing tours of the farm, and while the first course of the meal was being prepared and ready to be sent out, a Southern Nevada Health District employee came for an inspection.

"Because this was a gathering of people invited to our farm for dinner, I had no idea that the Health Department would become involved. I received a phone call from them two days before the event informing me that because this was a 'public event' (I would like to know what is the definition of 'public' and 'private') we would be required to apply for a 'special use permit.'" Despite Bledsoe's conviction that the event was private, and outside the authority of public health officials, she decided to be pragmatic and completed all the paperwork.

Unfortunately, the health inspector arrived right as the guests were mingling. It didn't take long for the inspector to declare "our food unfit for consumption and demand that we call off the event," for various "safety" reasons — for example, an absence of labels and receipts and the fact that it wasn't USDA certified, all explainable because most of it was produced on the Bledsoe farm. The inspector rejected Bledsoe's explanations, threatening to call the police and escort guests off the property. Bledsoe concluded that "the only way to keep our guests on the property was to destroy the food."

"I can't tell you how sick to my stomach I was watching that first dish of mint lamb meatballs hit the bottom of the unsanitized trash can.

"Here we were with guests who had paid in advance and had come from long distances away anticipating a wonderful dining experience, waiting for dinner while we were behind the kitchen curtain throwing it away! I know of the hours and labor that went into the preparation of that food.

"We asked the inspector if we could save the food for a private family event that we were having the next day. (A personal family choice to use our own food.) We were denied and she was insulted that we would even consider endangering our family's health. I assured her that I had complete faith and trust in Giovanni our chef and the food that was prepared (obviously, or I wouldn't be wanting to serve it to our guests).

"I then asked, if we couldn't feed the food to our 'public guests' or even to our private family, then at least let us feed it to our pigs . . . "

The result: "another negative response."

At this point, Bledsoe was moving from being upset to being angry. "So the food that was raised here on our farm and selected and gathered from familiar local sources, cooked and prepared with skill and love, was even unfit to feed to my pigs!?! Who gave them the right to tell me what I feed my animals?"

"To add insult to injury, we were ordered to pour bleach on it," making the food unfit for even animals to consume.

Bledsoe finally decided to call a lawyer from the Farm-to-Consumer Legal Defense Fund, who advised her to ask the health inspector if she had a search warrant or an arrest warrant. When it turned out she had neither, Bledsoe ordered her to leave the property, which she did. The inspector later returned with local police, who not only declined to issue any kind of citation, but asked the health inspector to leave when she couldn't come up with an explanation of what law had been violated.

"The wind taken out of the inspector's sails, Gio and his crew got cookin'. It just so happened that we had a cooled trailer full of vegetables ready to be taken to market the following day. An employee hooked on to the trailer and backed it up right next to the kitchen. Our interns who were there to greet and serve now got to work with lamp oil and began harvesting anew. Knives were chopping, pots of pasta and rice from our food storage were steaming, our bonfire was now turned into a grill, and literal miracles were happening before our eyes!"

She then explained the situation to guests and "offered anyone interested a full refund, and told them that if they chose to stay their dinner was now literally being prepared fresh, as [in] 'just now being harvested.' The reaction of our guests was the most sobering and inspirational experience of the evening. In an instant we were bonded together. They were, of course, outraged at the lack of choice they were given in their meal."

Things improved quickly with the health inspector now out of the way. "Before long we were seated at the beautiful table and the most incredible dishes began coming forth. It was 'loaves and fishes' appearing before our very eyes! We broke bread together, we laughed, we talked, we shared stories, we came together in the most marvelous way."[9]

The hard-earned happy ending Bledsoe experienced is more the exception than the rule, though. Even bake sales and lemonade stands aren't off-limits to the increasingly aggressive public health inspectors. In early 2012, a San Francisco public health inspector shut down a bake sale being held in Golden Gate Park to raise funds for a twenty-two-student nursery school.

In Hopkinton, Massachusetts, health inspectors shut down a lemonade stand set up in a homeowner's driveway at the start of the 2012 Boston Marathon. The stand had become an annual event, selling not only lemonade but banana bread and brownies. Proceeds went to charity — but no matter, the stand wasn't licensed and had to go. The Hopkinton run-in was one of a growing number involving lemonade stands — enough to spark creation of Lemonade Freedom Day in 2011. "In the recent past, bureaucrats and law enforcers have shut down lemonade stands for not having permits or licenses," organizers said on their website. At that time, "thousands of people across the world participated in Lemonade Freedom Day to show these bureaucrats and law enforcers that they could not shut down kids' lemonade stands."[10] So many participated that the organizers of Lemonade Freedom Day expanded their reach by teaming up with a group of raw milk proponents for the 2012 event.

What is behind the growing tension around food — more specifically, around privately distributed food that had long been off the regulatory radar? Part of it has to do with growing concerns about "safety" — not just food safety but an atmosphere stemming from the terrorist attacks on 9/11.

Immediately following the attacks, our government rounded up terrorist suspects from around the world and threw them into prison in Guantanamo Bay, Cuba. Authorities came up with a new term for these individuals — "enemy combatants" — and denied them the rights normally accorded those accused of violating American laws. In *The Rights of the People: How Our Search for Safety Invades Our Liberties*, a sobering assessment of how constitutional protections eroded after 9/11, Pulitzer Prize–winning reporter David K. Shipler states that "for over two centuries . . . America has enjoyed and endured an intriguing fluidity within the walls of its constitutional ideals. From time to time, courts and legislatures have enlarged or curtailed the scope of liberty . . . especially during times of national stress and fear, they have narrowed and compromised rights that are explicitly delineated by the Constitution. Later, to its credit, the country has looked back on the violations with shame."[11]

Shipler identifies "at least five periods before September 11, 2001, [when] the United States strayed from its principles dramatically. After the attacks on that day, we lost our bearings for the sixth time in our history."[12] The most notable previous examples have been before and during major wars — the Civil War, World War I, and World War II. Shipler's most prominent examples of how we have "lost our bearings" concern criminal investigations and terrorism. He points out how the courts have granted more authority to conduct searches, monitor personal communications, and carry out other enforcement to counter criminal and terrorist activities.

Former President Jimmy Carter complained in a 2012 *New York Times* op-ed about "unprecedented violations of our rights to privacy through warrantless wiretapping and government mining of our electronic communications. Popular state laws permit detaining individuals because of their appearance, where they worship or with whom they associate."[13]

Food didn't figure into either Shipler's or Carter's analyses, but it did figure into the post-9/11 terrorism equation, since America's food and water supplies were feared to be potential bioterrorism targets. In the days and weeks following 9/11, police and other security personnel were assigned to keep watch over water reservoirs and treatment plants.

Over a relatively short period of time, "food security" became a part of "food safety." Congress enacted the Public Health Security and Bioterrorism Preparedness and Response Act of 2002 (the Bioterrorism Act), requiring that all food facilities in the United States register with the FDA before the end of 2003. At the same time, the FDA published a document designed to provide food producers with guidance on "preventive measures that can be taken to minimize the risk that food under their control will be subject to tampering or criminal or terrorist actions."[14] The government sought to make food security a fixture in training associated with food safety. It helped fund the Western Institute for Food Safety and Security at the University of California in Davis in 2003. Kansas State University added a food safety and security program area to its Food Science Institute shortly after the institute's founding in 2001.

The concern about food security coincided with exploding public interest in all aspects of food — cooking, nutrition, gardening, and farming. Books like *The Omnivore's Dilemma* and *Fast Food Nation*, which questioned the integrity and health of America's factory food system, became top sellers. Acclaimed documentaries like *Food, Inc.* and *Fresh* showed cattle and pigs crammed into concentrated animal feeding operations (CAFOs) and chickens confined in cages that barely allowed them space to breathe.

The Food Network, which launched as a tiny cable network in 1993, expanded in popularity during the first decade of the 2000s. By early 2012, an estimated 1.3 million viewers were watching it each evening.[15] Publications like Martha Stewart's *Whole Living* and *Everyday Food* became big sellers, and hundreds of blogs devoted to various aspects of food sprang up. They chronicled debates over federal food subsidies, childhood obesity, and GM food, and one even monitored what the president and his family ate in the White House.[16] Farmers markets boomed, increasing in number from six-thousand-plus to seven-thousand-plus in just the one year from 2010 to 2011.[17] Winter farmers markets made up 17 percent of the total in 2011.[18]

During this time of renewed enthusiasm about food, troubling images also surfaced suggesting that the image many Americans had or wanted to believe about farms — bucolic images of healthy family farms, which often appeared on the labels and in the advertising of major food producers — was one that did not accurately represent most food being sold in supermarkets and other major retail outlets. There was an outcry when videos appeared showing "downer cows" (sick cows) being abused so they would stand up while being unloaded at the slaughterhouse, even though sick cows weren't supposed to be slaughtered for fear their meat might carry disease. Many Americans remembered the vivid television reports showing piles of dead farm animals in England in early 2001, when millions of cattle and sheep were slaughtered to rid the country of an epidemic of foot-and-mouth disease.

Indeed, the bucolic images people had of farms had become far removed from even the reality of those few bucolic farms that remained. Americans seemed to have collectively forgotten that farms are not just places where cows and sheep graze on emerald pastures, but also places where chickens poop in the barnyard and spiders spin webs around the barn and field mice scurry about at night among the bales of hay — and droughts kill crops and animals alike.

Over generations of urbanization, many of us had grown ever more distant from our food and how it is produced — including officials being asked to rule in food-regulation cases. One such case involved a dairy in upstate New York that sold unpasteurized dairy products, on a private basis, to shareholders of its limited liability company. In 2008, New York regulators not only challenged the dairy owners' contention that they were selling their food privately (charging they were selling without a license), but claimed that they were also allowing unsanitary conditions at their farm.

A hearing officer for the New York State Department of Agriculture and Markets, Susan Weber, said in her ruling in favor of the agency that a barn wall was "caked with old manure, chickens were found roaming free in the milking barn," and there were flies, mouse droppings, and spiderwebs to boot. Even though she allowed that "the department offered no evidence that there was any actual injury to the public or any intent to deceive consumers by offering product which was not what it was purported to be," the agency's claim about unsanitary conditions "was the most compelling" to her.

What seems to have been lost in our collective memory is that farms have, for ages, had spiderwebs, mouse droppings, and chickens intermingling with cows. It didn't seem to matter that none of the shareowners from the nearby Ithaca area had become ill or complained about the cleanliness of the farm. Weber's conclusion was dire: "The department's evidence establishes beyond doubt that the conditions at Meadowsweet in October of 2007 were not sanitary, that the products produced, processed and manufactured there may have been contaminated with filth or rendered diseased, unwholesome or injurious to health."[19] I visited Meadowsweet Dairy in early 2008, and to me, the faint smell of manure in the barn and barnyard was normal farm smell. If there was manure on barn walls, it didn't stand out as much different from what existed at several dozen other old farms and barns I had visited in recent years.

The hearing officer's view that dangerous germs lurked everywhere on a farm where manure was visible and chickens hung out was indicative of not only the expanding distance between consumers and their food, but a growing need to hide how food is produced. While most small farms that sell directly to consumers, including Meadowsweet, actively encourage their customers to visit and learn about how their food is produced, large corporate producers often try to keep shocking images of vast crowded animal holding areas off-limits to public scrutiny. After several videos of farm animal abuse were publicized, a number of states with a substantial number of farms owned by major corporations — Iowa, Utah, Florida, Illinois, and Minnesota — actually promoted legislation that would make it illegal for anyone to film CAFO farms undercover. As of late 2012, Utah and Iowa were understood to have implemented such bans, while Illinois tabled such a proposal. (Kansas and Montana had enacted similar bans in the 1990s.)

The New York hearing officer's view was also indicative of growing fears about food safety — fears that focused most heavily on conventional pathogens that cause food-borne illnesses such as salmonella, campylobacter, *E. coli* O157:H7, and listeria. In actuality, food safety includes other problems, like antibiotic residues in meat from the drugs used to prevent disease among overcrowded animals in CAFO facilities, antibiotic-resistant pathogens, potential dangers from GM foods, and cancer and other serious illnesses arising from bisphenol A (BPA) or mercury-tainted corn syrup. Several studies have even suggested that chicken may have infected many women with antibiotic-resistant forms of urinary tract infections.[20]

Fears about GM foods moved into the spotlight in 2012, when California residents voted on Proposition 37, which would have required food producers to include information about GMO ingredients on food labels. Corporate food and seed producers like Monsanto, DuPont, and Dow Chemical Company put up an estimated $46 million, outspending proponents by eight to one according to some sources, to argue that the new rules were unnecessary and would raise food costs. The ad campaign worked, and the proposition was defeated with 53 percent of the vote against, but the issue seems likely to remain a bone of contention that will come up in other election cycles.

The nearly exclusive food-safety focus on pathogens was so powerful that at the end of 2010 national politicians considered legislation designed to expand the FDA's power to crack down on food producers. It gave the FDA vast new powers to inspect any company's records at will (with no cause having to be shown or search warrant obtained), to require all producers to have detailed safety plans (so-called hazard analysis critical control points or HACCP plans, with the FDA having arbitrary power to approve or disapprove), and to implement "produce safety standards" that would for the first time allow the government to regulate farmer growing and production practices.

When the Food Safety Modernization Act finally passed a lame-duck Congress in early 2011 and was signed into law by President Barack Obama, it contained an amendment (the Tester-Hagan Amendment). Pushed hard by proponents of sustainable food, it exempted farms and food producers with less than half a million dollars in sales (adjusted for inflation) that sell more than half of their products directly to consumers or local restaurants/retail establishments from the most onerous requirements of the legislation, such as having to prepare full HACCP plans and be subject to the "produce safety standards."

While the exemptions for the smallest producers were hailed as a victory for small farms, the reality of what would happen once the new legislation was fully enacted was unclear. It appeared that small farms and food producers wouldn't need to register with the FDA to prove they qualified for the exemption. But the presumption may well be that they should have registered under the 2002 bioterrorism law. Moreover, half a million dollars was not, for many food producers, necessarily a huge amount of revenue for those selling popular high-priced items like specialized cheeses, honey, and maple syrup. And when the FDA finally, in early 2013, issued the first proposed new rules for produce — covering such matters as making compost and preventing wild and domesticated animals from coming into contact with produce — it specified that the time to comply with most of the rules would be four years for farms with less than a quarter-million dollars in annual revenue and three years for those with less than half a million dollars in revenue.

The intense debates over the Food Safety Modernization Act, and particularly over whether to exempt smaller producers, highlighted a related trend: national efforts at the state level to exempt small food producers from onerous regulations requiring equipment and inspections. These efforts involved legislative campaigns to enact state "cottage food laws," sometimes referred to as "baker's bills," which cover producers of items like jams, jellies, and baked goods — and sometimes allow church suppers and farmers markets — but exempt private sales of meat and dairy products. While the new state laws, enacted in more than thirty states by 2012, reduced the up front costs and encouraged more people to start locally based food businesses, they did not ease tensions over more intense food regulations — in particular, the rights of individuals to access food on a private basis.

For people who were interested in buying or selling food on a private basis, a long-extant legal void has not helped matters. While there is legal precedent, including at the U.S. Supreme Court level, protecting the rights of Americans to associate privately for the purposes of providing legal advice or to promote unpopular causes like white supremacy, there is little precedent about extending such protections for people to access the foods of their choice on a private basis.

Indeed, the U.S. Constitution contains not even a single mention of the word *food*, perhaps because the distribution and consumption of food wasn't a matter of conflict in the late 1700s. When a right isn't addressed by the Constitution or the Bill of Rights, it becomes subject to the broad interpretation of lawmakers and judges.

The little judicial interpretation that does exist seems to grant the federal government wide latitude under the U.S. Constitution's so-called commerce clause, which gives the federal government authority in matters of "interstate commerce." That clause has been applied in a huge range of cases, from price fixing by Chicago meatpackers in the early 1900s to the Civil Rights Act of 1964, which banned segregation and discrimination against African Americans. According to an article from Cornell University Law School, "The Supreme Court found that Congress had the authority to regulate a business that served mostly interstate travelers in *Heart of Atlanta Motel v. United States*. . . . It also ruled that the federal civil rights legislation could be used to regulate a restaurant, Ollie's Barbeque, a family-owned restaurant in Birmingham, Alabama because, although most of Ollie's customers were local, the restaurant served food which had previously crossed state lines."[21]

The U.S. Supreme Court also used the commerce clause to rule, in the 1942 case of *Wickard v. Filburn*, that a farmer could be prevented from growing wheat for his own personal use under federally established wheat quotas.[22] In the case of food rights, it has come to be used in restricting producers of raw dairy products. For example, a tiny Washington State producer of award-winning raw milk cheeses, Estrella Family Creamery, was barred by a federal judge in late 2012 from selling its cheeses outside the state because the FDA said it found evidence of listeria contamination (though no illnesses) in its production facilities; it wasn't even clear whether the cheese maker would be allowed to sell within the state if any of its ingredients came from outside Washington.

In recent years, several organizations have sprung up to help individuals organize and protect what they consider to be their right to privately access the food of their choice. One of the first was Right to Choose Healthy Food, which was set up in the early 2000s by a California nutritionist who advocated the benefits of raw food, Aajonus Vonderplanitz. Vonderplanitz organized several dozen food clubs around the country that established lease agreements with farmers giving the clubs exclusive access to the farms' meats, eggs, and dairy products. Hundreds of consumer members paid a twenty-five-dollar annual membership fee and signed an agreement that positioned the club as outside the conventional food system.

One such agreement stated in part: "I demand access to food that 1) is produced without exposure to chemical contaminants such as industrial pesticides, fertilizers, antibiotics, cleansers or their gases; 2) is not subjected to artificial temperatures above 99° Fahrenheit (F.), dairy not above 104° or below 40° F., and meats not below 38° F. ; 3) is complete with its natural unadulterated enzymes intact; 4) may contain microbes, including but not limited to salmonella, E.coli, campylobacter, listeria, gangrene and parasites; 5) the cows and goats are grazed and grass-fed; 6) fowl are pastured and/or free-range outdoors and not fed soy products; and 7) the eggs are unwashed and may have bacteria and poultry feces on them. I fully understand that these features represent a different paradigm for food preparation, storage and safety than those that are currently enforced by all local, state and federal government agencies."[23]

The Farm-to-Consumer Legal Defense Fund sprang up on July 4, 2007, to protect the rights of farmers and consumers being prosecuted for dispensing foods privately. One of its first cases involved defending Meadowsweet Dairy, which I described earlier in this chapter. In early 2010, it challenged the FDA in a federal court suit on behalf of ten plaintiffs, arguing that the agency's ban on interstate shipments of raw milk interfered with individual rights to privacy and due process. The case was notable for prompting the FDA, in a motion to dismiss the case, to declare that Americans have "no absolute right to consume or feed children any particular food."[24] Its rationale? "Comprehensive federal regulation of the food supply has been in effect at least since Congress enacted the Pure Food and Drugs Act of 1906, and was strengthened by the passage of the FDCA [Food, Drug and Cosmetics Act] in 1938. Thus, plaintiffs' claim to a fundamental privacy interest in obtaining 'foods of their own choice' for themselves and their families is without merit."[25]

Government control went even beyond food, though, according to the FDA: "There Is No Generalized Right to Bodily and Physical Health," it headlined the second section of its brief. "Plaintiffs' assertion of a 'fundamental right to their own bodily and physical health, which includes what foods they do and do not choose to consume for themselves and their families' is similarly unavailing because plaintiffs do not have a fundamental right to obtain any food they wish."[26]

A Wisconsin judge put an exclamation point on the FDA's argument in late 2011, when he ruled against two farmers who challenged the state's Department of Agriculture, Trade, and Consumer Protection (DATCP) efforts to restrict their private distribution of raw milk to members of their food clubs. Wisconsin prohibits most sales of raw milk, except on an "incidental" basis.

When the Farm-to-Consumer Legal Defense Fund asked the judge for a "clarification" on his ruling as to whether the cow owners could milk their own cows, the judge became irritated. He said his decision translated further that "no, Plaintiffs do not have a fundamental right to own and use a dairy cow or a dairy herd . . . no, Plaintiffs do not have a fundamental right to consume the milk from their own cow."[27] And in a verbal banging of his gavel, he added: "no, Plaintiffs do not have a fundamental right to produce and consume the foods of their choice."[28]

The legal uncertainty over private food rights, and the FDA's stance, quickly became apparent to Daniel Allgyer, the Amish farmer. The day after FDA agents searched his farm, he received a "warning letter" from the agency threatening him with "seizure and/or injunction" if he didn't discontinue shipping unpasteurized milk across state lines to his food club members in Maryland.[29]

Allgyer made a quick decision of his own, which he communicated via a handwritten letter to his Maryland food club members five days later: "As you probably know by now, the FDA is trying to shut me down based on the Interstate commerce clause. We usually thought a private contract does not fall under their jurisdiction and deep down I still think that way. But . . . due to my religion on non resistance and the fact that I spend every hour trying to produce good food for you, I feel that the fight should be in somebody else's hand."[30]

Allgyer then alluded to a Pennsylvania Mennonite raw dairy farmer, Mark Nolt, whose farm was raided three times between 2007 and 2009 by Pennsylvania agriculture officials, aided by FDA agents, because he turned in his Pennsylvania permit allowing him to produce raw milk, contending that he didn't need it since he was selling his food products privately. "I talked to Mark Nolt's wife and she said that Mark didn't do any farming for a whole summer. I personally don't want to go looking for somebody to run my farm while I fight. Last but not least is the amount of stress it would create on my family to see Dad and husband used like a real criminal."[31]

Allgyer's allusion to putting the "fight . . . in somebody else's hand" was Allgyer's way of saying he had decided to sign up with Aajonus Vonderplanitz's Right to Choose Healthy Food organization to help him further privatize his arrangement with the Maryland food club in a way he hoped would stand up to legal scrutiny. Right to Choose Healthy Food, which was at that time known best for one of its food clubs (Rawesome Foods in Los Angeles), would lease his cows, pigs, goats, and chickens so as to counter potential charges of illegal food "sales." In this structure, the food being received by the members was already owned by them. The money they paid the farmer was for boarding their leased animals. The members of the Maryland food club Allgyer served would join Right to Choose Healthy Food, pay an annual twenty-five-dollar membership fee to share in the food from the leased animals, and hopefully gain some measure of protection as a result.

Would the new arrangement work? Allgyer didn't speculate. "I will close with a prayer that we can continue to provide our family's [sic] with healthy, nutritious food," the letter ended. "Sincerely, your farmer, Dan Allgyer."[32]

CHAPTER 3

THE HUNDRED-YEAR WAR AGAINST RAW MILK

In the struggle between Americans and our government over the right to choose what we eat, raw milk is a sort of crucible. Government regulators have spent more than one hundred years trying to rid our society of it. In the early years, they had some good reasons; in recent years, far fewer.

In the late 1990s, raw milk had all but vanished, only to see a revival of consumer demand. Within ten years, it had become a hugely popular food. Growing numbers of consumers began to appreciate it as a delicious and nutritionally wholesome alternative to pasteurized milk and wanted to benefit from what growing research indicates is its ability to alleviate chronic health conditions like asthma and allergies. Sally Fallon, the head of the Weston A. Price Foundation, an organization that encourages consumption of so-called nutrient-dense foods (more on those later in this chapter), has called raw milk "a magic food."

As raw milk has become emblematic of the growing interest in unprocessed wholesome foods, it's also become more controversial — some might even say polarizing — in our society. Professionals in the medical, agriculture, and public health communities mostly hate it, seeing it as a highly risky food and potentially dangerous carrier of food-borne illness, especially for children. The head of the FDA's dairy division, John Sheehan, has stated that "drinking raw milk is like playing Russian roulette with your health."

A memo to state public health officials from the CDC distributed in 2011 put it this way: "The role of raw milk and other unpasteurized dairy products in the transmission of infectious diseases is well documented. Raw milk was recognized as a source of severe infections over 100 years ago, and pasteurization of milk to prevent these infections is one of the public health triumphs of the 20th century."[1] While the CDC memo's distillation of history seems tidy, the reality is more nuanced and includes a significant amount of history and symbolism, and a number of important "firsts."

Milk, of course, is nearly everyone's first food — dispensed by mothers — and has been since the beginning of time. Even after they stop nursing, most children graduate to milk from cows and goats. One of our best historical resources on the role of milk in mankind's early history is the Bible. It makes frequent references to milk, at least half a dozen with a promise of the divine — as in Exodus, to bring the freed Israelites "into the land . . . which he swore to your fathers to give you, a land flowing with milk and honey." It was a respected and desired food, equal to wine as a symbol of celebration, as in the Song of Solomon: "I came to my garden, my sister, my bride, I gathered my myrrh with my spice, I ate my honeycomb with my honey, I drank my wine with my milk. Eat, friends, drink, and be drunk with love!"

Interestingly, there are no concerns expressed in the Bible (at least that I could find) over raw milk's safety. That isn't the case with respect to other foods. Pork, in particular, is repeatedly disparaged — as in Leviticus: "And the pig, because it parts the hoof and is cloven-footed but does not chew the cud, is unclean to you. You shall not eat any of their flesh, and you shall not touch their carcasses; they are unclean to you." This prohibition is generally understood to be a reference to pork's danger as a source of the infectious disease trichinosis. (Other off-limits foods included shellfish like shrimp and lobster.)

The contrasting views on raw milk and pork are intriguing and ironic; then, pork was viewed in the culture as inherently unsafe, while milk was a sustenance of life. Yet today raw milk is viewed by much of the culture as inherently unsafe, while pork is a staple food, the basis of a huge industry.

The Bible also expresses that a cow's owner has unrestricted access to its milk. "Who serves as a soldier at his own expense? Who plants a vineyard without eating any of its fruit? Or who tends a flock without getting some of the milk?" A far cry from the Wisconsin judge's declaration that in the so-called Dairy State, cow owners don't have an inherent right to the milk of their cows.

Raw milk enjoyed a long and unexamined tenure in the human diet until the middle of the 1800s, when hundreds of thousands of people migrated from the countryside to rapidly growing industrial cities like Boston, Philadelphia, New York, Chicago, and Milwaukee. These were cities where the power of coal and fast-flowing streams and rivers were being utilized to drive the steam engines that powered machine tools, lathes, and milling machines for the mass production of screws and nails, clothing, sheets, and blankets.

But while there were innovations in using labor, machinery, and energy to mass-produce consumer and industrial goods, little was known about the spread of infectious disease and how crowded conditions could make dangerous mass outbreaks of life-threatening diseases like tuberculosis, diphtheria, and typhus nearly inevitable. Because there was so little understanding, there were few sanitation efforts to prevent transmittal of disease — among not only people but animals as well — through water, sewage, manure, and food.

As masses of people migrated from the countryside to the city in search of jobs, businesspeople also brought grains and cows in from the country to provide basic commodities — alcohol for adults and milk for children. First, distilleries fermented corn and barley to make vodka and whiskey. The leftover grains, their nutrients depleted, would be fed to cows housed in adjoining buildings.

These were the first feedlots, the first major effort at agricultural industrialization based on exploiting farm animals on a large scale to maximize profits. Robert Hartley, an advocate for the poor who investigated the urban dairy industry, described the situation in the early 1840s, for anyone who was "still skeptical as to the pernicious quality of the milk":

> If the wind is in the right quarter, he will smell the dairy a mile off; and on reaching it, his visual and nasal organs will, without any affectation of squeamishness, be so offended at the filth and effluvia which abounds, that still-slop milk will probably become the object of his unutterable loathing the remainder of his life. His attention will probably be first drawn to a huge distillery, sending out its tartarian fumes, and, blackened with age and smoke, casting a somber air all around. Contiguous thereto, he will see numerous low, flat pens, in which many hundreds of cows, owned by different persons, are closely huddled together, amid confined air, and the stench of their own excrements. He will also see the various appendages and troughs to conduct and receive the hot

slush from the still with which to gorge the stomachs of these unfortunate animals, and all within an area of a few hundred yards.[2]

Hartley described how the cows at first didn't care for the distillery slop. The dairy owners would deprive them of water, so the cows ate the slop to satisfy their thirst. For a few months, their milk production soared, but eventually they became diseased and unable to stand. At that point, they were sold for slaughter, and their meat sold as beef. Because there was so little understanding about the connection between animal health, sanitation, and communicable disease, few people objected to the animal abuse. But even without scientific evidence, people like Hartley felt certain the connection was there.

> Let the parent who feeds his children with milk from the dairies at Brooklyn, visit those places and look for once into the buildings where the cows are crowded together with scarcely space enough between them to allow a milkman to pass; let him take two long breaths of that filthy atmosphere, from which the poor animals are not permitted to stir for weeks and months; let him smell of the heart-sickening rum-broth upon which these abused creatures are compelled almost exclusively to feed — each drinking from fifteen to thirty gallons a day; let him examine the stumps of the teeth corroded down to the gums by the acrid fluids generated from the unwholesome food; let him learn that some of these animals, becoming in a single season unfit for the dairy, are fattened partly upon the same poisonous composition, and killed and carried into market to be eaten by himself and family; and then let him say whether he will patronize such nefarious establishments.
>
> Nothing can be more certain, than that the quality of the milk is greatly influenced by the state of the health of the animal producing it; and where such immense quantities of a mischievous material as fifteen or thirty gallons are made to pass through the organs of a single animal in twenty-four hours, it is impossible that the functions of the organs should be performed in a perfect manner. The milk thus produced might almost as well

be taken directly from the distillery, without the ceremony of straining it through the blood-vessels of a sickly cow.[3]

Hartley followed up these descriptions with examples of individuals becoming ill from drinking the distillery milk — individuals who had consumed milk from rural farms without problems.

Enter Louis Pasteur, the father of microbiology who is credited with the principle that has guided much of medicine since the 1860s — the germ theory of disease, the idea that microscopic bacteria are responsible for making us sick. Of course, he is also credited with the development of pasteurization, a method of using heat to reduce microbial pathogens in food, though the process actually dates back centuries as a way of preserving beer and wine.

Pasteur isn't even thought to have worked with milk; commercial application of his principles stemmed from the scientist's attempts during the 1860s to help the French wine industry prevent spoilage during transport. Pasteur identified bacteria that contributed to the spoilage and developed the technique of heating wine without air to between 60 and 100 degrees Celsius (140 and 212 degrees Fahrenheit) for a short time to slow the microbial growth.

Despite demonstrations intended to prove that the pasteurized wine tasted better after shipping than nonpasteurized wine, there were acrimonious debates in France about whether heating altered the taste of the wine. A blue-ribbon panel finally sided with Pasteur in determining that the wine's taste wasn't adversely affected. Nevertheless, France's wine industry grew disillusioned with pasteurization within a few decades — and pasteurization's uses would change as well:

> The experiments with heating wine succeeded because heating does kill microbes. Yet, applied to wine, pasteurization had neither the success nor the scope Pasteur anticipated. By the end of the century, phylloxera [insects that destroy grape vines] was to do more harm to French wine and wine trade than the diseases of cloudiness and bitterness that Pasteur had been able to control. The practice of heating fell into disuse among the vintners, who experienced far greater distress. . . . [But] the heating process was soon to be applied to other foodstuffs, as well as to other beverages, first and foremost to milk and beer.[4]

Actually, Pasteur's most notable accomplishments came nearly twenty years after his wine pasteurization project when he moved on from pasteurization to vaccination. Arguably his most famous experiment occurred in 1881, when he inoculated twenty-four sheep, one goat, and six cows against anthrax and then injected live virus into both the inoculated animals and a control group. The experiment went as he'd expected — the inoculated animals did not become sick; the control group's animals were dead or dying.[5] Pasteur's experiment helped kick off "the golden age of bacteriology" from 1880 to 1900, during which time more than a dozen important pathogens were identified — including malaria, tuberculosis, cholera, diphtheria, and tetanus.[6]

Despite excitement surrounding these discoveries, some of the most prominent scientists of the day (nearly all of whom were French) disagreed with Pasteur's germ theory. Antoine Béchamp argued for the cell theory in an attempt to explain why pathogens don't make everyone sick. In his view, some people's cellular systems were better able than others to fight off these pathogens and thereby avoid illness.

Likewise, the French physiologist Claude Bernard argued for "the milieu interieur," described by Ron Schmid in *The Untold Story of Milk*, as "the internal environment the individual brings to the battleground of infectious disease — that which creates resistance, inner strength and, for some, complete immunity. The great debate in science and medicine during the latter half of the nineteenth century was about microbes versus milieu in the etiology of infectious disease. At center stage stood Bernard and Louis Pasteur."[7]

Patrice Debre's 1998 biography of Pasteur describes a Bernard physiology course that Pasteur audited: "Pasteur did not pay sufficient attention to one of the most important concepts put forward by Claude Bernard, that of the internal environment. The notes he had taken on this subject when he audited the physiologist's course did not trigger anything in his imagination; and so he did not push his studies in this area any further, although this might have led him to discover the antibodies or the immune system in general."[8] As Debre summarizes, "On Pasteur's side is an exogenous concept, in which the microbe invades the body. On Bernard's side, disease is due to a disturbance of the internal environment."[9]

Perhaps the most significant voice of dissension came from Russian immunologist Élie Metchnikoff. During the 1880s, Metchnikoff developed a radical theory: that certain white blood cells could engulf and destroy harmful bodies such as bacteria. Most leading Western scientists, including Pasteur, scorned Metchnikoff and his improbable theory.[10] Pasteur nevertheless offered his rival an appointment at the Pasteur Institute, where Metchnikoff remained for the rest of his life. Lending support to his seemingly radical theory about immunity was the Nobel Prize he won in 1908.

As a new century unfolded, however, Pasteur's vision became more dominant, and those of Bernard and Metchnikoff less influential. Meanwhile, the basic conditions that allowed tainted milk to be widely distributed — lack of refrigeration, disease-carrying milkers, and the absence of basic sanitation tools like chlorinated cleaners — didn't change appreciably in big cities with the new century. Although scientists had made strides in identifying pathogens (and began working on vaccines) and the value of sanitation started to become clear, fundamental standards for producing clean and safe raw milk in an industrial setting still eluded most producers.

As a result of these circumstances, milk would become our first processed food in the years to come, although it would take a while. Despite the respect accorded Pasteur, his heat treatment was slow to catch on for milk, in significant measure because of the faith people had in the nutritional power of raw milk. The forerunner of the Mayo Clinic, the Mayo Foundation placed great emphasis on raw milk as an antidote to many illnesses. A physician described his approach in a 1929 article that ran in a dairy magazine: "For fifteen years the writer has employed the certified [raw] milk treatment in various diseases and during the past ten he had a small sanitarium devoted principally to this treatment. The results obtained in various types of disease have been so uniformly excellent that one's conception of disease and its alleviation is necessarily changed."[11]

But as outbreaks ravaged large cities during the first decades of the twentieth century, people began turning to pasteurization. The first city to begin requiring it was Chicago, although "it took eight years of political contestation for Chicago to mandate full pasteurization in 1916," according to one local history.[12]

In New York, a philanthropist named Nathan Straus began establishing "milk depots" to make pasteurized milk available to the poor as early as 1893. When a thousand people were sickened or killed by an epidemic of typhoid allegedly caused by raw milk in 1913, followed by an outbreak of foot-and-mouth disease in 1914 also blamed on raw milk, the city's health commissioner had seen enough. He ordered the pasteurization of the entire milk supply, with the exception of certified raw milk — milk officially sanctioned as produced under sanitary conditions. There were only thirty-seven certified dairy farms that supplied New York City with raw milk, guaranteeing shortages and turning pasteurized milk into the default choice. ("Certified" raw milk had the approval of the American Association of Medical Milk Commissions, which was a quasi-regulatory organization established in the early 1900s to oversee the production of safe raw milk around the country.) Boston, Philadelphia, Milwaukee, and San Francisco followed soon after. The accelerating demand for pasteurized milk led enterprising farmers and businesses to start up and invest in plants and equipment to handle the heat processing. A new industry was emerging.

To the CDC, all this was inevitable, regardless of a different direction history could have taken with sanitation and refrigeration standards. A historical summary it published doesn't acknowledge that raw milk has historically been recognized as a healing food and that it was the advent of industrialization that called its safety into question. Instead, the CDC's version of history interprets pasteurization as a slow but inevitable reaction to disease outbreaks:

> Pasteurization of milk . . . was also adopted slowly over many years. At the turn of the last century [1900], cows' milk was recognized as the source of a large number of different infections, including typhoid fever, bovine tuberculosis, diphtheria, and severe streptococcal infections. . . . However, pasteurization was opposed because it was believed that it might be used to market dirtier milk and also because of fears that it might affect the nutritional value of milk; therefore, the technology was implemented slowly. For some, the best way to prevent infections spread through milk was to pay scrupulous attention to the health of animals and to create sanitary conditions for the milk production process. This "certification movement" led to substantial improvements in dairy conditions. However, recurrent outbreaks of illness traced to some certified dairies clearly indicated a need for pasteurization. Initially, different jurisdictions adopted either improved sanitation or pasteurization.

The requirements of the Public Health Service Standard Milk Ordinance in 1927 combined the two strategies: first, milk was to be graded based on a variety of sanitation measures; second, only Grade A milk could be pasteurized. By the end of the 1940s pasteurization was heavily promoted throughout the industry and became the norm. Now, 99% of fresh milk consumed in the United States is pasteurized, Grade A.[13]

The assertion that "pasteurization was heavily promoted throughout the industry" means milk processors exploited the call for pasteurization to establish processing plants around the country. The emerging industry would eventually add homogenization — a means to prevent cream from floating to the top of the milk — to processing during the 1930s and 1940s. It was promoted as the modern and convenient way to drink milk. In an early example of an industry and regulatory joint effort, public health workers regularly condemned raw milk; during the 1930s, officials claimed that raw milk caused 25 percent of all food-borne illness.[14]

Finally, in 1947, the inevitable occurred: Michigan became the first state to require pasteurization of all milk, in effect outlawing raw milk. Over subsequent years, other states followed, including Ohio, Maryland, and Virginia. They made no concessions for certified milk or other means of distributing raw milk such as sales off the farm. Eventually, twenty states in all outlawed raw milk. About twenty others — including New York, Massachusetts, and Pennsylvania — limited allowances to dairy farms with raw milk permits.

Despite raw milk being for many centuries one of mankind's most important foods, its seventy-five-year downfall during the chaos of the Industrial Revolution resulted in it becoming not only the first processed food, but the first food in American history to be banned or sharply limited in its raw form. Because the restrictions occurred gradually (over a period of more than half a century) and the evidence seemed so convincing, the enormity of what happened — that an important precedent had been set that allowed public authorities to ban or curtail foods deemed "dangerous" so as to "protect" us — went largely unnoticed. (Also nearly unnoticed was that the system for mass-producing milk would become the forerunner for mass-producing beef, hogs, chicken, and eggs.)

For people who loved raw milk, there was still some hope in the post–World War II years. Ten states still allowed retail sales, including America's cultural trendsetter and most prolific agricultural producer: California. Not only did California have a large contingent of loyal raw milk consumers, it was also home to the largest producer of raw milk in the country: Alta Dena Dairy, producer of Stueve's raw dairy products, named after the three Stueve brothers who founded it in 1945. The dairy grew from a few dozen cows when it was founded after World War II to thousands, and it supplied much of the country (via health food retailers) with raw milk and other raw milk products like yogurt, butter, and ice cream during a time when bans and limitations were taking hold in many states. Fortunately for Alta Dena, the least restrictive states for raw milk sales tended to be in the West, in states like Oregon, Washington, Arizona, and Nevada.

Alta Dena's success made it a target of California's public health establishment for nearly fifty years. Ron Schmid, author of *The Untold Story of Milk*, contends that during that time California public health officials created crises around Alta Dena's milk. During the 1960s, they accused Alta Dena of selling milk contaminated with *Staphylococcus aureus*, a widely prevalent and not-so-dangerous pathogen, and *Coxiella burnetii*, a more dangerous one that causes Q fever. During the 1970s, there were charges that their milk contained brucella bacteria (also dangerous), even though Alta Dena cows, like most in the United States, were vaccinated against the pathogen. In the 1980s, salmonella led to one or more deaths among immune-depressed individuals thought to have consumed Alta Dena milk shortly before they died.

While Schmid contends that the public health establishment fabricated or exaggerated these crises, it's difficult in hindsight to verify to what extent the claims might have been true. The reality is that Alta Dena was a CAFO, which meant that its thousands of cows were kept confined in conditions that were inevitably unsanitary with the huge volume of manure they produced. So when serious outbreaks involving dozens of individuals occurred, and significant numbers had consumed milk from Alta Dena, the public health officials had a case.

In 1981 and 1982, the CDC reported 116 cases of *Salmonella dublin* in California — a type of salmonella that tends to hit immune-depressed adults — and found that nearly a quarter of the victims had consumed raw milk. In 1983, California had 123 cases of *Salmonella dublin*, the most ever, and found that more than 40 percent of the people affected had consumed raw milk. Because Alta Dena's milk was being shipped elsewhere in the United States, the problem went with it, implied the CDC: "In 1979–1980, *Salmonella dublin* infections in the remainder of the United States were similar to those in California in 1983 in many respects, including the strong association with consumption of raw milk, indicating that this problem is not localized to California."[15] (In its research reports the CDC doesn't identify food producers associated with illness, but raw milk proponents of the day assumed Alta Dena was the target; it was front and center in political disputes with California regulators, and it produced a substantial amount of California's raw milk, and much of the raw milk was used in neighboring states.)

Partly as a result of the ongoing controversy over Alta Dena's line of raw dairy products, several consumer groups at the national level went on the war path against raw milk. During the early 1980s, when the availability of raw milk was entirely a matter of state regulation, veteran consumer advocate Ralph Nader formed Public Citizen, a consumer rights group that lobbied for the FDA to clamp down. At that time, the FDA saw raw milk regulation as a state matter and resisted active involvement.

When the FDA failed to respond with a ban on interstate sales of raw milk, the organization filed suit in federal court. A Public Citizen official was quoted in the *New York Times* as claiming that "since 1980 there have been more than 1,000 cases of human infection and more than 20 deaths from drinking unpasteurized milk, certified or not."

The rabidly anti–raw milk website Quackwatch expresses the frustration felt by medical and public health officials who thought the federal government should have clamped down in advance of a suit being filed. "The FDA had stayed a proposed ban in 1973 and had begun to draft regulations again in 1982, but stalled — the president at the time, Ronald Reagan, favored limiting federal regulation as much as possible — until prodded by Public Citizen's health research group (HRG). HRG petitioned the agency in April 1984 and, together with the American Public Health Association (APHA), filed suit in September 1984 to force a response."[16]

The FDA held hearings in 1984 on regulating raw milk at the federal level, and a number of raw milk proponents testified, according to Quackwatch.[17] Citizens questioned the public health intentions of authorities, a pediatrician testified that his patients' health was better with raw milk, and a physician maintained that pasteurized milk was "dead milk, which will rot on standing."

No matter. A federal judge ruled in favor of the plaintiffs, ordering the FDA to implement regulations banning interstate sales of raw milk — making it illegal for Alta Dena to ship outside California. Even with a devoted California market, things went steadily downhill for Alta Dena in the 1990s. A 1991 suit by Consumers Union halted production for months, in 1997 Los Angeles County essentially banned raw milk, and in 1999 Alta Dena decided it had had enough of debilitating legal challenges and shut down its raw milk operation.

From there it was downhill for raw milk, even in California. By the turn of the century, there was only one tiny licensed producer of raw milk in the state — Claravale Farm, which had operated out of northern California since the 1920s. While many southern Californians simply went without, a core group of raw milk enthusiasts worked hard, sometimes secretly, for its availability. Two of those individuals were James Stewart and Aajonus Vonderplanitz, a couple of longtime health food advocates. Both of the men, then in their fifties, were searching for bigger things in their lives — and that bigger thing became raw milk.

Stewart, a lanky, handsome man, was an aging hippie rebel with long hair and a goatee. Growing up in the Northeast, he was so much a nonachiever that his parents shipped him off to boarding school. He came of age during the late 1960s, as the Vietnam War raged, and extricated himself from possible service by showing up for an army draft physical high on LSD.

He drifted to California, became interested in health and food in the 1970s, and for many years worked as a vegetable distributor and managed a number of health food stores. By the late 1990s, he began thinking that the soy-based vegan diet he had maintained for thirty-three years might be behind growing difficulty he was having with his balance — getting dizzy walking up the single flight of stairs to his one-room Venice apartment — and a bad case of acne. He feared the onset of multiple sclerosis, but "all the doctors wanted to do was prescribe cortisone." Stewart refused to go that route. A chiropractor friend Stewart consulted with thought he might benefit from the unusual nutritional approach of Aajonus Vonderplanitz.

The man with the strange name and the movie-star looks was also a rebel who had become fascinated as a young man with the effects of nutrition on health. He was born John Richard Swigart, and he recounts growing up autistic during a time when autism wasn't talked about. As a result, he had endured little understanding at home, and even less at school. At age eighteen, and still Swigart, he met a man who encouraged him to try raw milk and raw carrot juice. Several weeks on that combination brought him out of his distant state and "cured" him of his autism, he says. But around the same time, he was diagnosed with stomach cancer and underwent radiation therapy. He didn't realize until then, he told me, that "raw meat can reverse any medical condition."

A few years later, at age twenty-two, Swigart began learning the ways of the legal system when he challenged a traffic ticket in Los Angeles. He says he made a remark during a court break about the judge's "Gestapo tactics" that the judge happened to hear, and before Swigart knew it, he was sentenced to five days in jail for contempt of court. He was sent to a rural minimum-security jail "where they had raw milk and raw butter. I said, 'This is heaven.'" When he refused to shave his beard, he was placed in solitary confinement, where he was served soup and lettuce: "I lost eight pounds in four days." More importantly, "I got a taste of what the legal system was about."

The experience inspired Swigart to take a several-months-long bicycle trip through the Southwest—where he decided, among other things, to accept the suggestion of a two-and-a-half-year-old girl who called him "Aajon" to add "us" to it. Later, his father told him the family's last name in Europe generations earlier had been Vonderplanitz; "I loved the name," he says, so much so that he changed his name from John Richard Swigart to Aajonus Vonderplanitz.

The jailing also inspired an interest in the law, and during his free time Vonderplanitz began reading the briefs and decisions of various legal cases. He spent most of his time, however, promoting his budding nutritional expertise at a small table on Venice Beach (not far from James Stewart's apartment) among the purveyors of beads, posters, and paintings. He had an umbrella to protect him from the sun, and a sign: NUTRITIONIST. His niche was raw food. He had come to the belief that cooking food kills essential enzymes and good bacteria.

Stewart and Vonderplanitz met in 1998, when Stewart was experiencing his unsettling physical conditions and fearing the worst. Vonderplanitz remembers being introduced to Stewart, by the chiropractor the two knew in common, at a lecture on raw food nutrition that Vonderplanitz gave: "He was a very skinny vegetarian, six feet three inches, 143 pounds, with severe depression and chronic fatigue. He was unable to work and in serious debt, and there were warrants for his arrest for unpaid child support. After listening to me, James told his friend that I was incredibly fantastic, out of my mind and full of bull. However, James saw how his friend was doing eating a lot of foods on my diet. James began drinking raw milk, then eating raw meats. He gained weight for the first time in his life." Stewart recalls as well that his health improved significantly. The two men would become a team, a kind of modern-day version of Butch Cassidy and the Sundance Kid, in a corner of the food world made rough from the years of battle over raw milk (which had led to its near extinction), unpredictable local regulators, and raw dairy owners hardened by the unstable and unpredictable environment in which they tried to survive.

Stewart, for his part, became so enamored of raw milk that he became a distributor in southern California for the state's only dairy with a permit to produce and sell raw milk at retail stores, Claravale Farm. "Claravale was the last dairy standing, with eight cows," recalls Stewart. Thanks to Stewart's hustle, thirty stores in Los Angeles County, Orange County, Ventura County, and San Diego County were soon selling Claravale milk; the dairy's owner, Ron Garthwaite, was adding cows as quickly as he could. Unfortunately, raw milk was illegal in Los Angeles County as a result of the tumultuous Alta Dena years, despite being legal for retail sale in most of the rest of California. Los Angeles County health regulators began visiting food stores and forcing them to remove the Claravale milk from their shelves. Stewart was losing stores faster than he could replace them, and losing money in the process.

Coincidentally, Vonderplanitz was in the midst of a campaign to legalize raw milk in Los Angeles County, even as he was building his nutrition consultation business. He involved Stewart in helping organize protests and demonstrations. At one point in 2001, they mailed out 1,200 envelopes promoting a demonstration in favor of raw milk in downtown L.A.; five people showed up, including Stewart and Vonderplanitz.

They were an odd couple: Stewart, the engaging and chatty front man who liked to flirt with pretty women, and Vonderplanitz, the handsome but reserved and awkward cerebral guy studying legal texts in his free time.

While Stewart talked up the issues, Vonderplanitz assembled volumes of evidence and testimony attesting to raw milk's nutritional benefits and safety. He threatened possible legal actions if the L.A. County Board of Supervisors didn't agree to legalize raw milk.

By the end of 2001, the L.A. County Board of Supervisors had voted to give Los Angeles County residents the same access to raw milk as most of the rest of California, and the two men felt the satisfaction of a victory that also strengthened their friendship. Yet the two men also had a number of disagreements along the way, most frequently over the perceived quality of the raw dairy products from Claravale, recalls Stewart. "Sometimes Aajonus would call and say that certain dairy products were not up to 'the Aajonus approach.' I said, 'This is my distribution company.'"

Stewart's main problem, though, was that Claravale couldn't provide enough milk for the burgeoning demand that had grown out of the highly publicized hearings to get raw milk approved in Los Angeles County. In 2001, Stewart received a call from Mark McAfee, a second-generation Central Valley farmer, who was converting his organic dairy supplying milk for pasteurization into a raw milk dairy. Stewart immediately traveled north to Fresno to visit the farm, Organic Pastures Dairy Company. He liked what he saw — especially the many dozens of cows. He also liked McAfee's stated commitment to producing organic raw milk. Stewart encouraged Vonderplanitz to become involved. He did and loaned McAfee fifteen thousand dollars. Other members of the Los Angeles raw milk community the two men were in touch with also became involved. One of them, a real estate investor named Larry "Lucky" Otting, advanced seventeen thousand dollars. The family of actor Martin Sheen also became supporters.

Based on Stewart's success expanding Claravale's distribution, the promotion-minded McAfee wanted him to handle Organic Pastures' distribution in southern California. For his part, Stewart felt Organic Pastures could solve the chronic supply problems he was having with Claravale.

It seemed an opportunity neither could pass up. Stewart abandoned Claravale and took on the Organic Pastures line. The abrupt move nearly put Claravale out of business and embittered owner Ron Garthwaite. But Stewart had his increased supply; within three years he had eighty-nine stores regularly buying the Organic Pastures raw milk, yogurt, butter, and cream. The survival-of-the-fittest raw milk market hijinks would eventually catch up with Stewart — everything was great, he recalls, until McAfee brought distribution in-house in 2004.

Out of the raw milk distribution business, Stewart decided to devote himself full-time to a private raw milk buying group he and a few other raw milk aficionados had launched out of a garage in 2001, known to members simply as "The Garage." When the L.A. Department of Building and Safety began investigating complaints of people lining up outside the garage in the quiet neighborhood two days each week to pick up their milk, the garage's owners evicted Stewart and his friends.

For the next eleven months, the group operated their raw milk service out of a truck. Because they weren't distributing the milk at a retail establishment, the operation was considered illegal by local authorities (though in Stewart's view, the fact that he was distributing the milk privately, to individuals he knew who regularly sought him out, placed the arrangement outside the boundaries of the regulatory system). Sometimes Stewart and friends would be under police surveillance, so they'd load the truck up from a garage and distribute the dairy products at different locations around town, spreading the word by telephone.

In 2003, the group, which had grown to about two hundred regular buyers, moved to a vacant lot on Rose Avenue in the Venice area of Los Angeles (owned in part by Stewart). They put up a metal corrugated fence for privacy and brought in a huge shipping container for shelter. Stewart named the club "Rawesome" ("awesome with an R in front"). "We told everyone to be very quiet about what was going on," remembers Stewart.

Despite the low-key effort, Rawesome was soon caught in the wave of interest in organic and natural foods — a wave that was coming to include raw milk. Stewart's many years in food distribution and health store management became invaluable. So did Vonderplanitz's study of the law and his base of nutrition clients. As Vonderplanitz remembers it, he wrote the club's membership agreement and helped solicit members from his client base.

Because Rawesome was operating as a private organization, without any permits, it inevitably ran afoul of regulators. In 2005, inspectors from the L.A. County Department of Public Health came around, and they didn't like the absence of building and health permits. "One of them asked me, 'What's your name?'" recalls Stewart. "I said, 'James.' I refused to tell him my last name. He left me a notice to appear at a hearing."

On the advice of Vonderplanitz, Stewart ignored the hearing. Instead, Vonderplanitz explained the situation in a letter to the L.A. County Department of Public Health:

> I am the elected President of Right To Choose Healthy Food's Rawesome Club. I represent the Club in all matters. Right To Choose Healthy Food's Rawesome Club is not open to the public. It is a members-only club. No one may enter the premises without having voluntarily and supportively signed the Membership Agreement (copy accompanying this letter). The Agreement explains in specific terms our pursuit of healthy life, liberty and happiness. We rejected, and continue to reject, any government health department regulations because they are harmful to our health. Therefore this club and its membership are out of your jurisdiction. All members have adamantly supported and signed the Agreement. Please understand and accept our choices for our pursuit of healthy life, liberty and happiness.
>
> Without intending to be antagonistic, we must face the legal implications regarding your trespassing onto that property clearly posted as no trespassing. Seven of the members testified that you entered the posted No-Trespassing premises without permission or warrant. Four of them testified that they told you to leave the property immediately but you refused and did not leave for about 30 minutes. That was antagonism and harassment against us. We are willing to forgive your trespass unless you and the county continue to harass us. Resultantly, the Hearing Notice is without legal merit. This letter and supportive documents have explained everything that you would have learned in a hearing and we choose not to attend.

The result, according to Stewart, was silence from the authorities. Vonderplanitz painted it as a victory for food rights: "The county failed to respond to the letter and dropped the citation, which was proof that government had no legal jurisdiction."

As the prospect of government interference faded, Stewart moved two more shipping containers onto the site, added more bins, and included more products, including raw honey, kombucha, eggs, chicken, beef, bison hearts and livers, and raw goat and cow cheese from small Missouri producer Morningland Dairy. Not long after that expansion in 2005, however, Stewart put out a notice to all members: "We are finding it difficult to meet our costs. The recent purchase of the lot and the high cost of our monthly mortgage payments has depleted funds. . . . Due to these rising costs we are asking everyone to chip in and help us by agreeing to a surcharge on all groceries. This surcharge will help all of us to meet our need to keep this community grocery alive and well. We appreciate your generosity and understanding in helping us to meet this need. If you cannot or do not wish to pay the surcharge please let us know and we will waive it."

The members rallied with the needed financial support, and Rawesome made it through the crisis. The main governmental interference over the next five years was annual notices from the city of Los Angeles inquiring about whether business was being transacted at the Rose Avenue property where Rawesome was located. Vonderplanitz handled those inquiries. In late 2007, he wrote that Stewart and the other owners "donate the lot at 665 Rose Avenue to Right to Choose Healthy Food's Rawesome Club. Our club is a private not-for-profit membership club that distributes particular food to its members. . . . No one conducts any commercial endeavor involving the public at 665 Rose Avenue. Therefore no license, registration or certificate is necessary under Los Angeles Municipal Codes."[18] Vonderplanitz expressed irritation over the fact that he had previously alerted city officials as to his view of the club's status: "We notified you of this arrangement in our letter dated September 28, 2006 . . . in which we included our membership agreement for clarity of our private purpose. Please cross reference your files so that you do not make this mistake in the future." As usual, he signed it, "Healthfully."[19]

Rawesome's growth — it would climb past one thousand members during those years — mirrored what was happening in the rest of California (and nationally). By 2007, Organic Pastures Dairy Company had become the largest raw dairy in the country, with more than three hundred cows making products available in more than four hundred stores around the state for in excess of fifty thousand customers, according to McAfee. Elsewhere around the country, small dairies were increasingly offering raw milk to individual buyers. Individuals with a few acres weren't just raising chickens — in many cases they added a few goats, or even a cow or two, and sold the milk to neighbors, who seemed to appear out of the woodwork when word spread in a suburban or exurban area that raw milk was for sale.

How many Americans were actually consuming raw milk? Anecdotal evidence pointed to rapidly growing sales by 2005, 2006, and 2007, but no one knows for sure since the FDA seemed determined not to explore anything related to raw milk — aside from pathogens. Sally Fallon, head of the Weston A. Price Foundation, estimated there were half a million to one million raw milk drinkers during that time period.

In 2011, some raw milk advocates discovered that there had in fact been government research into the number of raw milk drinkers. In 2006 and 2007, the CDC conducted a telephone survey through a professional survey company of more than seventeen thousand individuals in ten states (including each region of the country) about their eating habits — including raw milk consumption.[20] The survey showed that an average of 3 percent of the respondents said they drank raw milk in the previous seven days; Minnesota and Colorado were at the low end, with 2.3 percent and 2.4 percent of their populations; New York and Georgia were at the high end, with 3.5 percent and 3.8 percent each. Based on the U.S. population of a bit more than 300 million, regular consumption could now be projected at more than 9 million people — many times what even Sally Fallon estimated.

The good news was that raw milk wasn't anywhere near the scourge it had once been. Illnesses popped up occasionally, but they were a tiny proportion of food-borne illnesses. CDC data indicated that reported illnesses of all kinds from raw dairy amounted to between 25 and 175 cases per year during the first ten years of the new century. This put them generally at less than one percent of the total number of reported food-borne illnesses, which generally ranged from thirteen thousand to twenty-seven thousand per year.

New research also emerged suggesting that raw milk possesses important healing qualities. In 2006, the PARSIFAL (Prevention of Allergy — Risk Factors for Sensitization in Children Related to Farming and Anthroposophic Lifestyle) study of nearly fifteen thousand European school-age children concluded that "consumption of farm milk may offer protection against asthma and allergy." While half the families said they boiled their farm milk before serving it, the researchers thought that number was likely "biased due to the social desirability of responses because raw milk consumption is not recommended for young children."[21]

Nevertheless, John Sheehan, the head of the FDA's Division of Plant and Dairy Food Safety, dismissed the notion that the study offered any meaningful support for the idea that raw milk offers health benefits. Raw milk proponents, he said, had "mischaracterized" the study as one contrasting raw milk with pasteurized milk, when it wasn't clear whether the "farm milk" had been served raw or not.

In 2011, a study of more than eight thousand European children, known as the GABRIELA study, also pointed — this time more directly — to raw milk's health benefits: "The results of this large epidemiologic study add to the increasing body of evidence identifying consumption of farm milk (early in life) to be associated with a reduced risk of childhood asthma and allergies independently of concomitant farm exposures. The results indicate that the effect is due to the consumption of unheated farm milk. For the first time, associations between objectively measured milk constituents and asthma and atopy could be demonstrated." The authors emphasized that only the unpasteurized milk produced the asthma and allergy protection, stating, "Boiled farm milk did not show a protective effect."[22] Contrary to what many raw milk advocates assumed at the time — that the "good" bacteria in raw milk are mainly responsible for its healing properties — the study's authors said the real help likely came from certain whey proteins: "Milk processing, such as heating, does not affect heat stable caseins, whereas whey proteins, accounting for 18% of the total protein in cow's milk, are more sensitive to heat treatment and might influence the bioavailability of the proteins."[23]

Sheehan of the FDA didn't comment on the GABRIELA study, but he was clear in his dismissal of the study's conclusions when he testified on proposed legislation in Maine that would allow small dairies to sell raw milk without a permit. "Pasteurization does not destroy milk proteins," he claimed. "Caseins, the major family of milk proteins, are largely unaffected by pasteurization. . . . Any changes which might occur with whey proteins are barely perceptible."[24]

In 2012, in a follow-up to the GABRIELA study, researchers in the United States and Europe surveyed 157 American Amish families, about 3,000 Swiss farming families, and close to 11,000 Swiss nonfarm families. They examined allergy and asthma rates in children ages six through twelve in all these families. The Amish children had less than one-third the allergies of the nonfarm Swiss children. The researchers found that just 5 percent of Amish kids had been diagnosed with asthma, compared to 6.8 percent of Swiss farm kids and 11.2 percent of the nonfarm Swiss children. Why the differences? The authors said they didn't know for sure but speculated that raw milk likely played a role: "All the Amish children and the Swiss farm children had exposure to large animals and a significant percentage consumed milk directly from the farm. Recent studies have implicated a protective effect from farm milk."[25]

The International Milk Genomics Consortium (IMGC), based at the University of California in Davis and with ties to the conventional dairy industry, concluded in a footnoted article in its newsletter that the European research on raw milk did, indeed, come up with significant findings strongly suggesting health benefits from raw milk.[26] The IMGC's article acknowledged the CDC's stated risks associated with raw milk but also noted, "The data suggest that raw milk can cause both trouble and advantage to a human body. . . . To be sure, heating milk to 72°C for 15 seconds reduces the odds of a bad belly, but does it also destroy complex proteins and other components that could bolster human health? Apparently so."[27] The article went on to state that "there is strong evidence that [raw milk] benefits young children" and concluded that "the world needs studies testing whether large numbers of grown-ups suffering from asthma, hay fever, and similar medical problems see their allergies dampen down after drinking raw milk for a prolonged period."[28]

While health advocates have drawn a lot of attention to raw milk and its potential effects on allergies and asthma, people are beginning to pay attention to the potential healing properties of other foods as well. The Weston A. Price Foundation has helped popularize the notion that an array of nutrient-dense foods can significantly improve health. Besides raw milk, this includes fermented foods (which are rich in good bacteria) such as kimchi, sauerkraut, kefir, and kombucha. Nutrient-dense foods also include pasture-raised beef, pork, and chickens and their eggs — which appear to be richer in key nutrients like beta-carotene, linoleic acid, omega-3s, and other key components than factory-farmed meats and eggs.

Not everyone agrees on what "nutrient-dense" even means. The Weston A. Price Foundation took exception to the definition offered by the USDA in 2010, which by denigrating animal fats and encouraging low-fat and no-fat dairy products "provide[s] an awfully strange definition of the phrase 'nutrient dense' that leads them to advocate a diet that is anything but."[29]

All this may seem like verbiage over subtle technical distinctions until we begin applying these ideas to our daily lives — and realize the chain-reaction variety of changes that can occur. Accepting the notion that high-quality fats of the sort found in avocados and grass-fed meat and raw milk butter are likely healthier than portrayed and improve vitamin and nutrient absorption often leads people to reduce consumption of low-fat foods like pastas and potatoes, and their inherently high sugar content. A focus on fermented foods like sauerkraut and kombucha may well substitute for fried snack foods or high-sugar fruit juices. Eggs may move from forbidden foods because of worries about their cholesterol content to highly prized protein sources when they can be sourced from farmers who allow chickens to scrounge for bugs and grass.

When people sense themselves becoming healthier as a result — perhaps because they are getting fewer colds or flu episodes, or because they notice a chronic condition like acid reflux or hayfever clear up — they often delve deeper, questioning the significance of cholesterol readings and attaching more importance to the results of blood-sugar tests while wondering even more about the relationship between food and health. Eventually, like members of the Grassfed on the Hill food club who turn to acquiring their food privately from farmers like Daniel Allgyer, they may well become skeptical not only of the entire conventional low-fat, low-cholesterol, food-system pyramid as promoted by the USDA, but of the bulk of what is turned out by the nation's factory-food system and sold via mass-market supermarkets and box stores. It's not much of a stretch, then, to see the regulatory actions against people like Allgyer as official interference with their personal food supply, and even an assault on their health.

That was the reaction among many Grassfed on the Hill members when the FDA in its 2011 warning letter ordered Allgyer to detail a plan for ending milk shipments from Pennsylvania across state lines to Maryland. The letter gave him fifteen days to let the agency know about "the specific steps you have taken to correct the noted violations, including an explanation of each step being taken to prevent the recurrence of similar violations. If corrective actions cannot be completed within 15 working days, state the reason for the delay and the time within which corrections will be completed."[30]

Allgyer, who had come to see himself as being key in providing for his members' good health, ignored the letter and continued going about his business.

CHAPTER 4

"WE HAVE JUST BEEN ... HANDED A FANTASTIC CASE!"

The research that came out of Europe suggesting that raw milk's whey proteins could help protect against childhood asthma and allergies was actually a subset of a huge and potentially revolutionary research thrust taking shape around the world focused on the human body's own ability to fight disease. This shift in focus has been most publicly apparent in reports of new cancer treatments based on stimulating the body's immune system.

At a more fundamental level, however, scientists are trying to make sense of the human body's complex communities of microbes — the trillions of bacteria and other microorganisms that inhabit our stomachs, intestines, noses, mouths, and other organs and orifices. Inspired in part by the Human Genome Project that launched in 1990, in which scientists mapped the human body's twenty-five thousand genes over a period of thirteen years, the National Institutes of Health launched the Human Microbiome Project in 2008 with the goal of sequencing the microbiome and understanding its relationship to human health.

In a 2010 front-page article the *New York Times* described the implications of such research: "In addition to helping us digest, the microbiome helps us in many other ways. The microbes in our nose, for example, make antibiotics that can kill the dangerous pathogens we sniff. Our bodies wait for signals from microbes in order to fully develop. When scientists rear mice without any germs in their bodies, the mice end up with stunted intestines.

"In order to co-exist with our microbiome, our immune system has to be able to tolerate thousands of harmless species, while attacking pathogens. Scientists are finding that the microbiome itself guides the immune system to the proper balance."[1]

The international business magazine *The Economist* weighed in two years later with a cover article featuring a futuristic drawing of a human headlined, "Microbes Maketh Man." It called emerging research about the microbiome "revolutionary," noting that "the world's leading scientific journals, *Nature* and *Science*, have both reviewed [the microbiome] in recent months . . . it will help the science and practice of medicine . . . yielding new insights into seemingly intractable medical problems, and there is a good chance cures will follow."[2]

A number of research reports suggest the benefits of having the right array of microbes in place to fight disease. One research report suggested that people may have three different types of microbe, just like they can have four different blood types. A researcher speculated that doctors "might be able to tailor diets or drug prescriptions to suit people's entero-types, for example. Or . . . doctors might be able to use enterotypes to find alternatives to antibiotics, which are becoming increasingly ineffective. Instead of trying to wipe out disease-causing bacteria that have disrupted the ecological balance of the gut, they could try to provide reinforcements for the good bacteria."[3]

A study out of Yale and the University of Chicago found that mice exposed to "good" stomach bacteria had lower rates of type 1 diabetes.[4] Another study associated lowered CRP readings (a gauge of inflammation in the body) with high levels of good bacteria. A scientist involved in the research said that "higher levels of microbial exposure in infancy were as-sociated with lower CRP as an adult."[5] *Reader's Digest Canada* reported in a 2012 article about the expanding interest in the microbiome as an area of research, saying that "during the 1990s, only a few hundred academic papers a year addressed the impact of beneficial bacteria; last year [2011], well over 7,000 articles were published."[6]

While more research is needed about the relationship between nutrition and the microbiome, the announcements validated beliefs about nutrient-dense foods and sparked interest — especially in fermented foods — among more mainstream consumers. Fermented drinks like kombucha and coconut-based beverages began showing up in Whole Foods and health food stores alongside fermented beets and carrots. Raw milk drinkers wanted not just milk but kefir and yogurt as well.

Most states that allowed the sale of raw milk — either from the farm or at retail — didn't allow the sale of fermented raw dairy products. This created a dilemma for many raw dairy farmers, since such value-added products are usually more profitable than plain milk. In a number of states that limited raw milk sales to farms, like Pennsylvania and New York, farmers responded to increased demand for fermented products by opting out of their states' raw milk permit systems and moving to distribute their products privately via food clubs, herdshares, or cowshare arrangements.

These developments created a dilemma for federal and state agriculture and public health officials determined to restrict raw milk distribution. From 2005 to 2008, their strategy for restricting raw dairy sales had been to target individual farmers for prosecution and/or administrative penalties. Farmers like Gary Oaks of Kentucky, Richard Hebron of Michigan, and Mark Nolt of Pennsylvania were hit with aggressive enforcement raids, interrogations, and fines, and/or their products and equipment were confiscated. But as demand and prices for their products soared, farmers weren't inclined to back off.

The expanding attention being paid to the microbiome may have been attracting a lot of interest from researchers and the media, but not from the food safety community — which remained focused on pathogens and seemed to have little interest (for example) in exploring why, in nearly all outbreaks of food-borne illness, most people who ingest food contaminated with a pathogen don't get sick. One explanation is that pathogens disperse unevenly in food and many people don't come into contact with the bacteria. But there have been cases in families in which everyone ate from the same tainted salad bowl or shared the same contaminated cantaloupe or jar of peanut butter, but not everyone got sick. Some people who ingested the same pathogens as those who became seriously ill or even died didn't have even minor symptoms.

The food safety community's main explanation is that some people have weakened immune systems — perhaps because they are elderly or are undergoing radiation treatment for cancer. Pregnant women are thought to be at higher risk — especially for certain pathogens like listeria, which have been known to cause miscarriages. But could people be encouraged to eat foods that might *improve* their microbiomes and, by strengthening their immune systems, make them less susceptible to food-borne illness? This has been an off-limits discussion for food safety experts. Even if there had been a champion within the food safety community for plugging into the microbiome revolution, that individual would have encountered resistance. That is because there were forces at work in Washington DC and elsewhere from 2008 to 2011 that kept the focus on pathogens.

⇒ THE CDC'S HEALTHY ⇐ PEOPLE 2020 INITIATIVE

Every ten years, the CDC sets goals for improving Americans' health — things like reducing cancer and diabetes, improving family planning and exercise, and improving food safety. For about three years in advance of the 2010 deadline for publishing the 2020 goals, public health officials spent time submitting goals and inviting public comment. In the early stages of establishing the 2020 goals, one of the goals under consideration was to restrict raw milk availability by reducing the number of states allowing access to raw milk.

That proposal eventually disappeared — likely it was considered too politically charged for what is supposed to be a nonpolitical process. But a major commitment focused on reducing the incidence of pathogens in food remained; the CDC sought to reduce the incidence of illnesses from various pathogens like campylobacter and salmonella by one-fourth to one-third over the coming decade.

⇒ PRESSURE TO PASS THE ⇐ FOOD SAFETY MODERNIZATION ACT

A number of highly publicized outbreaks of illness from peanut butter, ground beef, eggs, and other foods gave urgency to food safety. The Food Safety Modernization Act was supposed to grant the FDA powers it supposedly lacked to go after producers of tainted food. A number of organizations representing small farmers argued that the FDA already had plenty of power and was using it to focus unfairly on small farms, but the Food Safety Modernization Act had strong bipartisan support.

It passed in early 2011, after opponents managed to include a partial exemption for small farms, and was signed into law by President Barack Obama. Farms selling within a radius of 275 miles, with less than half a million dollars in annual sales, and with half their food being sold directly to consumers wouldn't have to draft food safety plans or comply with certain other provisions of the legislation. But they would be subject to anticipated more aggressive inspections and to safety rules after several years; in early 2013 the FDA issued more than five hundred pages of standards for produce, focusing on irrigation water and compost.

⇒ MORE ATTENTION TO ⇐ SANITIZING AMERICAN FARMS

This effort took several forms. Regulators devoted increased attention to eliminating pathogens from wild animals defecating on fruit and vegetable fields. A highly publicized outbreak of illness in 2006 from *E. coli* o157:H7 in bagged spinach that sickened more than two hundred and killed three was blamed at least partly on wild boars that invaded the growing area. The incident, which led to spinach being pulled off the market nationally for a few weeks and tens of millions of dollars in losses to growers, prompted the FDA and state public health agencies to focus on ways to keep animals away from vegetable fields. States and vegetable marketing organizations implemented regulations requiring farmers to erect fencing and eliminate brush around vegetable fields. At many established farms, old trees were cut down, ditches dug, and other costly measures taken to clear out areas around vegetable fields, in attempts to shield food from wild animals. "Concerns over the correlation between animal defecation in vegetable fields and potential *E. coli* infection has the entire vegetable industry searching for quick, yet accurate answers," said an article on the website of Western Farm Press, an information source for Western farmers.

In late 2010, Michigan's Department of Natural Resources issued an order (to take effect in April 2012) prohibiting the possession of feral pigs, supposedly to protect crops. But the matter turned into a controversy when the state began going after small artisanal farms that raised feral pigs as premium sources of pork and was accused of using the order to favor corporate pork producers. Even if they were kept confined, the pigs were still outlawed. Other states watched Michigan to determine if it made sense to implement a similar ban.

⤜ INSTITUTIONAL RESISTANCE TO CLAIMS ⤛
THAT PARTICULAR FOODS COULD IMPROVE HEALTH

To the FDA, the suggestion that a given food might improve a particular health condition, say by boosting immunity or reducing cholesterol, places the food in the realm of "medicine," subject to the same rules that apply to pharmaceutical companies before they can introduce new drugs — extensive and costly human studies and safety assessments. To food producers, the FDA seems overly rigid at times in its enforcement — Michigan cherry producers objected in 2005 when the FDA sent letters to twenty-nine producers warning that claims that the juice helped relieve gout and was an antioxidant amounted to marketing the products as medicine.

The FDA's strict interpretation of medical claims has even been blamed by some for inhibiting American research into the health benefits of probiotics. For example, a researcher with the California Dairy Research Foundation, a nonprofit established by the state's conventional dairy industry, complained in 2012 that researchers investigating the potential health benefits of probiotics were being driven to conduct their work outside the United States: "If you want to investigate a drug . . . you'd be crazy NOT to file an IND [investigational new drug application] if your intent is to develop a drug," stated Mary Ellen Sanders, an expert in probiotic microbiology. "But if your intent is to conduct research that will substantiate claims on a food (or dietary supplement), then an IND is an expensive, time-consuming, unnecessary task, that may lock your product into the drug category. . . . Consequently, companies are turning to ex-US locations for conducting probiotic food research."[7]

It was in this atmosphere of attentiveness to food-borne illness that the FDA seems to have begun reassessing its crackdown on small producers of raw milk. The 2007 CDC survey indicating that nine million Americans were consuming raw milk suggested that not only was the crackdown on farmers not working, but that the official warnings and negative publicity about raw milk were doing the opposite of what the regulatory establishment intend-ed — they were encouraging more, not less, production and consumption.

Small dairy farms have been mired in a financial slump since the end of World War II as a result of low dairy prices and consolidation of the in-dustry. The United States lost nearly 90 percent of its dairy farms between 1970 and 2006, even while the number of milk-producing cows declined only 25 percent. The fact that milk production per cow doubled made the obliteration of the small-dairy business nearly imperceptible, except to those dairy owners who were driven out of business and the surrounding communities whose economic vitality was sapped as a result.[8] In 2009, two California dairy farmers were reported to have committed suicide as a response to the continued downward pressure in dairy prices.[9] In 2010, an upstate New York dairy farmer shot fifty-one of his cows and then turned his rifle on himself.[10] In 2009, Farm Aid published a report on its website stating that conditions for dairy farmers had become so dire that "even the most tested farmers haven't seen anything quite like this."[11]

It's not surprising then that raw milk began looking like an attractive revenue option to dairy farmers. Processors paid farmers about $1.50 to $2.50 a gallon, while consumers buying directly from farmers paid between $5 and $10 a gallon. The extra money from raw milk consumers was often the difference between operating at an unsustainable loss and breaking even or making a profit. By one calculation, the number of Pennsylvania dairy farmers who were selling privately to consumers more than doubled between 2005 and 2008, from fifteen to thirty-one; many of those had given up their raw milk permits to be able to add yogurt, kefir, butter, and cream to their offerings.[12]

Likewise, the number of consumers flocking to private buying entities like Grassfed on the Hill in the Washington DC area seemed to be growing even more rapidly than the number of farmers who could supply the clubs. Membership at the Community Alliance for Responsible Eco-farming (CARE), a Pennsylvania buying club that launched with eighty-five members in 2005, skyrocketed to more than 3,700 individuals by 2008, each paying twenty dollars annually to shop on a private basis with mostly Amish and Mennonite farmers; by 2012, the number of members was more than six thousand, buying from more than forty farmers.[13]

So many farmers were getting into the raw milk business on a part-time basis that Organic Valley Family of Farms, a huge national cooperative of pasteurized dairy producers that had launched in 1988 to take advantage of the organic craze, began hearing complaints in 2006 and 2007 from some of its dairy farmers. They were upset that other dairy farmers were violating the standard contract between Organic Valley Family of Farms and its farmer members, which required the farmers to sell exclusively to the cooperative. Some of the farmers who complained told me they were worried that if people got sick from the raw milk sold by an Organic Valley Family of Farms supplier, the whole cooperative could be tainted. But others simply seemed jealous. By 2010, the cooperative decided to formally enforce a ban on raw milk sales — in effect, forcing raw milk dairy farmers to make a choice between selling their milk for pasteurization or switching all of their production to direct-to-consumer raw milk sales.[14]

In response to this trend, the FDA appears to have broadened its crackdown on raw dairies, extending it beyond farmers to consumers and managers of food clubs. I say "appears" because there were no formal announcements, such as when New York City began a "War on Graffiti" in the 1970s, or when Arizona passed a new law to usher in a crackdown on immigrants in 2010. An FDA "War on Raw Dairy Consumers" or "Crackdown on Private Food Clubs" wouldn't have been a smart public relations move, especially on the heels of the USDA's successful "Know Your Farmer, Know Your Food" campaign. Criminalizing ordinary consumers for their food choices wasn't something that had ever been tried before, aside from Prohibition during the 1920s and 1930s, so regulators would have undertaken their crackdown quietly. The FDA appears to have launched the campaign nationally with enforcement actions made to appear as if they were occurring randomly around the country, initiated by state regulators in an uncoordinated fashion.

But an examination of several aggressive actions shows evidence suggesting the FDA was involved. The FDA's initial involvement with private food clubs came in Wisconsin, targeting a food club manager there. He obtained raw dairy products, meat, and eggs from several farms in Wisconsin and then transported them to members of a food club he helped operate in Chicago. The Wisconsin authorities learned about the food club from public health officials in the Chicago area after a young boy there, who had consumed raw milk, became ill.

The Wisconsin food club manager was Max Kane, a husky thirtysome-thing who had spent much of his youth as a sickly kid with colitis. It was only after he switched his diet to raw milk and other raw foods that he became the bulked-up fellow he was by 2008, when I first met him. To dramatize his recovery, he rode a bicycle early in 2008 from Virginia to California — and said 85 percent of his nutrients came from raw milk. He bunked along the way at raw dairy farms and was warmly greeted at the finish in California by Mark McAfee — the owner of America's largest raw dairy, Organic Pastures Dairy Company.

In late 2008, the Wisconsin Department of Agriculture, Trade, and Con-sumer Protection (DATCP) began demanding information from Kane after learning that the Chicago-area boy showed some symptoms of brucellosis, a dangerous bovine disease that the CDC says can be passed to humans via consumption of raw milk, but which has essentially been eradicated in the United States. After extensive testing, the boy was found not to have brucellosis, but that didn't end the matter. State authorities in late 2008 and early 2009 continued demanding information from Kane's food club, Belle's Lunchbox. The agency wanted his list of members in Chicago and a list of the farmers in Wisconsin he obtained milk and other foods from.

Kane is a feisty guy, not one who takes well to being intimidated. He felt the requests for the names of his members and farmer sources represented a violation of his Fifth Amendment rights against self-incrimination, not to mention a potential risk for both the farmers who supplied him and his food club members. Kane showed up at a meeting requested by the Wis-consin attorney general's office with a video camera. He asked the assistant attorney general, Phillip Ferris, if he had read the U.S. Constitution. Ferris said he was the one who would be asking the questions. Kane left without answering anything. (A video of the encounter was posted on YouTube but has since been removed.)

That May, Kane began requesting DATCP communications related to his case under Wisconsin's Open Records Law, and he eventually received eight pages of e-mail communications that included summaries of conference calls between FDA officials, DATCP, and other Midwest state agencies. Robert Ehlenfeldt, administrator of the Wisconsin DATCP's Division of Animal Health, wrote on December 19, 2008, to several of his state colleagues: "I hope I don't come to resent making this statement but the brucellosis issue may have been the simplest part of this problem and could have been a pretty good lever to use to push the raw milk issue."[15] The e-mails also suggested that the FDA was involved in the communications around the Kane case: "Larry Stringer [of DATCP] spoke with CFSAN [FDA's Center for Food Safety and Applied Nutrition] about the raw milk issue. They indicated that raw milk sales are a high priority to them as a significant health risk." The e-mails also suggested a broader FDA-directed effort — including state agriculture and public health officials in Illinois, Indiana, and Michigan — to potentially target farmers in at least two of those states for possible raw milk violations.[16]

Eventually, Wisconsin's attorney general filed contempt-of-court charges against Kane for failing to provide the demanded information. On December 21, 2009, a bitterly cold day in the small town of Viroqua, Wisconsin, Kane went on trial following a rally that included more than one hundred supporters outside the courthouse. Kane opted to represent himself, but the judge was unimpressed with Kane's arguments that his constitutional rights were being violated. In pronouncing Kane guilty, Judge Michael Rosborough said that "a lawyer would not be questioning a judge about the constitution. . . . Your arguments about why these regulations are unconstitutional are primitive and undeveloped." Kane put off any immediate danger of going to jail by appealing his case.

On October 15, 2009, a couple of months before Kane's trial, the FDA became involved in an assault on Eric Wagoner's food club in Georgia. Wagoner is a rumpled-looking but hardnosed part-time farmer who had, over several years, built up a food club that supplied several hundred members with fresh meats and vegetables.

As a service to some of the members, the Georgia farmer would drive his truck east to a farm in South Carolina every week and pick up milk that his members had individually preordered and prepaid the farmer for. Wagoner insisted on the advance ordering and payment to head off any accusations that he was violating the federal ban on selling or commercially distributing raw milk across state lines. He was simply an "agent," he maintained, much like a grocery delivery boy who brings food to elders who are unable to go out to the store — and being paid a few dollars for the service.

"We don't even bring a single extra gallon back with us," Eric told me at the time. "Each gallon has to have a name tied to it."

Georgia consumers needed to acquire South Carolina raw milk because Georgia only allows the sale of raw milk for animal consumption and had hassled farmers suspected of selling it for human consumption. In 2007, the Georgia Department of Agriculture (GDA) came up with a plan to discourage people from drinking this "pet food" by proposing to require that farmers inject a black dye into raw milk sold for pets. The agency eventually backed off after hundreds of protesters packed a GDA hearing room during discussion of the proposal.

In South Carolina there was no such tension, since the sale from farms to consumers was legal. For five years, Wagoner had been making his trips to fetch milk from South Carolina without any problems. But when he returned from a South Carolina run this particular Thursday afternoon to a farmers market in Athens with one-hundred-plus gallons of milk for club members, three agents from the GDA were waiting for him.

"They told me it's illegal to cross state lines to sell or distribute raw milk, and distribute is the key word. They taped all my coolers shut and put a 'stop sale' notice on them." To forestall their confiscating his truck with the milk, they agreed he'd hold the milk until the following Monday, when the agents would come to his farm and watch him destroy the milk.

Wagoner alerted his members and requested they each come and destroy their own milk, since they were the owners. On October 19th, one of the most sadly bizarre scenes in the struggle over food rights — captured on video and placed on YouTube — played out on an empty field as dozens of consumers gathered at Wagoner's farm and carried out the GDA's order to destroy the milk. At once spirited and humiliated, consumers poured milk they had paid five dollars a gallon for onto the grass.

Why didn't the consumers simply take their milk and leave — and challenge the authorities to do something? Would the regulators have tried to stop mothers taking milk to feed their children? Those were questions that wouldn't be answered, at least in Georgia. But there was another troubling aspect to this raid. Who were the authorities in charge? Wagoner kept contending that the FDA had helped the GDA.

The answer goes beyond semantics because the FDA positioned itself as outside the fray. But the targets, and their supporters, were convinced that the local agencies were acting at the behest of the FDA. In other words, the raids on dairies — and now what seemed to be an initiative against food clubs and consumers — were part of a national campaign to reduce the appetites of Americans clamoring for raw dairy and other nutrient-dense foods.

There was no hard evidence of FDA involvement in the Wagoner affair until the Farm-to-Consumer Legal Defense Fund (FTCLDF) filed suit in U.S. District Court against the FDA in early 2010 and included Eric Wagoner as one of eight plaintiffs. (The other plaintiffs were consumers who had crossed from states that prohibited raw milk to buy it in states that allowed it and brought it back for their personal use — including Anne Cooper, a member of Wagoner's food club.) In its suit, the FTCLDF alleged that the FDA had been involved in the seizure of milk from Wagoner.[17] Lawyers from the U.S. Justice Department, in an early response to the suit, categorized Wagoner's contention of FDA involvement as "bizarre allegations."[18]

That denial led to an unfriendly legal back-and-forth between the FTCLDF and the U.S. Justice Department. The FTCLDF produced video shot by raw milk supporters showing Wagoner identifying a woman as an FDA agent during the raw milk pour-out at Wagoner's farm.[19] The video identification prompted the FDA to essentially change its story and admit involvement in the Wagoner affair. It provided a detailed account of the role of its agent, as a passive observer at the milk dumping, in a federal court brief in which it sought to have the FTCLDF case dismissed and also sought to minimize its own role. According to the FDA brief, the GDA had sole responsibility for the case, until the question came up of how and where Wagoner would dispose of his milk. "The embargo described above was carried out entirely by GDA under the authority of Georgia law. FDA played no role in the embargo of the Embargoed Milk and/or the discussions with Mr. Wagoner leading up to his decision to voluntarily destroy the Embargoed Milk."[20]

The FDA's shading seemed more like legalistic gymnastics than anything else. That was the FTCLDF's attitude as it challenged the FDA's effort to suggest its agent simply stood silently observing the proceedings. While admitting that the FDA didn't have any contact with Wagoner during the weekend between the embargo and the pour-out, the FTCLDF challenged the FDA's assertion that its agent didn't mention the ban on interstate sales of raw milk. "Ms. Willis was asked about the requirements of federal law and her response was that the raw milk must be destroyed. Ms. Willis also acquiesced in the GDA inspector's comment that changing the law required congressional action."

Wagoner, in a comment on my blog in July 2011, noted that it was only the existence of videos of the event that pressured the FDA to become more forthcoming. "It's thanks to that video that our case has been able to progress as it has. The FDA first claimed the dumping never occurred (calling my testimony 'bizarre allegations'). Now they admit it did happen, but that they were not involved *and* that it was done by me voluntarily. You don't need to watch all 20 minutes on the YouTube video to see how absurd both of those claims are."[21]

In late spring of 2010, another incident targeting consumers and food clubs unfolded in the Minneapolis area. Like the other enforcement actions, it began with raw milk.

Minnesota has restrictive, and vague, laws regarding raw milk and private food distribution. Its state constitution specifically allows farmers the right to "peddle" foods produced on their farms. But state law restricts raw milk, permitting it to be "occasionally secured or purchased for personal use by any consumer at the place or farm where the milk is produced."

For years, the state dealt with the inconsistency and vagueness by generally ignoring the handful of dairy farms that sold, and in some cases delivered, raw milk to private customers. That changed in May 2010, when eight people in the Minneapolis area became ill from exposure to *E. coli* O157:H7, associated with a farm about eighty miles from Minneapolis owned by Michael Hartmann. In such circumstances, whether it involves raw milk or any other food suspected of having made people sick, the investigation typically involves two components.

First, public health authorities seek out as many people as possible who may have become ill—identifying them, interviewing them, and trying to connect their illnesses to a particular food they consumed in common (making an "epidemiological" connection). Then, if the food is identified and a pathogen isolated, the public health and agriculture authorities focus on linking the pathogen to a farm or food-producing facility and determining what conditions at the farm might have led to the outbreak.

In this case, the genetic origins of the pathogens in the sick individuals were matched up to pathogens found in manure and hay in the barn of the Hartmann farm. The match was made via pulsed-field gel electrophoresis (PFGE), which is the "gold standard" method for genetic subtyping of food-borne pathogens. Once the link was made to the Hartmann farm, the state moved to shut it down. Hartmann objected, contending that because the offending pathogen wasn't found in his milk, an absolute connection to his milk hadn't been made. The Minnesota Department of Agriculture (MDA) countered by obtaining a court order in late May placing the Hartmann farm's products under embargo.

Once a farm is shuttered, that is typically the end of the story as far as it affects the public. It's up to the farmer or food producer to demonstrate that the unsanitary conditions that led to the outbreak have been cleaned up, and that there are no more pathogens lurking in the product or on the farm's premises. But in the case of the Hartmann farm, the court order shutting the farm was more the beginning than the end of the story.

Within days of the Hartmann farm shutdown, MDA officials took the unusual step of forcibly searching the home of one of Hartmann's Minneapolis-area customers, Rae Lynn Sandvig. The suburban mother of four was a loyal customer of the Hartmann farm; for the previous eight years she had regularly stocked up on the Hartmann farm's milk and meat to feed her family.

Trained as a teacher, Sandvig had homeschooled her children, and she gradually became enamored of nutrient-dense foods such as those Hartmann produced. She loved the Hartmann farm's products so much that she encouraged a number of her neighbors to buy as well, and eventually Hartmann began delivering to her Bloomington neighborhood (among a number of other drop sites) so his customers wouldn't have to travel the eighty miles to pick up their food. Sandvig allowed Hartmann to park his truck in her driveway every week when he dropped off milk and meat orders to her and forty neighbors and nearby friends. He followed the same routine at his other drop sites in the Minneapolis area.

On the morning of June 10th, however, a group of seven investigators — two Bloomington detectives, three officials of Bloomington Public Health, and two investigators with the MDA — arrived at the Sandvig home with a search warrant and forced their way in past Rae Lynn's husband, Greg.

The search warrant stated the "following grounds: The possession of, particularly the sale or distribution of raw, unpasteurized milk or milk products and the packaging or sale of other food products at a home, the property above-described constitutes a crime." As evidence, the warrant stated that "the MDA received the information regarding sale and/or distribution of the raw, unpasteurized milk and other food items including, but not limited to, custom processed meat, frozen fish, frozen vegetables, nut products and tea, from interviews and signed statements [the MDA investigator] conducted with individuals in the neighborhood who reported receiving the food products from Rae Lynn Sandvig."[22] An MDA agent had actually gone around Sandvig's suburban neighborhood, asking three or four residents to provide information about their neighbor who allowed a farmer to park his truck in her driveway. He even peeked into their refrigerators to see what foods they had acquired from the Hartmann farm.

Once in Sandvig's home, the investigators began quizzing Sandvig about her role in distributing food from the Hartmann farm. How much was she earning? Didn't she know it was illegal to resell food without a license? Didn't she know it was illegal to sell raw milk anywhere but on the farm?

She was defensive, explaining that she wasn't reselling anything, only making it more easily available to her neighbors. By reducing their travel to the Hartmann farm, she was helping reduce pollution and keeping mothers and their children safe from having to drive on busy highways. She explained further that her family neither handled money for the Hartmanns nor distributed any of their products. Nor were any products produced by the Hartmanns stored in the family's refrigerators or freezers other than products for their own use. As for the agents' questions about whether she sold foods from other nonfarm sources, Sandvig explained that she did buy food products like frozen vegetables and fish in bulk at sizable discounts that she then redistributed to their friends and neighbors. All products picked up at the residence were preordered. As compensation, she received occasional "extra" food from these distributors.

Perhaps her most effective argument came when one of the investigators went down a few steps from her kitchen into the garage and opened the refrigerator where Hartmann stored the milk and meat he dropped off each week. It was nearly empty, save for a half gallon of raw milk and a pound of ground beef, which the agent dutifully photographed and confiscated. Clearly, Sandvig wasn't keeping food from Hartmann's farm to resell. It had nearly all been picked up by neighbors shortly after it was dropped off.

Some months later, Sandvig was ordered to attend a hearing at the MDA, where a discussion similar to the one that occurred in her kitchen that June

morning took place. She was issued a "warning letter" to discontinue reselling food without a license and was threatened with criminal prosecution if
she didn't obey.

Five days later, MDA officials — led by John Mitterholzer, one of the investigators who entered the Sandvig home and those of her neighbors — en-
listed Minneapolis police for a new mission, this time a raid on Traditional
Foods Minnesota. This was a buying club begun in 2008 by two advocates
of nutrient-dense food, and it was located in a warehouse adjoining a lower-
middle-class area of the city. By 2010, Traditional Foods Minnesota had
about eight hundred members, who each paid a lifetime membership fee of
seventy-five dollars to access its locally produced foods. Just a month before
the MDA visit, the Minneapolis *Star Tribune* published a review under the
headline "A Warehouse with a Different Approach":

> In a bleak industrial sliver of Minneapolis, near a concrete
> plant and behind an automotive body parts shop, you can find
> some of the wildest, most interesting food in the Twin Cities.
> Traditional Foods Warehouse, a buying club, sells items you
> won't find in grocery stores or even at natural-food co-ops.
> There are racks of small-batch kombucha (a fermented tea)
> in beautiful indigo blue bottles, kimchi and fermented carrot
> salsa, freshly churned cream, fresh cottage cheese, kefir, fresh
> duck eggs, pickled quail eggs, frozen quail, pheasant, buffalo,
> and free-range pork, beef and bison. There's your choice of
> dandelion coffee, raw cocoa nibs, sun-dried zucchini and dried
> mushrooms. And there are infused salts, herb olive oils and
> vinegars, and a variety of nonfood items, including hand-spun
> yarn, organic soap and more. Much more. It's not a pretty
> space, all cinderblock and cement floor, but even on a dreary
> Thursday afternoon, there was a small, steady stream of shop-
> pers checking out products and chatting with the folks who run
> the place and sell their stuff.

But Monday, June 20th, would not be a good one for Traditional Foods
Minnesota. Kathryn Niflis Johnson, a health consultant, told me about
being at the warehouse that afternoon:

I live on the other side of the city and I hadn't been there for a really long time. I had completed my shopping, and was just getting ready to leave, when the Department of Agriculture people came in, accompanied by a uniformed Minneapolis police officer. There was the head of the dairy division and a few others. I know because they gave their business card to the check-out clerk. There were a few other customers there at the time, but they kind of scattered.

Niflis Johnson decided to call Pete Kennedy, the head of the FTCLDF, for advice, "and the bottom line, according to Pete, was that we shouldn't answer any questions."

That prompted Johnson to try to intercede. The agent in charge identified himself as John Mitterholzer. She says she told the manager that he was "not supposed to answer any questions. It's so difficult not to answer any questions when the questions seem so easy, like who owns this or what do you do here. I kept saying not to answer any questions. And finally Mitterholzer looked at the police officer and said, 'Get her out of here. She is interfering with my investigation.'"

Johnson objected to the Minneapolis police officer, but he agreed with Mitterholzer, who was already telling the officer to take down her license plate number and snap her photo. "Then the police officer led me to my car, and I took off. I called Pete and said, 'I tried. They made me leave.'"

Johnson was shaken by the experience. "It was scary and intimidating. I consider myself a law-abiding citizen. I've always felt police officers were my friends. I've never had any run-ins with the government or the law. I thought they were on my side. I had no idea about my rights. Later, people said, 'You could have done this, or that.' It changed my whole paradigm for the worst."

The MDA inspectors carted off a number of products and then taped a notice on the entrance stating that the store was "embargoed." Traditional Foods Minnesota has remained shuttered since that day in June 2010 despite efforts by one of its owners, Warren Burgess, to negotiate the appropriate licensing necessary to reopen. City officials have signaled their determination to keep the food club out of business. When some Traditional Foods Minnesota members gathered at the site for an informal farmers market—

type event featuring several farmers and food producers later that year, the MDA filed a complaint with the city.

Both events — the Sandvig residence search and the Traditional Foods Minnesota shutdown — received scant public attention at the time. The *Star Tribune* published a brief article about the closing of Traditional Foods Minnesota, noting that a sign on the door said "embargoed" and that the club "hoped to open soon." There was no mention of the police and agency raid of the site. Minnesota Public Radio had a brief item as well, mentioning that a consumer's home had been searched, but without any more detail. The Sandvigs were so shaken they decided to not speak with the media, so the only other reporting occurred on the FTCLDF's website and on my blog (with the family's name not included).

But the MDA still wasn't done. Among the food confiscated at Traditional Foods Minnesota that June afternoon was raw milk and frozen fruit supplied by Minnesota farmer Alvin Schlangen. He had no connection to the Hartmann farm, which was associated with the illnesses in May, but the MDA targeted him as well. Its agents obtained search warrants to confiscate business records from his farm in 2010 and thousands of dollars worth of food from his van as he made deliveries in St. Paul in 2011. In February 2012, Schlangen was charged with a series of misdemeanor counts by both his local district attorney and one in Minneapolis, both at the behest of the MDA, for selling raw milk and other foods without a license. The charges had the potential to land him in jail for more than a year. A trial would be scheduled for May of 2012.

What was the FDA's role in the Minnesota events? There is no smoking gun I could locate showing a direct connection between the MDA and the FDA in the Hartmann/Sandvig/Traditional Foods Minnesota/Schlangen investigations, as there was in Georgia or Wisconsin. But the Minnesota health and agriculture agencies are known to be close to the FDA. A little over a year after the MDA's crackdown, it issued a press release saying it had received a million-dollar grant from the FDA "to strengthen its capacity to respond to food-borne outbreaks and other food safety events."[23] A year later, the MDA was awarded six hundred thousand dollars in FDA grants "to enhance the state's food safety capabilities."[24]

In its report to Congress covering 2011 activities in various states, the FDA said it had seventy-four employees in Minnesota, along with contracts and grants with the MDA. The report alluded to a contract with the MDA to "conduct food safety inspections" as well as a grant for a "Food Safety Task Force to coordinate and address food safety and defense issues among regulated industry and regulators within the state."[25]

The FDA's ties to Minnesota agencies are representative of a national campaign to strengthen the relationship between states and the FDA. In its messages to Congress and the public, the FDA communicates the sense that it cooperates closely with state public health and agriculture agencies. It even has a Division of Federal-State Relations, and in a *Year in Review* report recapping its activities, its director, Joseph Reardon, stated that the FDA handed out to states more than forty-one million dollars in grants, contracts, and cooperative agreements in 2010.[26] Moreover, the FDA "commissioned 1,346 State and Local officials to assist FDA in traditional program areas such as foods and animal feeds."[27] According to Reardon, "The FDA and the States can equally benefit from the goal of a national food safety system."[28]

Why should anyone care about such a seemingly upstanding goal? Traditionally, state and local public health agencies have been independent, much like school systems and fire departments. We don't hear talk about "a national public school system" or "a national fire-fighting system," even though the latter have much to do with safety. The funding and statement suggest growing FDA control over local public health agencies to achieve federal goals.

The most dramatic example of the FDA's shift in tactics occurred with Amish farmer Daniel Allgyer, who was supplying the Maryland food club Grassfed on the Hill. As described near the end of chapter 1, the food club was growing rapidly—and with government employees likely part of the food club's membership, it's reasonable to speculate that information about it reached the FDA's dairy division.

Whatever the exact circumstance, by 2009 the director of the FDA's dairy division, John Sheehan, was receiving items from Grassfed on the Hill's information package, including the warning on sharing information with government officials. The material about the club was coming from a "source," he told colleagues, and he was captivated. In August 2009, Sheehan e-mailed some of the food club documents to two FDA colleagues with the message: "More very useful information from my source. I think we have just been basically handed a fantastic case!"[29]

Within two months, the number of FDA officials passing around information about Grassfed on the Hill had grown to a dozen, according to e-mails I obtained about the investigation from the FDA under the Freedom of Information Act. At that time, the Philadelphia office's director of the investigations branch, Karyn Campbell, sent an e-mail to the FDA's Baltimore office ordering it to assign an investigator to join Grassfed on the Hill as a member and begin ordering raw milk on an undercover basis.[30]

As if to signify the high priority of the Grassfed on the Hill/Allgyer investigation, in an e-mail two months later (in December) Campbell said to a Baltimore colleague that "the Region can help with funding"[31] if the local office's budgets should be strained by what would turn into a long-term investigation. That was code for saying that there was no need for any short-term worries about budget limits for this particular investigation.

By December 2009, an FDA investigator from Baltimore had become a member of Grassfed on the Hill via its online site and was placing orders for Allgyer's raw milk. Members picked up their food from refrigerators located in the garages or on patios of other members who had volunteered their homes as drop sites. This meant an FDA agent was entering the premises of various private citizens to pick up the contraband, which would immediately be packaged for shipment to a government laboratory for confirmation that it was unpasteurized and to test for pathogens.

Here is how the investigator described his/her activities (the investigator's name was blacked out, as were particulars like locations and certain dates): "I removed the [blacked out] containers of milk (ordered by Stephanie L. Shapley, CSO [for Consumer Safety Officer]) from the [blacked out], a residence located at [blacked out], MD. I then placed the [blacked out] containers of milk into an FDA cooler, with ice packs, which was located in the locked trunk of the government vehicle used for this assignment. The containers of raw milk were then transported to the BLT-DO (Baltimore district office) sample room."[32] Even the packaging of the samples was described in excruciating detail: The milk containers "were placed into a paper bag. The paper bag was taped closed and identified [sample numbers, some blacked out]. The paper bag was then officially sealed, [more numbers, some blacked out], Jesse Hardin, Investigator."[33]

There was much more, as the investigators apparently wanted to be sure they left nothing out of their documentation, presumably so they'd be prepared for a court case. They kept tabs on the temperature of the refrigerators in which the samples were stored, who opened and then closed various containers, even how many times a paper bag was folded closed and how many pieces of tape were affixed. The detail becomes mind-numbing, and I've included just a sample here so readers can appreciate how involved a serious FDA investigation becomes – down to the kind and number of pieces of tape and such . . . all for raw milk.

One segment records the actions of FDA Consumer Safety Officer Shapley: "CSO Shapley folded the brown paper bag closed 3 times, applied FDA 415a to brown paper bag & wrapped 1 cont. piece clear plastic tape around officially sealed bag 6 times. CSO Shapley affixed FDA 525 to officially sealed sample w/2 pieces tape. CSO Shapley placed officially sealed sample into large clear plastic bag w/zip closure + closed clear plastic bag. CSO Shapley placed closed clear plastic bag into white Styrofoam cooler w/7 blue ice packs. CSO Shapley secured cooler closed w/5 pieces tape. CSO Shapley placed closed clear plastic bag into white Styrofoam cooler w/7 blue ice packs. CSO Shapley secured cooler into a white cardboard box and taped the box closed. CSO Shapley documented the sample # on the upper left hand corner of the box and placed a 'Perishable' sticker on the upper right hand corner of the box. CSO Shapley affixed a FedEx US Air Bill to box, transported to BLT-DO security desk for FedEx p/u."[34]

There followed among undercover investigation documents a number of order forms from Daniel Allgyer, with the recipient and the amount of the raw milk sales blacked out,[35] and finally a number of photos of a MoneyGram money order used to pay for the orders, with everything blacked out except Daniel Allgyer's name in the "Pay to the Order of" line.[36] In retrospect, club administrators Karine Bouis-Towe and Liz Reitzig would realize that anonymous money orders should have been a tip-off of something amiss, since nearly everyone in the club paid with personal checks.

Another report, from December 23, 2009, contained the lab report on milk that had been so carefully packed, beginning with two common pathogens: "No Salmonella spp detected. . . . No Listeria monocytogeneses detected."[37] There were then readings for the presence of bacteria unlikely to be pathogenic, like *E. coli*, *Staphyloccus aureus*, and coliforms.

The FDA now had a two-front investigation involving Daniel Allgyer – of his farm and of the Grassfed on the Hill food club.

CHAPTER 5

LOCAL FOOD
AND SECOND CHANCES

It was just before 6:00 a.m. on a crisp, clear November morning in 2010 at a farm in southeast Pennsylvania when I began to understand some of the key drivers behind America's underground food war.

I had just walked out the front door of an Amish farmhouse, where I spent the night, to observe the early-morning farm activities. I was visiting the farm at the invitation of the owner, Amos Miller, and his wife, Becky, and I was amazed to be there. I had spent time at a number of farms around the country over the previous five years that I'd been writing about food rights, but never at one owned by an Amish family. Like many people, I had long been curious about the Amish and their commitment to an old way of life — reliance on the horse and buggy, doing without computers, and staying off the electric grid. Their private ways seemed only to heighten the aura of mystery among us "English," the term many Amish use to refer to non-Amish. I never expected I'd get any closer to their society than seeing them ride around in their horse-drawn carriages in the Lancaster, Pennsylvania, area where I traveled occasionally.

I had gotten to know Miller over the previous few years of attending conferences like Acres U.S.A. and the Weston A. Price Foundation's Wise Traditions. Miller always had a large booth at those conferences where he sold meats, fermented vegetables, yogurt, honey, and sausages.

I always found Miller to be an engaging guy who, unlike many Amish, liked to chat, and he acknowledged jokes or teasing with a slightly mischievous grin. I also appreciated his hustle and conscientiousness — he wanted to be sure I found the food I was looking for, and if he didn't have it on hand at his booth, he'd order it. I often had the feeling when I was with him that, if he wasn't a member of the Amish community — dressed in the standard dark blue shirt and black trousers with suspenders, and adhering to its strict requirements about doing without modern-day technology — he'd run a chain of fast-growing high-end food stores or serious gourmet restaurants.

Earlier in 2010, I had written a profile about Miller for the small business section of BusinessWeek.com (now Bloomberg BusinessWeek), in which I marveled that he was able to operate a successful farm, selling direct to individuals around the country, without most of the modern conveniences we take for granted, including e-mail, faxes, cell phones, automobiles, or copiers — not to mention a website or social media.[1]

Shortly after completing that article, I learned that Miller supplied a fledgling Boston-area food club I was interested in joining. When the Weston A. Price Foundation scheduled its Wise Traditions conference for 2010 in the Philadelphia area, about ninety minutes from Miller's farm in Bird-in-Hand, I decided to use the opportunity to visit his farm in advance of the conference and try to understand more about the dynamics of his operation.

So two days before the conference began early that November, I hung out at his fifty-two-acre farm to observe his farming operation in action. It was a mild afternoon for November when I arrived. As I stood around in the barn, in the fenced barnyard area, and out in the pasture, Miller's farm looked a lot like other small farms I had visited over the previous five years of writing about raw dairies. Some sixty cows grazed in the waning late-fall pasture; dozens of chickens clucked in the barnyard and in portable chicken coops in the pasture area. Maybe fifty pigs lounged in a muddy patch outside the barn. A couple of Miller's young blond children played tag and chased chickens around.

In the barnyard, I met Henry — a thin, almost gaunt young man with the standard Amish beard and bowl haircut. He told me that one of his jobs at the farm was to use traditional methods to slaughter a couple of cattle and three pigs each week for Miller to supply meat to his food club members. The tradition? A pistol shot between the eyes.

"You have to hit them in just the right spot," he said, motioning with his two thumbs and forefingers together to show the size of the spot — about the size of three silver dollars for a cow and two for a pig. "With the pigs, if you miss, the bullet bounces off the skull. They have a real hard skull."

Henry shoots the animals outside the barn and works fast, he said, to clean up the blood (especially with the pigs): "If you don't clean the blood up right away, the other pigs will roll around in it." A group of Mennonites were at the ready to skin the hides and take the carcasses to their own facility for butchering. This was the kind of meat the food clubs Miller supplied demanded — not only grass-fed, but custom-slaughtered and prepared outside the regularly monitored USDA system that some discerning consumers felt was unsanitary.

You didn't have to hang around at Miller's farm for long to appreciate that there were a lot of things going on there that were different from what happens at most quiet small farms. For one, there was a nearly continuous flow of trucks doing drop-offs and pickups. A white pickup pulled up in the late afternoon and a young Amish man, John, hopped out of the passenger side and worked with one of Miller's farmhands to unload twenty large boxes of frozen chickens. John ran a farm in the area and had hired a driver to help deliver to Miller. (The Amish hire drivers when they are in a hurry, need to travel a long distance, or need to transport a big load, since they aren't allowed by their community rules to drive motorized vehicles.) Because Miller's farm can't meet all the demand for chickens among the food clubs he supplies, he relied on relatives and neighbors like John. There was a brief exchange of handwritten yellow packing slips, and John was on his way. Not long after, a large refrigerated shipping truck pulled in the long driveway. Miller's Amish farmhands quickly loaded forty brown cardboard boxes destined for a buying club in Alabama. Next came a FedEx truck, its driver wondering if there was anything for him to pick up. Food intended for FedEx delivery wasn't yet ready, Miller explained, so the FedEx driver was on his way.

All of this activity took place in front of a long two-story building made of corrugated steel and cinderblocks, probably the length of a football field. On one side were two wooden cubicles, about twelve feet long and five feet wide, which each housed a small desk and two concessions to technology — a telephone and an answering machine. Outside the cubicles, a sign said CALL CENTER. Inside one of the cubicles, another sign deadpanned, I DO NOT REPEAT GOSSIP, SO LISTEN CAREFULLY.

A middle-aged woman wearing a black cotton scarf over her head and a black sweater over her traditional dark green cotton dress was on the phone at one of the desks. This was where orders came in from the outside world and Sadie, an employee, took them down in a notebook. Before she hung up, she'd dart inside the building briefly and come back with a FedEx tracking number to read to the food club member. When orders came in while she was on the phone or wasn't there, an answering machine picked up and recorded the order for later transcription.

The heart of the activity was at the front of the mammoth building — a high-ceilinged, high-energy packing and shipping area. This is where Miller spends most of his time, sorting and wrapping food items from his farm and neighboring farms and placing the items into brown cardboard boxes for shipping to individual food club members. This particular afternoon, he was munching one of his farm's products — raw chicken salad, from a plastic pint container. Becky, his dark-haired wife, sat at a desk arranging handwritten orders into notebooks.

Much of the food was prepared toward the back of the building, in the cheese and milk rooms. Indeed, I could see half a dozen Amish men in straw hats moving around and sealing plastic pint containers of cottage cheese that two women with ladles had just filled. Some of the products were produced on neighbors' farms. Miller's brother, Ben, supplied the cabbage used for the sauerkraut. A neighbor named Eli supplied the sheep milk that some customers ordered.

In this building the concessions to technology multiplied. There were powerful portable fluorescent lights so that as darkness descended around 4:30 p.m., Miller and his half dozen or so assistants could continue loading and sealing cardboard boxes. Parallel to the packing area and the milk and cheese production areas were two cavernous rooms — a massive cooler and a smaller but still sizable freezer measuring about fifty feet by twenty feet. Each contained shelves arranged nearly to the ceiling stocked with cultured butter, goat milk, cheddar cheeses, ground beef, beef hearts, fermented vegetables, and the 140 or so other products that made up the farm's selection of nutrient-dense foods. The power to run these rooms came from a large diesel-powered generator out back.

How do the technology-averse Amish justify this electricity? I never could get a clear answer. I was led to understand that the use of a generator is OK — you're still off the grid, after all — so long as the religious elders approve the use. An Amish community's religious elders are the group's most important decision makers; what they approve and disapprove can vary from Amish community to Amish community. Some are highly restrictive and others fairly liberal. In Miller's case, sending good wholesome food to people who value it was an approved activity, justifying the use of generators to operate coolers and freezers.

At about 6:00 that evening, Miller paused to join his family for dinner. His traditional-style farmhouse was steps from the packing-storage facility. I expected the absence of electricity to have turned his home into a primitive place, but far from it. As I joined him, Becky, and their four young children at the large wooden kitchen table, I couldn't help but notice the presence of a fairly up-to-date white refrigerator and stove. "Propane powered," explained Miller. More bright fluorescent portable lights countered the darkness. There were no signs of electrical outlets that I could see. Becky passed out slices of a homemade hamburger pizza. Rich with farm-fresh ricotta cheese, tomato sauce, and large amounts of ground beef, it was delicious and nutritious.

The guest room upstairs where I would sleep was spacious, with a comfortable bed, and a large flush-toilet bathroom was down the hall. If I woke up during the night, I'd have a portable light to help me make my way. But there'd be no thought of sleep for a while yet. After quickly downing a couple slices of pizza, Miller kissed his children goodnight and headed back to the packing and shipping area. There were still half a dozen or so boxes to pack. He asked me if I'd drive him to the local FedEx office to drop off some of them. Of course.

Along around 8:00 p.m., as he was still wrapping a couple boxes, I asked him if we shouldn't get going. The office was open till 8:30, he said, and was only ten minutes away. We still had fifteen minutes.

"What would you have done to get the packages over there if I wasn't here?" I asked Miller when we'd finally loaded half a dozen boxes into my small SUV and were driving to the FedEx office.

"I'd have taken the carriage and left ten minutes earlier," he said, referring to the horse-drawn carriage outside the packing facility. Yes, he had been down this road many times before.

The next cold and crisp morning, as I came out the front door of Miller's farmhouse, the first thing I saw off to my left was the implausible sight of a horse-drawn carriage rolling up the long farm driveway. Attached to the back was a small trailer carrying a single item — a fifty-gallon stainless steel drum. Maybe it was the astonished look on my face that caused Ben (there were a lot of Bens), the young Amish driver, to stop the carriage in front of the house. He told me this was his regular weekly delivery of milk to help Miller fill his delivery requirements to Rawesome Foods.

The enormity of what was happening gradually dawned on me as I watched that milk, along with milk from four or five other area farms, being bottled a couple hours later. Two Amish workers bottled it by hand, letting it flow out of a five-hundred-gallon stainless steel bulk tank in the milk room into one-gallon and half-gallon plastic jugs they held expertly under the flow, to be quickly sealed with red plastic tops.

There it was: milk from Pennsylvania was being prepared for shipment three thousand miles west to the number one dairy-producing state in the country — a state with a thriving raw dairy marketplace.

The fifty gallons of milk that arrived on a horse-drawn carriage that morning would be among two hundred gallons sent to California in a refrigerated truck that evening. Six gallons of cream, twenty-five dozen unwashed eggs (kept unrefrigerated), and forty-five pounds of beef — as well as raw dairy cottage cheese, crème fraîche, kefir, and yogurt — would also be on the truck. The products would be available to Rawesome members in two days, on Saturday — one of the two days each week that Rawesome was open. The food that showed up on the shelves wouldn't be inexpensive — milk at fourteen dollars a gallon, eggs at six dollars a dozen. Why would James Stewart and Aajonus Vonderplanitz go all the way to Pennsylvania to supply the tiny food club? You'd think similar food would be available in California with less hassle and risk.

I had assumed that the main reason Stewart and Vonderplanitz sought out Amos Miller's products had to do with the falling-out they each had had with Mark McAfee, owner of Organic Pastures Dairy Company. The largest raw dairy producer in California, and the nation, Organic Pastures had taken advantage of California's dairy laws allowing regulated raw milk, as well as backing from Vonderplanitz and Stewart in 2001, to become, as noted previously, a thriving multimillion-dollar business serving more than fifty thousand residents via four hundred retail outlets. For most Californians, no matter where they lived in the state, they weren't more than a short drive from a retail outlet carrying Organic Pastures milk, cream, kefir, and butter.

Stewart never forgave McAfee for terminating Stewart's southern California distributorship in 2004 with a year left on his contract. And he found it suspicious that Organic Pastures could produce enough cream and butter to satisfy so many consumers with only a few hundred cows and suspected McAfee was outsourcing for cream to produce those products. (McAfee would eventually admit that he outsourced for butter and cream, but not for milk — and discontinued all outsourcing by 2010.) Vonderplanitz, the obsessive food-quality overseer, had become convinced that McAfee had strayed from his organic roots and was feeding Organic Pastures' cows nonorganic feed. (California's only other licensed raw dairy, Claravale Farm, produced much less milk than Organic Pastures and, besides, made no bones that it didn't adhere to organic standards.) Vonderplanitz complained, further, that McAfee had failed to repay him the money he loaned Organic Pastures in 2001. McAfee denied both accusations.

The enmity may have driven Vonderplanitz and Stewart to seek out the Amish supplier, but there was a more significant reason Rawesome became dependent on Amish food; it likely had to do with the challenge of trying to find the same high quality of food — especially dairy, meat, and eggs — locally.

It wasn't that long ago, in the decades immediately following World War II, that a trip to the country from most urban areas in the Midwest and East meant scenes of cows grazing on pastures and chickens pecking in farm driveways. Those scenes have mostly been replaced by subdivisions and strip malls with fast-food joints and big-box stores like Wal-Mart and Home Depot. The dairy farms that once dotted the countryside are no more, their owners forced to sell their land and take up other occupations.

Yet as Americans have become more discriminating in their food tastes and farming has become cool, people have become attracted to farming. Young people are seeking out apprenticeships to learn the ins and outs of tending a farm. Some even go off on their own, leasing land and setting up a dairy or cheese-making operation, in hopes of eventually being able to acquire land of their own. Buying a farm? It's difficult given the high cost of land and often restrictive zoning requirements. Farmers who have had enough often sell out to developers, who will build subdivisions, rather than to aspiring farmers, who can't match the developers' offers.

Yes, there has been growing interest in locally produced farm goods in recent years, but much of the most readily available foods is limited to vegetables, fruits, honey, and maple syrup. If you go to most farmers markets, many of the stands are occupied not by farmers but by vendors selling breads, jams, pickled vegetables, and even caramel corn and tamales.

There has actually been an uptick in the number of farms, according to the USDA, on the order of 4 percent in a 2007 census, but many of those are part-time hobby farms and many owners have to hold nonfarm jobs to pay their bills.[2] There is still a dearth of high-quality dairy and beef production close to cities. Quality meat and egg suppliers like Joel Salatin in Virginia, who became famous when he was profiled in Michael Pollan's best-seller *The Omnivore's Dilemma*, quickly exhaust their supply; Salatin desperately acquired additional land to expand production.

Enforcement pressure in places like Maryland, Minnesota, Wisconsin, and New York hasn't helped matters, forcing buying clubs to source from faraway Amish farms. Sally Fallon, head of the Weston A. Price Foundation, who also runs a dairy farm in Maryland, has done some back-of-the-envelope calculations that her home state loses $90 million in farm food sales to neighboring Pennsylvania because of Maryland's restrictive regulations on raw milk. When you add the related economic activity associated with that $90 million circulating through the economy, the total loss to Maryland approaches $250 million, she calculates.

A number of organizations have sprung up to encourage local farming and food sovereignty — the production and local sale of food outside of regulatory parameters. One of these organizations is Food for Maine's Future, and its director, Bob St. Peter, speaks about "stopping the expropriation of knowledge, land, and our collective seed heritage for privatization, patents, and profit; and preserving a rural way of life that is economically, socially, and culturally vibrant."[3]

Aside from regulation, a key obstacle is economics: "The farther away you get from urban areas, the cheaper the farm land, but the closer you get to urban areas, the more expensive the land," says St. Peter. The more expensive land, of course, the more leverage (i.e., loans) required for farmers to buy the land, and thus the greater the financial risk for all involved. "Risk" is a word bankers don't like to hear, so obtaining mortgages to launch new farms near big cities can be a daunting task.

But where there is risk, there is also opportunity. The closer farmers are to urban areas, the higher the prices their products fetch at farmers markets and food clubs. Fresh farm-raised eggs that are $2 or $2.50 a dozen at a farm's roadside stand out in the country can be sold for $5 or even $6 a dozen at an urban farmers market. Gourmet raw milk cheeses that might sell for $12 or $14 a pound far outside the city can fetch $24 or even $30 a pound in an urban area.

The way Sharon Palmer remembers it, she first heard about James Stewart and Rawesome Foods in late 2007 while selling her farm's goat cheese at a Los Angeles–area farmers market: "I heard he wanted to find a steady supply of eggs. He also said he needed milk." She had become an expert at making top-quality cheese, and she had always wanted to raise goats. She got in touch, and thus began a long and complex business relationship.

Palmer is a pleasant, soft-spoken woman with shoulder-length black hair and closely set dark eyes, a bit matronly looking as she enters her fifties. She had come to California from New Jersey in 1990, at the age of thirty — a single mom fresh off a divorce in search of both financial opportunity and personal restoration. It was the start of the financially booming 1990s, and Palmer got caught up in the real estate part of the boom. She had done some work in real estate while in New Jersey, so a Los Angeles–area company that packaged mortgage loans for banks took her on. Before long, she was the company's chief loan processor for mortgages being packaged around the country.

Palmer became friendly with the owner, Edward Rostami; one thing led to another, and they were married. According to Palmer, she was on the outside looking in, both with Rostami's close-knit Armenian family and with his business. They had three children, and the business seemed to thrive. But appearances were deceiving; by the mid-1990s, things began to come apart.

According to Palmer, the problems arose when Rostami attempted to branch out from conventional mortgages to reverse mortgages. In the latter, a homeowner converts a portion of the home's equity into cash. The owner (usually elderly) gets retirement funds, and the mortgage company gains equity in the home, which can turn into an excellent investment when real estate values are rising. As Palmer tells it, her husband's mortgage company "made thousands of conventional mortgages and five of these [reverse mortgages]. All the reverse mortgages went bad."

"Went bad" is about as positive a spin as you could put on what happened. Banks and mortgage companies made allegations of fraud against the Rostami-Palmer mortgage company in suits filed against the two. They lost a number of the suits. "They took our home and cars," recalls Palmer. "I watched our lives unravel." This included her marriage to Rostami.

Palmer's father was a sport fisherman who had friends in Mexico. In 1998, she took her three children to Rosarito and moved in with a family her father knew. "Being in Mexico was probably one of the best things I ever did. I was living in a Third World country. It brings you back to basics, going to the lake for water every day, washing your clothes by hand."

Palmer says she didn't know that indictments were being prepared back in California charging her and Rostami with fraud in connection with one of the reverse mortgages. The state alleged that she and Rostami committed to providing a reverse mortgage to a seventy-six-year-old woman, Irene Schuler, who lived alone in a home in Santa Clara. In the process of ostensibly replacing an existing reverse mortgage Schuler had on her $450,000 home with a new, supposedly more attractive one, Palmer and Rostami forged Schuler's signature on checks and various statements and letters to instead use her home to obtain a $240,000 mortgage and $100,000 line of bank credit. Only Schuler never received the $340,000. In a reversal of fortune, instead of a new reverse mortgage — which would pay her income each month — she was on the hook for the $340,000 in loans, requiring her to make monthly payments. There was also a federal complaint against Palmer and Rostami involving an elderly Malibu woman, Eleanor Coppola. It made allegations similar to those of the Schuler case — that Rostami and Palmer altered her deed and took money intended for the home owner.[4]

In 1999, Palmer was arrested when she tried to bring a member of her Mexican host family over the border to San Diego for medical treatment. Bail on the California charges was set at an astronomical $12 million. Palmer says the authorities wanted to lock her up in hopes of convincing Rostami, who had gone into hiding, to surrender. For nine months she sat in jail, unable to post bail. Her mother and other family members came out to California from Pennsylvania to care for her children. Finally, when authorities nabbed Rostami, they offered Palmer a deal: Plead guilty to felony fraud charges and she could go free, with the nine months in jail counting as her time served. If she didn't sign, she'd be waiting another year in jail for a trial to begin. "I had three small children at home without their mom." She signed. Rostami went to jail for nearly four years on the state and federal charges.

Palmer went back to work for an online real estate firm, but she hated the long hours away from her children. The jail experience reminded her that "you can get a second chance. I wanted to bring the whole family together." That included her mom and three young children; her father had died in the meantime.

Palmer decided that farming was the best way to bring everyone together. "It didn't matter what we were doing in farming, it was that we were together." The family pooled its resources and bought a small farm for $1 million near the town of Fillmore, in Ventura County, north of Los Angeles. It was great, except for one problem: it didn't have a reliable water supply. "We had to bring in water for bathing and for the orange groves." In late 2007, she and her family stopped paying the mortgage and moved out.

But Palmer did make a name for herself with the goat cheese she was producing. Shortly after she met Stewart in late 2007, she gave him some, and Stewart passed some on to his good friend Larry "Lucky" Otting, the real estate investor who had joined Stewart and Vonderplanitz in support-ing Mark McAfee as he was launching Organic Pastures Dairy Company in 2001. Now, Otting marveled at Palmer's cheese. "It was the best cheese I'd ever tasted," he told me.

In early 2008, Palmer found a more attractive Ventura County farm, this one in Santa Paula. Not only did the one-time apricot grove have an adequate water supply and a location less than ninety minutes from Los Angeles, but the setting was so beautiful it might as well have been in an-other country. The area had something of a European flavor, with narrow, winding roads and pretty, rolling rural landscapes. It was easy to see why someone with an agricultural bent would want to settle here, within an easy drive to the Pacific Ocean and Los Angeles — as well as farmers markets whose customers were prepared to pay premium prices for good food. But those attributes also made it expensive; it was in one of the most affluent counties not only in California, but in the United States. Palmer's lease gave her the option to buy the farm within a year — for $1.975 million. She had a bit over $100,000 to put into the deal.

Where could she raise more than $1.8 million? The $1 million she and her family had sunk into the Fillmore farm was gone. The stress of that situation was so intense that Palmer's mom had bailed, moving back to Pennsylvania. While Palmer had filed suit on behalf of her mom against the realtor and the previous owner of the Fillmore farm for allegedly defrauding her by hiding the water problems, recovering damages could take years.

The answer to the question about raising money began to emerge as Palmer's links to Stewart and Rawesome Foods grew and strengthened. She quickly acquired egg-laying hens and some forty milking goats, and before long she was an important supplier of two essentials for Rawesome Foods — eggs and raw milk. This happened under a herdshare agreement whereby Rawesome owned the goats and the milking equipment, and Palmer boarded them.

Stewart liked what he was seeing from Palmer's farm and introduced her to Otting in hopes he could apply his real estate expertise, and deep pockets, to help her figure out how to acquire the farm before the purchase option expired. Otting quickly came up with an approach: he would use his credit to help obtain a $1.1 million bank loan as part of the payment; with Palmer's $100,000-plus contribution, the remaining $750,000 would also be Palmer's responsibility. Since she didn't have anything approaching that amount, she, Otting, and Stewart brainstormed about trying to attract financial supporters from within the Rawesome community.

Otting, a trim and tan California real estate executive in his mid-sixties who liked to start off his days making fresh vegetable juice in a blender, would retain ownership of the property and lease it to Palmer until she had completed the bank loan payments. "I saw myself creating a community farm where we were going to have food," he told me from his expansive Los Angeles condominium with a breathtaking view of Venice Beach and the Pacific Ocean. "We could feed the clubs," he added, referring to other food clubs in the area that were springing up. As Otting remembers it, there was discussion of ten acres on the property being set aside for Stewart as "a vacation spot" where he would build a yurt.

The three determined that the lion's share of the funding would best be obtained from well-heeled Rawesome members and other people who were sympathetic to their vision. That summer, a friend of Palmer's posted a flyer at the Rawesome Foods in Venice that drew heavily on the bucolic images many Americans have of farms and farming:

AWESOME RAWESOME INVESTMENT OPPORTUNITY

It has been a dream of many of us to have fresh, local foods and full control over the production and supply of those foods. You may have heard rumors about James, Sharon, and Lucky being involved in the purchase of a farm located about an hour north of Venice. Well, the rumors are true and we've begun to live the dream. ☺ After taking possession of . . . pristine farmland near Ojai two months ago, we've accomplished the following . . .

The flyer listed eight items being worked on, including building "secure housing areas for our 3,000 egg-laying chickens," restoring an egg-packing facility, installing water and electricity in the poultry housing areas, and completion of "a Grade A milking facility for goats and sheep." But funding was necessary to complete these projects:

We see no end to the possibilities for developing the land and within 1½ years intend to be producing an incredibly diverse array of foodstuffs. . . . Due to the conservative nature of the mortgage industry today, we are also in need of additional funds for the down payment of the purchase of our farm.

One individual who didn't share in the vision was Aajonus Vonderplanitz. It's difficult to know exactly what was bothering the introverted raw food proponent. He told me at different times that the eggs Palmer's farm was producing didn't agree with him. That was a potentially significant problem, since he consumed upward of a dozen or more raw eggs every day. He also told me he didn't fully trust Palmer, even though he had only spoken with her on the phone and never met her in person. Besides, his financial interests were separate from the day-to-day operations of Rawesome; his nonprofit organization, Right to Choose Healthy Food, collected the twenty-five dollar annual membership dues that Rawesome members paid for the privilege of obtaining their food from the club.

No matter. Enough other local food enthusiasts were captivated not only by the romance of what Palmer was doing, but by the local, community-oriented nature of the project — and visions of the nutrient-dense food that would come from it. One such Rawesome member was Wayne Markel. He had been involved in Rawesome pretty much from the idealistic early days of 2005. The investment and career advisor sometimes volunteered to help out at Rawesome, putting up shelves and cleaning up.

"I saw this as something where we could all bind together," he recalled of the Palmer farm. "It was sold as an opportunity to participate more fully in the food we get, plus provide for our future. James could have a house on the farm." In other words, the more milk and butter and cheese and eggs the Palmer farm could produce, the less that would be required to be shipped in from Amos Miller's farm in Pennsylvania.

The notion of a local food supply was personally very important to Markel, a tall, angular man who dresses in dark four-button double-breasted suits — not typical Los Angeles businessman dress. During his time with Rawesome, he had become a devotee of Vonderplanitz's raw food diet. He consumed mainly raw milk, raw eggs, raw meat, and bee pollen and spirulina, which he says helped him improve his health and energy levels to the extent that he needed only five and a half hours of sleep nightly rather than the seven or eight hours he had needed previously. He eventually became one of a group of at least seven outside backers, ponying up an unspecified amount.

Amazingly, some food enthusiasts who had never even met Palmer became intrigued enough with her local farm start-up effort to join the group of backers. At the Weston A. Price Foundation annual national conference in San Francisco in November 2008 — attended by nearly ten thousand foodies from around the country — two friends of Palmer announced at one session that a new farm outside Los Angeles was seeking funding.

Sitting in the audience that November afternoon when the speaker made the announcement about Palmer's new farm was Mary Hetherington, at that time a thirty-one-year-old mother of two young children. She had gotten caught up in the camaraderie of the conference and its outside-the-establishment feel. "Everyone is so like-minded," she recalled. "You are sharing stories about how you feed your family. We're all working against the grain. We were part of a larger group. Plus, we love our local farmers." Hetherington didn't know Sharon Palmer, but she liked her story. "This mom-farmer was working very hard to live this new life."

The financial opportunity at the farm coincided with a desire by Hetherington and her husband to invest $60,000 planned months later for doors and windows on a new home they were building north of Los Angeles. After speaking with Palmer, they decided to place the money in a six-month loan with Palmer; they would receive 10 percent interest, and at the end of the six months retrieve the funds to buy the windows. Two other conference attendees put in a total of $150,000. In a December 2008 e-mail to Rawesome members, Stewart stated that Palmer's friends "got the word out at the Weston A. Price Foundation's Conference in San Francisco over November 7–9 raising $210,000. WOW!"[5]

So anxious was everyone involved to help this single-mom farmer, and to secure a local source of milk and eggs, that they asked for little in the way of references and paperwork. As a result, most knew nothing of Palmer's criminal past — though she was certainly open in discussing it with anyone who asked.

Even if they knew about Palmer's past, it's doubtful these food enthusiasts would have changed their minds. They were, after all, operating privately — outside a public food system they profoundly mistrusted — and may well have seen Palmer as a victim of a corrupt system. And in their view, they were helping build a new kind of food system, untainted by mass-production corporate interests. The deal with Otting went through, and Palmer seemed to have her second chance.

One afternoon in mid-December, just a month after Palmer gained her new financial lease on life, a heavyset woman showed up at the farm (now named Healthy Family Farms) inquiring about buying some goat cheese for an upcoming holiday party. As Palmer would later relate the events, she told the woman the farm's state license prohibited retail sales and limited Palmer to selling her cheeses at farmers markets. So Palmer initially refused the woman's request. When the woman persisted, talking more about how important her upcoming holiday gathering was, Palmer decided to give her two pounds of cheese — and refused to accept payment.

The cheese she gave the woman — in fact, all the cheese at Healthy Family Farms — was produced at her old farm, the one in Fillmore that had the water problem, which she insisted was licensed by the California Department of Food and Agriculture (CDFA). She didn't yet have a license to produce cheese at Healthy Family Farms, however, so she was relying on inventory she had previously made and frozen in the old licensed facility.

Shortly after giving the stranger the cheese, Palmer left her farm to run some errands. About twenty minutes down the road, she was pulled over by a Ventura County sheriff and told she was under arrest in connection with illegal cheese production. She was handcuffed and placed in the police cruiser. It was then Palmer realized the woman asking for the cheese had been an undercover agent. Palmer was asked if regulators could inspect her facility. They didn't have a search warrant, but the implication was that if everything was OK, she would be released. She agreed.

The cruiser returned to her farm, where a caravan of about a dozen police and agency cars, including a crime unit van, were parked — representatives from five different state and county agriculture and law enforcement agencies. When Palmer was taken out of the police cruiser and her three children — two daughters (ages twelve and thirteen) and son (age nine) — saw their mom in handcuffs, they became hysterical. Officials taking videos didn't seem to care; they kept Palmer standing in handcuffs with her children for two hours while they searched her cheese-making facility.

The officials wanted to know where her pasteurizer was. She told them she didn't have one at this facility yet — all her processing had been done at her old facility. She said she showed them her license for the old facility (police removed her handcuffs temporarily so she could retrieve the documents), and she requested they call the regular CDFA dairy inspector who oversaw her facility to corroborate her version of the story.

A female official told Palmer that it was a felony to sell raw milk, she was under arrest, and she would have to accompany the sheriff's deputy for booking. They allowed her to call a relative to come over and care for her three children and feed her goats. At about 4:00 p.m. Palmer was placed (still handcuffed) in the cruiser, taken to a predetention facility, and placed in a cell. At about 4:00 a.m. she was released, and she was told to return at 8:00 a.m. the day after Christmas for arraignment.

The undercover agent who tricked Palmer into giving her cheese was Scarlett Treviso, a veteran CDFA investigator who prided herself on her toughness. Her specialty was finding wrongdoing at dairy farms in the state — violations of sanitation regulations, defective milking equipment, sick cows. She would later tell a judge in an affidavit that she had investigated more than five hundred dairy cases resulting in more than 120 criminal convictions.

Treviso was known among dairy farmers as a tough regulator who had a penchant for launching investigations independently without consulting superiors — such that detractors would come to refer to her as a "rogue." In the case of Sharon Palmer, she said she had received information from the Ventura County Sheriff's Department's Rural Crime Unit that Palmer was making cheese using a license that had expired the previous December, and not using the required equipment for handling the milk intended for cheese.

Amazingly, a month later, five deputies from the Ventura County Sheriff's Department showed up at Palmer's farm again, this time with a fourteen-page search warrant that, essentially, entitled them to take anything they wanted from her home, nearby barn, and car.

Five more deputies went to the tiny house of Palmer's grown daughter from her first marriage, who lived fifteen minutes down the road and whose major crime seemed to have been that she assisted Palmer at farmers markets. Using another search warrant, they rummaged through her home and car and confiscated her computer.

The sheriff's deputies spent two and a half hours at Palmer's place, videotaping goat cheese and chickens and sheep as well as carting off her computer and personal papers. What caused the regulators and police to come after Palmer so aggressively for what were, essentially, licensing violations? After all, she had been registered in California's agricultural system and had at one time all the necessary licenses. According to her, she had applied to renew the license that Treviso said had expired a year earlier, sent in her check, and never noticed that the renewed license didn't arrive.

Was it her criminal record from eight years earlier? Was it more recent accusations by Ventura County businesses that she had skipped out on several debts? There was a 2005 case filed in a Ventura County court by Ike's Pump & Drilling Inc. against Palmer; the court awarded Ike's $1,156 following a hearing.[6] In 2007, Palmer was one of three defendants in a suit filed by FarmTek, a farm feed and supply outlet; the following year the court awarded FarmTek $12,498.60 in principal, interest, court costs, and attorney fees.[7] In late 2008, Danny Miles eventually was awarded $2,800 against Palmer for bad checks.[8]

It seemed as if Palmer lived more on the edge financially — even assuming she had lots of unexpected expenses from having to leave one farm and launch another — than you'd want to see from a woman desperate for a second chance. Or was the offensive against her part of the national crackdown on private food? The fact that so many agencies had come together twice within two months to raid Palmer's farm implied a great deal of coordination.

I contacted both the sheriff in charge and the lawyer in the Ventura County prosecutor's office in charge of the case, but no one would speak with me about why they mounted such a show of force. Palmer said the officers wouldn't tell her what their probable cause was. "I'm so sad," Palmer told me the day after this second raid. "I'm trying to do something wholesome. . . . I said to my daughter, I must have been an awful person in a previous life. . . . If this keeps dragging on, I may not be able to keep the farm."

CHAPTER 6

THE VIOLENT BIRTH OF THE FOOD RIGHTS MOVEMENT

In retrospect, it's easy to understand why Daniel Allgyer signed up with Aajonus Vonderplanitz's Right to Choose Healthy Food (RTCHF) following the search of his Pennsylvania farm in the spring of 2010. Amish farmers may not have e-mail, Facebook, or Twitter, but that doesn't mean they don't keep up on the news that's important to them. They each have telephones with answering machines (or share telephones with other families), usually located in barns, and they leave each other long messages about family and community matters — and also about food regulatory developments that might affect them.

On this last score, Vonderplanitz's accomplishments in standing up to government regulators had become well known over the previous few years. They began in 2005 when Vonderplanitz and Stewart pushed back at Los Angeles public health officials who were trying to force Rawesome Foods to obtain permits, which would have made distribution of many of its products impossible. Five years later, when Allgyer endured the FDA search and follow-up warning letter, Rawesome was thriving — without having endured any further official hassles. And, much to the liking of the Amish, Vonderplanitz had done it all without involving lawyers.

Moreover, Vonderplanitz had created a financial model for the private distribution of food from farmers to consumers. The way it worked was that RTCHF negotiated lease agreements with suppliers on behalf of food clubs whereby the RTCHF clubs gained exclusive access to a farm's production.

It's a more direct arrangement than large retail food cooperatives, which usually operate like conventional grocery stores, obtaining their food from a variety of producers and distributors. Shoppers who become members (for, say, a fifty- or one-hundred-dollar one-time membership fee) are like shareholders and may receive a portion of the cooperative's profits based on how much food they buy each year, sort of like a small rebate. While the cooperatives may commit to buying as much food as possible from local producers, the members don't have a direct stake.

Under a RTCHF lease with an Amish farmer, RTCHF paid the farmer a token yearly lease fee of one hundred dollars; food prices to members for milk and meat were linked to boarding, milking, and bottling fees spelled out under the lease agreement — the farmer's costs plus "what is fair and reasonable."

The contract also prohibited the farmer from actually selling milk to anyone outside the RTCHF clubs to emphasize the private contractual nature of the arrangement, completely different than commercial sales. Further differentiating the arrangement was a clause in the agreement that encouraged the farmer to apply different quality standards than corporate milk processors might want. While existing standards both for conventional milk destined for pasteurization and for raw milk sold under state permits or regulations emphasize low counts of various naturally occurring harmless bacteria, the RTCHF agreement promoted the opposite. Based on Vonderplanitz's belief that bacteria in all forms (including pathogens) are helpful in building immunity, his lease agreement with farmers stated that "limiting [what] the natural bacterial counts are is moot because all Club members prefer high bacterial counts for better health." All of the farmers I spoke with who have been part of RTCHF don't necessarily buy fully into Vonderplanitz's theories and maintain high standards of conventional safety in an effort to avoid pathogens in their milk that could sicken members.

To Vonderplanitz, these leasing agreements were preferable to the herdshare or cowshare arrangements that were being established in various parts of the country, many of them under the guidance of the Farm-to-Consumer Legal Defense Fund (FTCLDF). These agreements, whereby the consumer purchases a share in a milk cow or goat or dairy herd, were attractive, states the FTCLDF, because "such contracts are legal and valid, as guaranteed by the Constitution of the United States of America. The consumer does not buy milk from the farmer. Rather, they pay the farmer for the service of keeping the cow or goat and his labor for milking and processing the milk into value added products such as butter, cream, cheese, etc. However, they may directly purchase other products from the farm, such as eggs, vegetables and meat."[1]

To me, the two approaches—lease agreements and cowshares/herdshares—didn't seem all that different from each other. Both involved paying the farmer-boarder for food from the animals covered by the agreement. But to Vonderplanitz, there was a big difference: "Leasing has 85 years of business precedence behind it, while herdshares have almost no precedence behind them," he told me. "If you lease anything, you have full responsibilities, as if you were owner. However, herdshare agreements are arguable as to ownership. You can own a stock but have nothing but the right to receive dividends—no ownership in the company or property. One judge in Wisconsin argued to herdshares, 'What part of the cow do you own? The ass? If so, you get the fecal matter, not the milk!'"

In RTCHF arrangements, there was a second legal component (apart from the farmers) that involved the food clubs, which received food from their leased animals. These were private organizations in which members paid an annual membership fee — typically twenty-five dollars a year — and signed agreements swearing off the conventional food system for its supposedly dangerous food in favor of the private food club with its unpasteurized milk, unwashed and unrefrigerated eggs, and meat not fed antibiotics or injected with hormones. I signed one of these when I joined a food club in the Boston area.

There was a certain tension between Vonderplanitz and the FTCLDF lawyers over their divergent approaches. The tension stemmed partly from the fact that Vonderplanitz was seen as infringing on the FTCLDF's territory—he wasn't a lawyer, yet he was drafting legal agreements for farmers and consumers. The Amish may have appreciated Vonderplanitz's absence of a law degree, but the FTCLDF lawyers didn't.

To boot, Vonderplanitz's approach appeared to be working, in the sense of keeping regulators at bay. In June 2006, the Pennsylvania Department of Agriculture issued Amos Miller a court summons for selling raw milk without the necessary state permit; Pennsylvania allowed raw milk sales directly to consumers for farms with the requisite permit, but since Miller was producing milk for private RTCHF clubs, he saw himself as outside the publicly regulated system and not required to hold a permit.

Vonderplanitz wrote a legal brief on behalf of Miller that the Amish farmer sent to the Lancaster County District Court, where the case was due to be heard in August of that year. The accusation of selling raw milk illegally, Miller stated, "is not possible. Since January 2005 I have leased my herd to a private club, 'Right To Choose Healthy Food's Rawesome Club' that owns all of the milk production on my Amish farm. I sell the club my services of tending, milking, bottling and processing the milk production for the private club to their standards established in our signed agreements and contracts. . . . Secondly, the citation states that I refused to obtain a milk permit. That is not a violation of law in this case. Since the private club owns all milk production, there is no commerce involved."[2]

On August 15, 2006, Amos Miller drove his horse-drawn carriage the ten miles or so to the Lancaster courthouse for the scheduled hearing. As he was sitting in a parking lot outside the courthouse, a clerk came out and told him he didn't need to come in. According to Amos, "He said there wouldn't be a hearing and I should just leave. That was the last I heard of it."

That sounded mysterious to me, given the aggressive regulator actions against so many other farmers, so I did a search through Lancaster County court documents and, sure enough, Amos Miller's citation came up. It was issued June 2nd; on July 20th, a trial was scheduled before Judge Denise B. Commins for August 15th. The outcome? On August 15th, the case was "withdrawn," according to the docket records, with no explanation provided.[3] Vonderplanitz interpreted the withdrawal as validation of his leasing approach. In his view, the officials had concluded that Amos Miller was in the right and decided to withdraw the legal action rather than risk a precedent-setting court defeat.

Later in 2006, a second RTCHF Amish farmer, David Hochstetler of Indiana, found himself in a potential legal thicket over his distribution of raw milk to consumers in Michigan. Hochstetler worked with a Michigan farmer, Richard Hebron, to serve food clubs in Ann Arbor and Detroit — Hochstetler providing the milk and Hebron the meat, eggs, and vegetables. Hochstetler also served other food clubs in Indiana and Illinois.

The food club had been a saving grace for Hochstetler, a tall, bearded, soft-spoken man in his early fifties. The father of eight children, four boys and four girls, he had watched four grow up and leave the farm in Middle-bury, Indiana, for other lives. But his fifth child, a son in his early twenties, had shown "a big interest in the farm and taking over when I retire," Hochstetler told me. Making his dairy's milk available directly to consumers via the cowshare arrangement had enabled the farm to triple its revenues of a few years back, when Hochstetler instead sold his milk to processors.

The new economics enabled Hochstetler to begin dreaming of handing the farm over to his son someday. He also experienced tremendous satisfaction learning about the health benefits his consumer members attributed to the milk. "My son and I, we ride along to the drop-off points in Chicago, and we get to meet these people" who are consuming the milk. "A lot of mothers say how their children had asthma and allergies and they tried everything the medical profession had to offer and nothing worked till they tried raw milk." The most touching story he heard came from a man whose wife had multiple sclerosis. "She's tried everything that medical science has to offer, and none of it works. Her physical therapist told the husband that every time she drinks raw milk, she is stronger. He told me, 'This is all I've got.'" As Hochstetler summarized, "Hearing all the appreciation they have shown for this product has put new meaning into our occupation. They thank us from the bottom of their hearts."

In October 2006, when the Michigan Department of Agriculture and Rural Development confiscated seven thousand dollars worth of raw milk and other food from Hebron while he was on his way to deliver the products to Ann Arbor food club members, agents from the FDA came calling on Hochstetler, too.

Shortly after that, Vonderplanitz wrote a letter to the FDA, explaining that Hochstetler's milk had been produced as part of a private contractual arrangement. In language similar to what he used to argue on behalf of Amos Miller, Vonderplanitz stated that Hochstetler and Hebron had "been accused by FDA employees of selling and buying raw milk. That is not possible." He argued that the FDA had no jurisdiction: "Since the club members own all of the milk produced by Cooperative's herd that Mr. Hochstetler boards and tends for Cooperative, there is no commerce involved."[4] The FDA's only response was to issue Hochstetler a warning letter in February 2007, demanding he discontinue raw milk shipments across state lines.[5] Hochstetler ignored the warning.

Everything was fine for Hochstetler until March 2010, when twenty-five food club members he and Hebron supplied in Michigan, Indiana, and Illinois got sick from campylobacter. Public health authorities in those states used epidemiological evidence — the fact that nearly all the victims had consumed raw milk before becoming sick — to pin the blame on Hochstetler's dairy. However, extensive and sophisticated testing of milk, including at a CDC lab — both from samples preserved by victims of illness and from Hochstetler — showed no signs of campylobacter. ("We were unable to confirm the presence of Campylobacter in any of the seven unpasteurized dairy products that were collected for testing, despite having the samples tested in three labs," explained a report from the Michigan Department of Community Health.) Hochstetler even shut down his dairy for a week to conduct private testing for campylobacter, and those tests all came back negative as well, he says.[6]

Once again, however, FDA inspectors visited Hochstetler. Shortly afterward, the farmer says agency representatives threatened legal action to pressure him to end his shipments to out-of-state club members. He involved the FTCLDF to engage in negotiations on his behalf about a possible agreement whereby Hochstetler would withdraw from supplying food clubs in Illinois and Michigan and confine himself to those in his home state of Indiana.

"They [the FDA] wanted me to go away," Hochstetler told me. "We came very close" to an agreement whereby he would limit his distribution to Indiana, he said. But the FDA wouldn't grant him immunity for past transgressions, such as those detailed in the agency's 2007 warning letter. While the FTCLDF was encouraging Hochstetler to come to terms with the FDA, Vonderplanitz advised him to reject the agreement. Finally Hochstetler asked the FTCLDF lawyer to end the negotiations.

Without an FDA commitment to leave him be, Hochstetler concluded, there was no reason to discontinue his normal operations, which he and Vonderplanitz always felt were legal to begin with. "We felt because of our private contracts [with buying clubs and their members], geographical barriers did not pertain to private contracts."

There was one other factor at work that kept Hochstetler with RTCHF, according to Vonderplanitz. He says that at the time of the negotiation with the FDA, he informed Hochstetler he couldn't walk away from his food club members. "I told him that since he was under contract, that if he stopped producing milk from our cows, RTCHF would collect the cows and board them elsewhere until the contract ended," says Vonderplanitz. So Hochstetler walked away from the FDA instead to fulfill his contractual obligations, Vonderplanitz suggests.

Regardless of Vonderplanitz's seriousness about enforcing the contract, the underlying message was important because part of the legal argument against food clubs, lease contracts, and herdshares is that they are sham agreements designed to circumvent restrictions on raw dairy. Judges had in a few instances sided with this view. The fact that Vonderplanitz was prepared to take legal action to enforce a leasing arrangement added potentially important legal legitimacy to such arrangements.

Once again, the regulators seemed to shrink away in the face of a strong stand by a RTCHF farmer. Vonderplanitz was ecstatic: "I rescued another farmer," he told me. Vonderplanitz's aura of success prompted a Wisconsin farmer in hot regulatory water to contact him. That farmer, Vernon Hershberger, was feeling the heat many raw dairy farmers in his state were experiencing as the state Department of Agriculture, Trade, and Consumer Protection (DATCP) began cracking down in 2009 and 2010. Wisconsin law prohibited all but "incidental" sales of raw milk, and its definition of "incidental" shifted over the years according to which regulators were in charge.

In 2009 and 2010, the state moved into one of its strict interpretation periods. Hershberger, who has a farm of about thirty-five cows about an hour outside Madison — and who sold dairy, meats, eggs, and other products to a couple hundred regular customers — asked Vonderplanitz about a lease agreement with RTCHF. Vonderplanitz agreed to put together lease and membership agreements covering Hershberger's farm and turning his customers into a food club.

For a few months in early 2010, Hershberger, who had been born into an Amish community but left to live a more conventional life, let the proposed contract sit unsigned on his desk. Then, on June 2nd, agents from the Wisconsin DATCP raided his Grazin' Acres farm and placed yellow and red seals on the refrigerators in his small store to prevent distribution of any food. He was operating without a retailer license and a dairy license, the regulators said. The fact that a retailer license and a dairy license for the sale of raw milk didn't exist was irrelevant. The fact that he wasn't open to the general public — but was selling directly to private customers of his farm — didn't matter either.

The day after the raid, in a public show of civil disobedience, Hershberger cut the DATCP seals and defiantly reopened for business. Other farmer friends had tried to dissuade him, encouraging him instead to go to court. One expressed fear that Hershberger could lose everything. But, in the Amish tradition, Hershberger decided his religious beliefs precluded him from filing an administrative appeal and he'd "place [himself] in God's hands." That day, he decided to sign the contract with RTCHF. The deal was "simple" in Hershberger's mind and, besides, "I think Aajonus knows what he's doing," he told me.

Vonderplanitz followed up by sending a letter, even more strongly worded than his letters for other farmers, to Wisconsin's DATCP explaining that Hershberger "is not engaged in commerce. His farm animals are leased to Right To Choose Healthy Food's Grazin' Acres Farm Coop Club who owns them. . . . Since no commerce of buying or selling raw milk and our other products to the public is involved, or distributed in public places, government agencies have NO JURISDICTION over the production, labeling and use of the club's products consumed by its members, nor is any permit required. . . . It is shameful for [DATCP] to try to prevent us from producing and distributing our health-giving raw milk and other farm products to our members by threatening and imposing false warrants, seizures, and arrests of our property. Since you were duly warned that this was a private club and you had no jurisdiction over it, your actions were criminal stealing, kidnap, and trespass."

Though DATCP agents returned to the farm twice more over the next few months with search warrants — the last time taking Hershberger's computer, checkbook, and other records — no criminal or other charges were filed against the farmer. Life returned to normal for Hershberger and his family.

By this time, messages recounting Vonderplanitz's exploits had been left on any number of Amish farmer answering machines in the East and Midwest. He was the guy who knew how to keep them where they always wanted to be — outside the legal system. If the Amish had engaged in street talk, they would very likely have affirmed that Vonderplanitz had "cred," that he was "the main man" allowing them to distribute the farm-fresh milk, meat, and eggs the government opposed to growing legions of eager consumers.

So when Daniel Allgyer opted to turn his animals over to RTCHF in April 2010 and delivered his handwritten note to members of Grassfed on the Hill (described in chapter 2), he concluded, "so . . . attached to this paper you will find a club membership agreement. [RTCHF] will be leasing my dairy cows, steers, pigs, chickens, etc., so that everything that is produced on this farm is owned by the club and that means in order to obtain any food after May 8, 2010, you must join this club." The change made Allgyer comfortable enough that he ordered his driver to end night–time deliveries to Maryland — begun after the first FDA search in February — and resume driving in broad daylight.

By the time Allgyer signed up with Vonderplanitz, about eighty RTCHF clubs had sprung up around the country. Some were just one hundred or two hundred members, while a few had more than one thousand members.

When Vonderplanitz wasn't putting out fires for Amish farmers, he was promoting himself as a kind of holistic, antiauthoritarian nutritionist. He spent much of each year traveling the United States and other parts of the world, promoting not only his "primal diet" but himself as a sort of Lone Ranger standing up to evil corporate and government forces. He gave lectures in the homes of devotees — a "Primal Potluck for Aajonus" — where attendees would bring various raw food concoctions like raw ground beef, raw pizza, and raw chicken salad.

I attended one such event in 2010 at a home in Carlsbad, just north of San Diego, along with about fifteen other people who seemed to range from their twenties to their seventies. At the end, a number stayed for three-hundred-dollar-an-hour consultations with Vonderplanitz on their diets and health. It was a beautiful sunny afternoon when Vonderplanitz appeared, as people were chomping on the pizza and chicken salad. He took a chair on the grass just beyond the patio. He was wiry, with close-cropped, wavy, brown-gray hair — youthful-looking for a man in his sixties. He didn't need to explain who he was, since everyone was familiar with him; a number had attended other such events. He immediately launched into a tale of how he was "abducted in my hotel room" in Thailand a year earlier, blindfolded, and held down by mysterious assailants. "I was injected three times. I had mercury, barium, and chromium readings off the charts after that."

He then pulled up a pant leg to show large red sores that he said were part of the assault. As sweat accumulated on his brow under the hot sun, he proceeded to remove his shirt and sat bare-chested for the rest of his presentation. He speculated that the hotel-room assault was retribution for radio interviews he had done criticizing flu vaccines. "This is an $8 billion business," he said, proceeding to apologize that the hotel-room injections had sapped his health. "As you can see, I've aged a good deal in a year and a half. I lost three inches on my arms. I am never one to work out, but all that muscle is gone." He had since tried to throw corporate and law enforcement enemies off his path. "My cell phone is not on. Sometimes I buy a ticket and don't get on a flight. I have a Taser. . . . They are out to stop me wherever I am."

I looked around at the faces of his audience, expecting to see a few smiles, raised eyebrows, or looks of skepticism — but everyone else was watching him intently, and some were nodding in approval. An attendee asked about the wisdom of eating raw meat from wild animals. Wonderful stuff, suggested Vonderplanitz. "A friend of mine hunted a deer a few years ago. I butchered it. I got 38 pounds of meat, he got 40 pounds. I put the glands into a blender with milk and ate those right away. I was up for three days. I was picking up my girlfriend at the airport, and I was wide awake. We had sex for five hours. She was tired. So I gave her a half a cup of the glands and milk. We were up for another two days having sex." Once again, no snickers. Just serious looks, and I suspect some sense of awe.

Afterward, one attendee, seventy-year-old Joe Manfredi, a patient of Vonderplanitz for the previous eight years, told me he was worried that the supposed hotel attack had taken a toll: "Those injections he talked about really made a mess of him. He always looked so much better. He's aged a lot. His hair has gotten gray really quickly. It happened just like that."

While it seemed like Vonderplanitz was on a roll, the reality was that his leasing and private membership models hadn't been tested in the courts. If they were tested, however, the United States' long tradition of respecting privacy might be expected to work to Vonderplanitz's advantage.

While the Constitution doesn't mention "privacy," the respect is strongly implied in the First Amendment's guarantees of the right to assemble and worship free of government interference. Under those freedoms, political organizations — like white supremacist groups — can recruit, organize, and even conduct public demonstrations. Americans have private houses of worship, private investment clubs, country clubs, sewing clubs, hunting clubs, even cooking clubs. In some cases, these private organizations have violated antidiscrimination laws, as many country clubs and hunting clubs do. In 2000, the Boy Scouts of America were allowed by the U.S. Supreme Court to bar gay scout masters — in effect, to violate a state's anti–gay discrimination law — given its status as a private organization, part of whose mission prohibits the active involvement of homosexuals.

The Fourth Amendment's restrictions on "unreasonable searches and seizures" add another layer of privacy protection. Regulators who object to activities of a particular organization need to obtain a judge's approval for a search warrant before they can confiscate computers or rummage through records and e-mails.

But there isn't a lot of case law concerning private food organizations, especially those that challenge regulations. One of the biggest wins came in late 2006, when an Ohio judge ruled in favor of farmer Carol Schmitmeyer, who had established a herdshare. Schmitmeyer was among a half dozen or so farmers targeted by the Ohio Department of Agriculture — though the agency hit her especially hard by revoking her Grade A dairy permit, which meant she was barred from selling milk to processors for pasteurization. By prohibiting her from having a herdshare and from selling milk to processors, the regulators were effectively putting her out of business. She went to court to challenge the herdshare ban and to get her license back.

The judge agreed with Schmitmeyer's argument that the Department of Agriculture had been inconsistent in its rationale for banning herdshares while allowing farm owners and family members to drink raw milk on the farm. He took the agency to task over "the failure of the Department to articulate specific problems with the cow share agreement" involving Schmitmeyer and her herd's 150 shareholders.

In his analysis, the judge raised a number of important questions that exposed the arbitrariness of the Department of Agriculture's cowshare crackdown: "Does the Department allow herd owners and their children/family members to consume raw milk? Or must the children/family members reside in the farm household? Or must the children/family members also be active participants in the milking operation in order to 'legally' consume raw milk?" Further, "if the cows are owned by a partnership, can all partners consume raw milk? Or must the partners be family members? Or must the partners consuming the raw milk reside on the farm? And if the cows are owned by a corporation, the same troubling questions apply with even more shareholders being involved in the equation." The judge provided his own answer to the questions when he stated "the Department . . . argues that the 'herd share agreement' is a transparent attempt to circumvent the law. If the herd share agreement is a circumvention of the law, so is the Department's inexact practice of allowing owners and their families, etc. to consume raw milk."[7]

Ohio decided not to appeal and suddenly about-faced from a state that banned raw milk to one that allowed it via herdshares. Following the raid on farmer Richard Hebron as he was bringing Indiana Amish farmer David Hochstetler's milk and other food to an Ann Arbor food club, Michigan's attorney general also allowed herdshares — another about-face from the first state in the country to have banned raw milk.

Another favorable decision came out of Canada in 2009 when a judge ruled that farmer Michael Schmidt's herdshare arrangement was legal. Canada's provinces have more strict laws on raw milk than most American states. The judge, in this case, distinguished between the public and private domains. He said Ontario's restrictive dairy laws were fine for the public, but that Schmidt's herdshare members had the right to make their food choices privately, outside the public system.[8]

And out of Colorado there was a 2005 legislative decision to legally sanction herdshare arrangements, which gradually took shape in the years that followed. By 2010, there were fifty-five dairies under the umbrella of the Raw Milk Association of Colorado, committed to its "testing protocol and bacterial limits for product distribution."[9]

Those decisions were encouraging for people in Ohio, Michigan, Colorado, and Ontario, but what about the rest of the United States and Canada? (Indeed, even in Ontario, the ruling would come into jeopardy; since there is no prohibition in Canada on convicting someone who's been acquitted, the government appealed Michael Schmidt's exoneration of charges he violated Ontario's dairy laws, and an appeals court reversed the exoneration on appeal. As of this book's publication, Schmidt had appealed the ruling a level higher.)

Elsewhere in the United States, there were some troublesome negative rulings. In the Meadowsweet Dairy case in New York, dairy owners Barb and Steve Smith filed suit in late 2007 to challenge the state Department of Agriculture and Markets' efforts to restrict the dairy from providing items like raw milk, yogurt, and butter and making deliveries to its shareholders in Ithaca. Courts all the way up the to the state's supreme court failed to undo a lower court decision against the dairy. There, a judge ruled that the LLC shareholders were completely subject to the dictates of the Department of Agriculture and Markets — indeed, they couldn't even give raw milk away.[10]

Similar rulings came out of Wisconsin. There, a judge ruled in 2012 that private herdshare and food club operations run by two different farms violated the state's retail and strict dairy laws — using tough language, quoted in chapter 2, that there is no right even to drink the milk of your own cow if it isn't licensed.

Even in those states where the rulings went against them, farmers continued to operate in their gray areas. Meadowsweet Dairy in New York switched after its appeals ran out in 2011 from being an LLC to reorganizing as a herdshare. Dairies in Wisconsin continued to make raw milk available to food club members from farm stores while their cases continued on appeal.

Whether it was the legal victories in the Midwest and East that gave regulators new confidence is uncertain, but in any event California regulators in mid-2010 were back on the private food hunt. They renewed their investigation of single-mom farmer Sharon Palmer — and in the process (seemingly by accident) wound up honing in on their old nemesis, Aajonus Vonderplanitz, and his food clubs.

In March 2010, after a fourteen-month hiatus since the massive search at Sharon Palmer's Ventura County farm, Scarlett Treviso of the California Department of Food and Agriculture (CDFA) was once again pursuing Palmer, who was selling eggs and chickens at various Los Angeles–area farmers markets and using the farmers markets to deliver raw milk and cheese to members of a community-supported agriculture (CSA) group she serviced.

Eleven days after receiving an alert from Ventura County officials, on March 27th, Treviso visited a Santa Monica farmers market held on Saturdays on a string of closed-off streets stretching several blocks through the main part of the bustling oceanfront downtown. Treviso planned the same come-on at Palmer's farmers market stand that she had used fourteen months earlier at Palmer's farm in convincing the farmer to give her cheese — that Treviso "was having a party and really needed some," according to her investigative report. This time, instead of approaching Palmer she approached Victoria Bloch, a woman who worked for Palmer part-time handling the farmers market stand. When Treviso asked to purchase some cheese and cream, Bloch told her the cheese was presold to members of the CSA.[11]

Scarlett Treviso and other investigators weren't so easily put off by Victoria Bloch's membership rules — a "private" arrangement Palmer had set up following the January 2009 raid on her farm, ostensibly to keep regulators off her back. Their view was that all food, including dairy, fell under government regulation. There was no distinction between private organizations and public outlets. The investigators would simply join undercover as members, as they had with the Grassfed on the Hill food club in Maryland, and make their "buys" that way.

Just in case Bloch was suspicious of her, Treviso had another CDFA agent, Robert Donnalley, join the CSA on April 5th, according to Treviso's subsequent narrative to justify a search warrant. "At 1012 hours, Donnalley received an email response from Victoria [Bloch] of Healthy Family Farms with the CSA membership application attached."[12]

Once he joined the CSA via e-mail, Donnalley went to the Healthy Family Farms stand at the Santa Monica farmers market on April 17th to meet up with Bloch. She accepted his fifty-dollar membership fee and gave him a CSA membership card. He picked up the items he had ordered — a half gallon of raw goat milk, eight ounces of raw feta, eight ounces of raw soft cheese, and a container of raw cream — and paid forty-two dollars for the items. He then handed the goods off to Treviso "at a prearranged site." She turned the dairy items over to a state lab, which confirmed that they were all made with unpasteurized milk.

Treviso was then determined to acquire more Healthy Family Farms raw dairy to make her case and upped the intensity of the investigation. On May 13, 2010, she went to a farmers market in South Pasadena where Healthy Family Farms had a stand, and this time she brought along a larger investigative party — two L.A. County District Attorney investigators, Ken Ward and Ted Holst, together with Robert Donnalley and herself from CDFA. There was a fifth person as well, a sound lab technician.

The reason they needed so many people together at one farmers market? Because this time they were going to secretly record the happenings on video and audio, using highly sophisticated equipment. According to a report filed by investigator Ward, "Sound Lab Technician Fred Scott provided Investigator Treviso with a black purse equipped with audio/video capabilities. I remained in the van parked on El Centro Street in South Pasadena with technician Scott to monitor the conversation."[13] As Treviso proceeded with her special purse to engage the young man working the Healthy Family Farms booth that day, Ward and technician Scott watched the live video feed in the van. "In addition, the video showed two Hispanic females working inside the vendor's area behind the folding tables. In the video, Investigator Donnalley was seen and overheard completing his purchase with the Hispanic female."[14]

But unlike agent Donnalley, Treviso still hadn't bothered to join the CSA — and so was refused yet again in her effort to purchase cheese. The fact that Treviso didn't fill out the membership form and pay the fifty-dollar fee suggests she was trying to demonstrate that Palmer was selling raw milk and cheese publicly, and not just to CSA members.

But in rejecting Treviso, the Healthy Family Farms employee, Chris Gerard, revealed new and intriguing information to the investigator. He inquired about where Treviso lived, and when she told him she lived in Santa Monica, he asked her if she knew about Rawesome Foods in neighboring Venice. When she said she didn't, he wrote down the address for her and "briefly explained Rawesome was well known for having the 'best of the best from around the world' in raw foods."[15]

Gerard went on, in the investigator's telling: "Rawesome is a private membership club and had no web site because they wanted to stay under the radar. Treviso asked where Rawesome got their products. Gerard answered 'from all over the world' and they carried [Palmer's] Healthy Family Farms products also. He explained everything in the store was raw. 'It is very off the radar.'"[16]

Two days later, investigator Ward initiated another secret farmers market recording session — this time wearing a special shirt outfitted with recording equipment — when he went to pick up Healthy Family Farms dairy products he had ordered undercover at a farmers market in Santa Barbara. "Sound Lab Technician Fred Scott provided me with a green short sleeve shirt with a button cam equipped with audio and video capabilities."[17] Again, Treviso was there to transport the dairy items he picked up to a laboratory for analysis.

Treviso put her newfound information about Rawesome Foods to immediate use in expanding the Palmer investigation. On May 19th, four days after Ward's button-cam recording session, the action shifted from farmers markets to Rose Avenue in the seaside Los Angeles community of Venice, the home of Rawesome Foods.

The section of Rose Avenue where Rawesome was located was a busy residential and retail area, about six blocks from the Venice beach, just down the street from a huge Whole Foods store, and next door to a large coffeehouse. Rawesome itself was nondescript, the kind of place you could easily walk past if you didn't know it was there, behind a ten-foot-high corrugated steel fence.

Though it had been five years since the club encountered any official surveillance, owner James Stewart had been unnerved by the 2008 and 2009 raids on Palmer's Healthy Family Farms, which was supplying goat milk to Rawesome members under a herdshare arrangement. A few days after Palmer's arrest in December 2008, Stewart put out a memo to everyone involved with Rawesome recounting Palmer's arrest, and ordering that every nonmember or potential member "will be escorted into Rawesome premises by another member."

The new protocol seems not to have been strictly enforced with Treviso when she arrived. "Sound Lab Technician Fred Scott [had] provided Investigator Treviso with a black purse equipped with audio and video capabilities," according to the report filed by investigator Ward. He and Treviso signed up at Rawesome for day passes at one dollar apiece to gain entry, and an employee briefly explained where different products were located before letting them loose to explore on their own.

As Ward described it, "Inside the market, Treviso read a bulletin that Rawesome sold milk products from the Amish community in Pennsylvania for 'Miller's Organic Farms.' . . . Included among different listings on the bulletin board were the prices of Healthy Family Farms dairy products. As we walked through the market, Investigator Treviso and I entered a freezer compartment containing various dairy products labeled as raw from different providers. Inside the freezer, Healthy Family Farms had a section for their unpasteurized products such as goat milk, goat cheese, goat whey, goat kefir and goat yogurt. The video [being recorded by the camera in the black purse] showed Rawesome Foods was selling a product labeled 'Amish Goat Yogurt.'"[18]

From the investigators' viewpoint, they had hit pay dirt. The investigation would quickly move into overdrive. Presumably because dairy products from states outside California were available at Rawesome, the California investigators involved the FDA. When it was found that Rawesome didn't have any food retailing permits, the L.A. County Department of Public Health was called in. On June 22nd, L.A. County District Attorney investigators filmed video of the alleyway behind Rawesome and drew by hand a "Search Warrant Location Schematic" showing offices, storage areas, and open shopping areas as part of an in-depth undercover reconnaissance mission to assemble a detailed plan of the club's layout, inside and outside.[19]

Five weeks after Treviso's initial surveillance of Rawesome, at 7:45 on a Wednesday morning, June 30th, all was at the ready for a team of eight investigative agents from the L.A. County District Attorney. A search warrant had been obtained from L.A. Superior Court judge Ronald Corabest the day before. The watch commander of the L.A. Police Department's Pacific Division had been notified moments before that the operation was about to commence. Tactical gear, including guns and bulletproof vests, were checked once again.

"The search team approached the rear of the business, which had its electronic rear gate closed," recalled Ted Holst, the tall, gray-haired L.A. County District Attorney investigator. "We could hear employees working inside the rear yard and I identified us by stating, 'Police, we have a search warrant for the business.' A male voice from inside the business acknowledged my presence and within one minute the electronic gate was opened. The search team then entered the business and directed the six employees inside to walk to the rear gate area while the rest of the business and office was safely cleared."[20] Holst and three other agents drew their revolvers and entered the main business area. They paused every few steps to lift their revolvers and assume a battle-ready pose, as if they expected to encounter resistance. (Their actions were recorded by the Rawesome security camera and are posted on YouTube.)[21]

Needless to say, the L.A. County District Attorney agents didn't encounter any resistance. That meant it was time for yet more agents to descend on the tiny outlet. According to Holst's written account again, "Once LADA

[L.A. County District Attorney] investigators safely cleared the location, investigators from the CDFA (California Department of Food and Agriculture), Los Angeles County Health Department (LAC Health), and the U.S. Food and Drug Administration (FDA) were notified they could begin their search of the foods and dairy products."[22] That brought in Robert Donnalley and John Yao of the CDFA; Emoke Csengeri, Michele LeCavalier, and Teresa Villasenor of the health department; and Marco Solorio, Anita Liu, and Celene Ngo from the FDA.

While these other agents rummaged through the food inventory, Holst and his colleagues questioned Jerel Winterhawk, the husky, long-haired manager of the food club. Winterhawk told them, according to Holst, that he had been with Rawesome for three years "and has never seen any permits or licenses. . . . Rawesome Foods is a private membership business. Any customer who wants to enter the store must read and sign an agreement acknowledging that the produce for sale is organic and/or raw. They must also pay a $25.00 yearly fee or a $2 fee every time they enter." (It's not clear why he alluded to a two-dollar daily fee, and Treviso said she paid a one-dollar daily fee.) He also explained that, while he managed the location, "all ordering is done by James Stewart . . . who owns the business." He added that "most of" the club's products came from California, but that it "receives shipments of dairy foods from Amish farms in Pennsylvania."[23]

Nearly six hours after they arrived, the eight members of the search team prepared to depart. "Most of the food refrigeration units were closed and 'red tagged' by the LA County Health Department and Rawesome employees were told the food was not to be sold," according to Holst's account.[24]

Not surprisingly, Rawesome didn't open that Wednesday from noon to 8:00 p.m. as scheduled. At least eight thousand dollars of food had been confiscated, and a sign posted on the front door said that Rawesome was closed by order of the L.A. County Department of Public Health. The health department officials also left a summons for James Stewart to attend a hearing the next morning.

Stewart complied with the order and arrived with two other people the morning of July 1st — Tony Blain, a Rawesome member who served as the buying club's lawyer, and Cathy Jones, another Rawesome member who was handy with a video camera. Vonderplanitz was in Thailand at the time, tending to his nutrition consulting affairs.

Awaiting Stewart and his two companions in the health department conference room were six enforcement officials led by Terrance Powell, the longtime director of the department's Bureau of Specialized Surveillance and Enforcement (which has responsibility for milk and food, along with street vendors). Three of his subordinates were there together with Ken Ward, one of the investigators with the L.A. County District Attorney, and Terrance Nguyen, an FDA consumer safety officer. The fact that Powell was leading the session, and was joined by representatives of both the district attorney and the FDA, signified its importance to the officials.

Not surprisingly, the hearing wasn't an amicable or conciliatory affair from the get-go, according to the terse department report written after the session. "Mr. Blain presented California identification for himself, but refused to provide identification for his clients Mr. Stewart and Ms. Jones. Mr. Blain identified Mr. Stewart and Ms. Jones as such. Ms. Jones requested to videotape the hearing and the request was denied."[25]

It didn't get any better. "Mr. Blain stated that his presence at the hearing was to represent his clients and to inform the hearing officer of his objection to the Department's jurisdiction over Rawesome Foods," the report continued. "As Mr. Blain held that the Department had no jurisdiction over Rawesome Foods, he stated that his presence was a courtesy."[26] When Powell sought to question Blain about city and county permits, things deteriorated. According to the report, "Mr. Blain refused to answer any questions regarding government permits of any kind. Mr. Blain reiterated that he did not recognize the Department's jurisdiction/authority and refused to provide information on the source of the food products. Furthermore, Mr. Blain declared that the club would not recognize the closure and would continue to operate as usual. . . . Mr. Blain and his clients walked out of the hearing without making a statement."[27]

On a separate "complaint report," someone handwrote: "Possible continued illegal operation after closure. . . . Adesina shall conduct surveillance on Sat. 7/3/10 to verify if operation is ongoing."[28]

A few metropolitan papers, notably the *Los Angeles Times*, took cursory notice of the Rawesome raid, describing the mysterious multiagency search and confiscation of food on June 30, 2010.[29] None made mention of the fact that Sharon Palmer's Healthy Family Farms property had been raided the same day by a search party from the Ventura County sheriff and the CDFA. They confiscated business records and computers and questioned her about the herdshare she maintained with Rawesome to provide goat milk.

For the expanding number of online media with a conspiracy orientation, the Rawesome raid was a godsend. One, called "Survive and Thrive TV," included lots of dramatic music around an interview with James Stewart as he recounted the surprise entrance of enforcement agents and regulators — and how they made off with huge amounts of food.[30]

Rawesome members spoke out as well and seemed more saddened than anything else. Tommy Rosen, a yoga teacher, wrote a Huffington Post article that Thursday headlined, "What's the FBI Doing in My Milk?": "Many of the foods sold at Rawesome — fruits, vegetables, nuts — can also be found at most any other market. The difference at Rawesome is that the quality is often better as is the possibility of finding heirloom varieties of one's favorite produce. There is also the fact that people who shop there have this 'in the know' grin on their face as if they are hip to some special thing that will make a difference in their lives."[31] Rosen promised to return to Rawesome when it hopefully reopened on Saturday, July 3rd.[32]

Aajonus Vonderplanitz wasn't able to stay as rational about what occurred. In an e-mail from Asia two days after the raid, he stated: "Our food-club Rawesome was raided by federal, California State and Los Angeles County Health Officials and Police with guns drawn and threatening . . . those government agents trespassed and kidnapped volunteers and members for the entire time that they seized the property, about 5 hours. Also, they stole, under the term confiscate, thousands of dollars worth of members' FOOD that was private property, mostly raw dairy products and honey. Two individuals identified themselves as FBI and Canadian government agents but they did not show their badges."[33]

Stewart and his colleagues scrambled the rest of that Thursday and Friday to restock Rawesome for its scheduled Saturday hours. The food club reopened on Saturday, July 3, 2010, without incident — with many dozens of members showing up to shop.

Everyone present that Saturday at Rawesome was relieved and happy to see the food club reopen so quickly — except for one individual. That was Kunle Adesina of the L.A. County Department of Public Health, who wrote this note on a department complaint report: "7/3/10 Upon investigation I observed various individuals coming and going into this establishment. . . . People walking in without products or produce but coming out with products, produce, grocery bags. . . . Premises was definitely open."[34]

Vonderplanitz's outrage about the raid freaked out the authorities – to such an extent that on July 7th, a week after the raid on Rawesome, they asked an L.A. Superior Court judge to "seal" two sixteen-page documents providing details of the investigation leading up to the June 30th raid. These court documents, which provided the chronology of the undercover investigation carried out over eighteen months involving both Rawesome Foods and Healthy Family Farms, were intended to convince a judge there was sufficient evidence of lawbreaking to justify a search warrant.

Ken Ward, the investigator with the L.A. County District Attorney, said in a filing with the Los Angeles court that he was prompted to make the request based on "numerous articles and other 'postings' [that] have been placed on various websites and blogs naming some of the search warrant participants."[35]

He made reference to claims from Vonderplanitz about the nature of the raid and who was involved. "These online notices have said that people at the locations were 'kidnapped' and have misrepresented what took place, including claims that the FBI and Canadian officials were involved. One posting asked that supporters come to the Venice, California location to challenge the closure by the County Health Department."[36]

His fear? "If the information contained in these affidavits and in related search warrant documents is made public, it would compromise this investigation and make it impossible to continue. The informants and other sources of information referred to in this affidavit would no longer be able to gather information, particularly those acting as undercover agents. . . . Additionally, their lives and safety would be put into jeopardy."[37] Judge Michael D. Abzug signed an order that same day, sealing the search warrant supporting material as requested for ninety days.

In late September, just before the ninety days were up, though, Ward would be back before the judge asking him "to extend the sealing" of all the search warrant documents for at least another sixty days. Investigators needed more time to review all the documents they had collected by virtue of their search, including "information garnered from several internet service providers . . . more than 11,000 entries."[38]

It turned out that, in addition to executing search warrants on Rawesome and Healthy Family Farms, the investigators had executed search warrants to obtain access to the e-mail accounts of Sharon Palmer, Victoria Bloch, and Aajonus Vonderplanitz.

The judge signed the extension.[39]

James Stewart resumed his role of running Rawesome Foods, opening to members each Wednesday and Saturday.

Vonderplanitz remained in Asia for the rest of the summer, as planned.

Of course, neither of them knew about the judge's approval of the L.A. County District Attorney's request to seal the key search warrant documents. Not only would the details of the investigation leading up to the June 30th raid remain secret, but the investigation would continue — and include e-mail surveillance of Vonderplanitz and the others.

As angry as Vonderplanitz and Stewart were — they were even considering suing the state or federal agencies involved in the raid — the two men figured that if Rawesome could get another five years of peace, as it did following its 2005 run-in with authorities, then the eight thousand dollars of food confiscated might become a not-exorbitant cost of maintaining the club's private status. Would that life were so straightforward.

CHAPTER 7

SINCE WHEN ARE
WE AFRAID OF FOOD?

It's never easy being on a raw food diet, but it's especially difficult when you are traveling. I got a sense of just how challenging it is when I was out to dinner a few years back with Max Kane, the Wisconsin food activist who was investigated by state and federal authorities in connection with supplying raw milk to a Chicago food club. As part of his recovery from Crohn's disease while in his midtwenties, Kane adopted the raw food regimen advocated by Aajonus Vonderplanitz. Kane eats four to six raw eggs — along with raw beef, chicken, or fish — and drinks several glasses of raw milk each day.

We were with several other people at an upscale restaurant in Charlottesville, Virginia, that specialized in Southern cooking with an emphasis on local ingredients. (We were in Charlottesville in connection with a food rights fund-raising event the next day at celebrity farmer Joel Salatin's farm.) When it came time for our party to order, Kane asked the waiter for one of the chicken dishes appearing on the restaurant menu — served raw.

The waiter was taken aback, said he'd check with the chef, and within a minute or two returned with the restaurant's chef in tow. The chef was a young amiable fellow who explained without hesitation that, no, he couldn't — or rather wouldn't — serve Kane raw chicken. Kane might be defiant with government regulators, but in a social setting he is good-humored and even-tempered. Kane politely offered to sign any legal waiver the chef might have, or even draw one up himself. Nothing doing, said the chef: "I just can't take the chance." The chance, of course, was that Kane might get sick and sue the restaurant.

But why was the chef so fearful about Kane getting sick? The discussion never got that far, but more than likely the chef was aware that most chicken in the United States — between 60 and 80 percent according to *Consumer Reports* — is contaminated with campylobacter and/or salmonella, pathogens that can cause an upset stomach but on rare occasions become more serious. That's part of the reason many food experts warn people to cook chicken thoroughly, since the heat kills off such pathogens.

Kane wasn't ignorant about the prevalence of contaminated chicken. The chicken he ate when at home in rural Wisconsin came directly from small farms he knew. But he was willing to risk eating raw food when he traveled because he was confident he had built up immunity to any pathogens that might be lurking in the raw chicken or other foods he ate on the road.

In the end, the chef and Kane compromised. The chef would soak the chicken in lime juice for twenty minutes, ceviche style, essentially cooking it minimally. Not only would this make the chicken more tender, but it would likely kill off at least some pathogens. And Kane would get something that was closer to raw than heat-cooked chicken.

The episode was telling in a number of ways. Had the incident occurred before the turn of the century, the chef might have inquired into what kind of crazy guy wanted his chicken uncooked, but he would have consented to serve the meat as requested, perhaps with a mumbled, "If that's the way you want it, that's the way I'll give it to you. Just don't come crying on my shoulder if you get sick."

Has our food really become so much less safe that we must live with ever more fear-laden restrictions on what we can access and how? If so, why? What is it that has made our food so much less safe? Or made us so much more afraid?

Yes, over the last several years, there have been highly publicized outbreaks involving ground beef, cantaloupes, raw spinach, peanut butter, and other foods; some have resulted in deaths. But if you look at the CDC data on reported cases of food-borne illness, not only has the trend not shown any alarming blips during the first years of the new century, it has shown signs of declining. From 2006 to 2008, reported illnesses from state public health agencies declined from 27,000-plus to 23,152.[1] Then, in 2009, the number plummeted, by nearly 50 percent from the 2006 number, to 14,586. In 2010, the number was slightly higher: 15,685. That was still nearly a one-third decline from 2008.[2]

❧

As it turned out, the unfolding Rawesome Foods drama shed important light on the growing fear of food, although the food safety aspect of the Rawesome raid didn't become apparent for nearly two months after the June 30, 2010, events.

Indeed, there was no official word from any of the agencies that participated in the raid for weeks as to what had happened and why. Even though the Internet and newspapers were full of descriptions of the June 30th events, from the view of Rawesome-associated individuals, regulators and law enforcement personnel involved in the raid were silent — save for the L.A. County Department of Public Health's printed order to close Rawesome, which had been temporarily attached to the front door on June 30th.

When word finally came, it came in a roundabout way, via two government press releases issued in late August, more than eight weeks after the raid. If you didn't know about the Rawesome raid, you could easily have missed the connection. The first press release, issued by the CDFA, didn't even mention the raid in its statement that a pathogen, listeria, had been discovered in two varieties of cheese produced by a Missouri cheese company, Morningland Dairy, and distributed at food outlets in San Diego, Mendocino, Santa Cruz, and L.A. Counties. Consumers were asked to "discard the cheese or return it to the place of purchase." In any event, "no illnesses have been reported."[3]

Four days after the CDFA's announcement, the FDA issued a similar press release about Morningland Dairy and its supposedly tainted cheese, except this one stated that all the dairy's cheese production already sold during the first eight months of 2010, nearly sixty-nine thousand pounds, had been recalled. And in the sixth of seven paragraphs, the Rawesome name was finally uttered publicly by authorities: "This regulatory sampling of Morningland Dairy cheese, which was taken from the Rawesome store in Venice, California, revealed the Morningland Dairy Hot Pepper Colby and Garlic Colby Cheeses contained the bacteria. Morningland Dairy has suspended the production and distribution of all cheese, as FDA, the Missouri Milk Board, and Morningland Dairy continue their investigation as to the root cause of the problem."[4]

In those two releases, with just the briefest of allusions to Rawesome, a partial explanation for the chaos created by the armed agents during the June 30th raid began to come into focus. Until then, the main clues consisted of the lists of documents, equipment, food, and other items the agents had confiscated. Agents from three of the agencies left handwritten lists of what they took, as required when a search warrant is executed.

According to a receipt signed by four L.A. County District Attorney agents, those individuals made off with order forms, supplier receipts, "one phone poster of employees and suppliers," "one folder labeled tall grass beef," $4,980 in cash (mostly in twenty-dollar bills), and Rawesome's computer.[5]

The CDFA left a long list of confiscated foods — some eighty-four items — including goat whey, colostrum, goat milk, salted Swiss cheese, unsalted cheddar cheese, and raw unsalted sheep cheese. There were even listings for "Amish Organic Whole Milk" and "Amish Heavy Cream." Next to each item listed was a number, like five or eleven or thirty, presumably to detail the number of items taken. Near the end of the CDFA's list, item #79 was Morningland Dairy Hot Pepper Colby Cheese, and #80 was Morningland Dairy Raw Milk Cheese Garlic Colby.[6]

The FDA left a shorter list, only seven items, including "ten bottles of Amish yogurt and Amish Goat Cheese Mozzarella." The last item on the FDA's list was a "mild cheddar raw milk cheese from Morningland Dairy."[7] What the lists didn't say was that all of the confiscated food had been sent for extensive testing in CDFA laboratories scattered around California. The news blackout was likely intentional. If all the tests came back negative, then the silence around the Rawesome raid could continue. But if the investigators hit a "bingo," then press releases could be issued and, in an official sense, the raid could begin to be justified as something related to food safety.

The minimal references in the official press releases issued by the CDFA and FDA to Rawesome suggested that there was, in fact, more to the Morningland Dairy component of the Rawesome raid than the regulators would have wanted to discuss. For the Morningland Dairy experience said more about the changing nature of food safety enforcement in the United States than any statistics ever could.

Morningland Dairy was as distant from Rawesome's home in Venice, California, in both setting and culture as one could imagine. The cheese facilities consisted of nondescript one-story structures — a barn, a milk parlor, a cheese-making plant, offices, and a refrigerated cheese storage facility — arranged almost like a small village on thirteen acres of woods and fields off a dirt road, way off a main road. It was miles even from the center of Mountain View, a tiny speck of a town three hours south of St. Louis in the Missouri Ozarks. The peaceful rolling hills are green and inviting in warm months. It's the kind of quiet rural setting where people swim in the rivers during the sultry summer and go to church on Sundays, and where it would be easy to imagine a close-knit family growing and thriving.

That's exactly what attracted Joseph and Denise Dixon, a couple in their midfifties, to the place. They acquired Morningland Dairy in 2008 from Jim and Marge Reiners, who for years had longed to retire if they could sell their raw cheese operation to the right people — the right people being those who shared their vision of producing high-quality and healthy specialty raw milk cheeses. To the Dixons, buying Morningland was a case of being in the right place at the right time. The Reiners had nearly given up finding a buyer for the operation, which is a combination farm, dairy, and cheese-making plant.

"We have twelve children," Denise Dixon explained to me. She is a handsome woman, with gray hair and soft but penetrating eyes. "We wanted to raise the children in a healthy atmosphere." The children ranged from their teens to their twenties and the couple had the same desire most farmers have: "We wanted them to be able to earn a living without having to go off to the city."

Making cheese is more like producing fine wine than producing milk or making butter or yogurt. It requires careful attention to subtleties and technique, practicing how to mix and heat and stir and cool and cut and age the different varieties of cheese. The Dixons were so intrigued by the notion of taking over the cheese-making operation that Denise spent two years at Morningland as an unpaid apprentice in 2007 and 2008. Joseph tended to the family's ninety-five-acre farm about thirty miles to the west, in Cabool, Missouri, where they milked sixty-five goats. It was a conventional milking operation in that the milk was pasteurized before it was canned and sold to box store retailers.

That farm was a low-margin operation, as are most businesses of any type that sell to box stores. Joseph had grown up with raw milk and always felt it was a healthy food, and he knew the market for raw dairy products was growing rapidly. "If you can get a good raw milk product, you can do very well," he concluded.

Denise Dixon loved her cheese-making lessons at Morningland. Moreover, she sensed that a business opportunity beckoned as well. The Reiners were doing between $400,000 and $500,000 in annual revenues. "They were in a holding pattern," in Denise's view. "They were tired."

The Dixons and Reiners negotiated a deal for the Dixons to buy Morningland's buildings, land, cheese-making equipment, existing inventory, and fifty cows for $355,000. The Dixons financed the transaction via loans from family and friends, financing from the Reiners, and funds from a retirement account Joseph had long ago established while working as a railroad electrician.

It was "a big stretch," according to Denise, but it seemed reasonable, representing as it did less than one year of revenues. In most industries, financial experts will tell you, acquiring a going business with real assets like land, animals, and buildings and operating with marginal profits for the equivalent of one year's revenues is generally a decent deal.

It quickly looked like a very good deal, as the Dixons injected new energy into the operation and added flavored goat cheeses like Italian, hot pepper, and garlic and chive that were well received by the dozens of retail and private food club buyers that were the business's customers. James Stewart and others at Rawesome, which was an existing customer, "were real excited about the new cheeses," recalled Denise.

Morningland's reputation for interesting high-quality cheeses had spread as well to Jefferson City, Missouri's capital, three hours to the north. When would-be cheese producers contacted Gene Wiseman, the executive secretary of the Missouri Milk Board — which oversees the state's dairies and cheese makers — he'd often refer them to Morningland. "They are unique," he would say some months later in a court case involving Morningland. "They utilize both cow and goat milk, so I was familiar with them. There are few places in the state like them, where people could find a goat-milk cheese operation."

As the summer of 2010 rolled around, the Dixons felt as if they were making headway. Revenues were tracking at $500,000 to $600,000 annually. With many of their cows due to go into a sixty- to ninety-day "freshening" period during August and September — when they would be giving birth to calves and wouldn't be producing milk for commercial purposes — the Dixons built up the company's inventory to a record (some 30,000 pounds, with a value of about $200,000). With the company's reputation expanding, and demand for raw milk cheese in general soaring, according to Denise "all the inventory was committed." It looked like money in the bank, the first payoff from a lot of preparation, risk taking, and old-fashioned hard work.

"We were just getting ready to pay ourselves back" on the $60,000 from Joseph's retirement fund that had been loaned to Morningland, Denise recalled.

It was late in the afternoon of Wednesday, August 25, 2010, just as he was preparing to end his day, that Gene Wiseman of the Missouri Milk Board received an urgent telephone call from Stephen Beam, head of the dairy division of the CDFA. Beam is a tall, youthful-looking man with light brown hair who had made a name for himself in the world of raw milk regulation by leading the CDFA's initiative in 2008 to get the California legislature to adopt tough new standards governing raw milk quality. His success prompted an outcry of opposition from raw milk drinkers before it was finally upheld, via a veto by then governor Arnold Schwarzenegger of legislation to eliminate the standards.

As Wiseman described the conversation with Beam, "He said samples of cheese from a Missouri plant had been analyzed in a California lab and they were found to contain pathogens." Later that evening Beam sent along an e-mail with attached lab reports and photos covering two samples of cow's milk cheese from Morningland Dairy — one the hot pepper Colby and the other the garlic Colby. The next morning, Thursday, Wiseman and Beam had another conversation. "Dr. Beam said [the Morningland cheese] showed positive for two pathogens — *Listeria monocytogenes* and *Staphylococcus aureus*."

Listeria monocytogenes is one of the four most common pathogens that taint food. (The others are campylobacter, salmonella, and *E. coli* O157:H7.) While staph aureus, as it's commonly referred to, is also a pathogen capable of causing what's commonly referred to as "food poisoning," it's not generally considered by the public health community to be especially dangerous. Unlike *E. coli* O157:H7, where just a few cells can cause serious illness, staph aureus has to be present in significant numbers before it can create problems. Moreover, staph aureus is pervasive not only in food, but on our bodies — in our nostrils and on our skin — where it may cause pimples or other dermatological reactions.

Wiseman expressed confusion to Beam about some of the photos he had sent along — a few seemed to be of products that had nothing to do with Missouri. "Dr. Beam told me there were a large number of products that were sampled and went through the lab at that time. The samples were broken up. The samples weren't necessarily tested together." What Beam was telling Wiseman was that the California labs had been very busy testing the twenty-seven coolers of cheese, milk, yogurt, whey, colostrum, honey, and so forth seized in the Rawesome raid. Not only did it take a long time, but when the results came through, foods from various producers were mixed together in the official reports.

When questioned in court, Wiseman would indicate ignorance about most of what was going on in California with Rawesome and its aftermath. He said he didn't know anything about the conditions under which the Morningland cheese had been stored during those nearly two months between the raid and the report of contaminated cheese, nor what protocols had been observed in the testing process — matters that could shed light on whether the storage conditions might have been such that a few pathogens could have been stimulated into spreading into the cheese. There wasn't any indication in his testimony about whether Beam had mentioned the seriousness with which the FDA took this case. Nor any mention about whether they had discussed the fact that no one had become ill from Morningland Dairy cheese that had been on the market immediately before and after the raid on Rawesome Foods on June 30th.

Nonetheless, when Wiseman got off the phone with Beam, the Missouri regulator moved swiftly and decisively. "I dispatched Don Falls [a dairy inspector] to the Morningland plant. We needed people on the ground to do that investigation. I instructed him to drop everything else and go there to condemn, seize, and embargo the cheese."

His immediate decision to restrict Morningland's entire inventory of cheese from sale — as opposed to other less drastic actions, such as ordering Missouri regulators to carry out their own tests of the thirty thousand pounds of cheese in Morningland's storage facility, or withholding just the two types of cheese California authorities had informed him contained pathogens — was notable. He would say it was based on his conclusion that Missouri law was being violated via the sale, or "offering for sale," of products "from an animal . . . that produces impure or unwholesome milk." It was also the most restrictive decision he could have made.

Denise and Joseph Dixon weren't even at their dairy when Wiseman dispatched the veteran inspector Don Falls to the dairy. The Dixons were in Seattle, attending the annual convention of the American Cheese Society, a fast-growing organization of artisanal cheese producers, and getting a welcome respite from the daily grind of the dairy. Out in Seattle that Thursday afternoon, Denise Dixon received a call on her cell phone from Jedadiah York, the Morningland plant manager. "He called to say Don Falls was on his way out because there was a problem."

"We told Jedadiah to be helpful," recalled Denise. She and Joseph knew Don Falls — he had been inspecting cheese and dairy plants for the Missouri Milk Board for sixteen years — and had always had a cordial relationship with him when he conducted annual inspections of the dairy and cheese plant. He hadn't found any serious problems since the Dixons acquired the operation.

Even though Don Falls placed a signed red tag, what the Milk Board refers to as "a condemnation and seizure card," on the door of the long fifty-three-by-ten-foot cooler containing the thirty thousand pounds of cheese, his demeanor wasn't at all confrontational or tense. The embargo sticker was merely a precaution, he suggested to the plant manager. Jedadiah York, just twenty-nine, had only been on the job ten months and so had never before met Falls or the colleague who accompanied him, but the situation seemed nonthreatening. "Their attitude was this was no big deal. They wanted to see if we had any more of the inventory from what had tested positive."

That Thursday afternoon, York had been planning to ready shipments to go out the following Monday. "I asked, 'What are the odds of being able to ship Monday and Tuesday?' They said, 'Count on it.' They were there primarily to make sure we didn't have any more of the product in our storage facility and to get information on the stores we sold to in California."

None of the cheese from the production blocks of the cheese the CDFA said was tainted remained in inventory. York provided the names of three California outlets that had received the cheese — Rawesome and two others. Within an hour, Falls and his colleague left, promising to return the next morning.

The Dixons didn't wait till the next morning to decide to leave the Seattle conference and drive back to Missouri. Despite Falls's assurances, they felt it necessary to be on-site in case things didn't proceed as smoothly as he thought they would.

It didn't take long for their concerns to be realized. At about 10:00 on Friday morning, Don Falls received a call on the Morningland Dairy phone from Michele Thompson of the FDA. She was the district recall coordinator for the Midwest area that included Missouri.

York, the manager, remembers it well. "That was when the entire tone changed." When he got off that call, "Falls said, 'Don't plan on shipping Monday.' There would need to be a product recall and FDA agents would need to take environmental swabs."

The Missouri Milk Board had alerted the FDA about the embargo of the thirty thousand pounds of Morningland Cheese, and now FDA officials were pushing for yet another step in the process besides quarantining the unshipped cheese — a recall of Morningland Dairy cheese distributed in the previous eight months. But should it be a recall of the two questionable cheeses, or of all Morningland's cheeses?

More often than not, when state authorities find pathogens in food or a food-production facility that serves multistate markets, FDA officials are notified and they push for a recall. Technically, there are three kinds of recalls the FDA can select from: firm initiated, FDA requested, and FDA ordered. Most recalls are of the first variety, firm initiated or "voluntary"; but in reality, such recalls are much like the proverbial call for volunteers in the military — "you, you, and you, clean the latrines."

The rules governing FDA recalls are contained in a seventy-five-page chapter within a larger rule book, known as the *Regulatory Procedures Manual*.[8] While the existence of a detailed rule book implies consistency, the reality is that the scope and timing of so-called voluntary recalls vary widely. Based on a review of other food company recalls carried out around the same time as Morningland Dairy's, the actions are generally limited to the product thought to be contaminated.

For example, in November 2010, the FDA announced that Del Bueno of Grandview, Washington, was recalling four different varieties of cheese — Queso Fresco Fresh Cheese, Queso Panela Fresh Cheese, Requeson Mexican Style Ricotta Cheese, and Queso Enchilado Dry Cheese — "because they have the potential to be contaminated with Listeria monocytogenes."[9] There was no mention of the company having to halt production or recall other varieties of cheese.

In June 2011, the huge vegetable and fruit producer Dole announced via an FDA press release that it was recalling about 3,300 bags of two kinds of bagged salad because Ohio regulators had discovered *Listeria monocytogenes* in one bag. Once again, no mention was made of an interruption to Dole's business or any other penalties.[10]

When the Wisconsin Department of Agriculture, Trade, and Consumer Protection discovered *Listeria monocytogenes* in some smoked trout and smoked salmon produced by Rushing Waters Fisheries in November 2010, a recall was ordered — but only of 225 pounds of the fish. "Only the smoked fish spreads with the matching lots and dates are being recalled; no other Rushing Waters Fisheries LLC products are included in the recall," the company said in its press release.[11]

For Morningland, though, the process wasn't so forgiving. Later that Friday morning, Michele Thompson called York and explained that the FDA wanted Morningland to "voluntarily" recall all the cheese it had sold in the previous eight months of 2010, not only the hot pepper Colby and the garlic Colby cow cheeses from the Rawesome raid that had tested positive for *Listeria monocytogenes*. That made the total amount of cheese to be recalled in excess of sixty thousand pounds. Of course, there was no way anywhere near that amount would be returned, since most of it would have been consumed by that point.

York was directed to write a press release to be both sent to the Associated Press (America's largest news service, which is subscribed to by nearly all daily newspapers in the country) and issued on the FDA's website announcing the recall. It was all rush-rush, with Thompson pushing for the release to be sent out that Friday afternoon; she said in an e-mail to Morningland that she had the contact information for the Associated Press. Back and forth went the drafts that Friday. At Denise Dixon's suggestion, York included in one draft a statement that Morningland had been forced by the FDA to carry out the recall. The FDA didn't like that and removed it.

Also unlike most other companies forced into voluntary recalls, Morningland was prohibited from continuing production, according to the release. "Morningland Dairy has suspended the production and distribution of all cheese, as FDA, the Missouri Milk Board, and Morningland Dairy continue their investigation as to the root cause of the problem."[12]

The only potential positive for Morningland was this statement, in all caps: "NO ILLNESSES HAVE BEEN REPORTED TO DATE."[13]

When Denise and Joseph returned to work that Monday morning, not only had the release been issued, but the FDA was true to its word that it would "continue their investigation as to the root cause of the problem."

As it turned out, the FDA was conducting a lot of cheese plant inspections during 2010. Earlier in the year, the agency had embarked on a thorough review of its long-established policy on raw milk cheese — which was fairly permissive, considering the agency's antipathy to raw dairy in general.

Since the late 1940s, such cheese had been legal for sale, so long as it was aged for sixty days — the logic being that sixty days would be enough time for any pathogens to die. The policy wasn't as liberal as that of France or Quebec, which specialized in gourmet soft cheeses that weren't aged at all, but it also wasn't a ban — and allowed for the production of gourmet cheeses for America's increasingly sophisticated food marketplace. Demand for raw specialty cheeses climbed despite cost, which often run from twenty to thirty dollars a pound. The American Cheese Society saw its membership nearly double from 776 in 2003 to more than 1,300 by 2011. Entries for raw milk cheese in its annual competition during that period increased from 762 cheeses to 1,462.

But throughout 2010, many American Cheese Society members reported FDA inspections — three-fourths of the 130 members who completed a survey questionnaire developed by the organization had been visited by FDA inspectors during the year, versus less than 10 percent in previous years. Moreover, the inspections were more thorough than the cheese producers expected: "Beyond the obvious inspection spaces such as make rooms and aging rooms, respondents reported that inspectors are examining intake and receiving areas, storage areas, brine rooms, milking rooms, barns, kitchens, bathrooms, packaging areas, and retail spaces."[14]

But none reported anything distinctive about the appearance of the visiting inspectors on the order of what Morningland Dairy experienced. There, two FDA agents arrived at the tiny dairy on Monday morning, August 30th — dressed in military fatigues.

Unbeknownst to most people, there is a U.S. Public Health Service Commissioned Corps, which is part of the U.S. Defense Department. In addition to providing health services to underserved citizens and participating in global health emergencies, it is also charged with "ensuring that . . . food is safe and wholesome."[15] Its website describes the corps as "an elite team of more than 6,000 well-trained, highly qualified public health professionals dedicated to delivering the Nation's public health promotion and disease prevention programs and advancing public health science."[16] The members are scattered among ten federal agencies, including the FDA.[17]

At 10:55 that morning, August 30th, two FDA agents, Audra Ashmore and Diana Guidry, walked into the Morningland Dairy office dressed in camouflage uniforms with their last names stenciled on the right-hand side of their shirts and USPHS on the left — and combat boots. The apparel turns out to be one of six sets of uniforms the Public Health Service Commissioned Corps can wear, technically known as "battle dress uniform."[18]

Anticipating the worst about the unfolding regulatory process, the Dixons had as a first step asked one of their sons, Isaac, to videotape the Monday-morning proceedings with the FDA inspectors. They took this step based on advice from other farmers and food producers who had encountered regulatory pressure — to videotape regulators conducting a search or inspection at one's farm or food plant. That way, there's less chance for misunderstandings later on, and also less likelihood the regulators are going to be inappropriate or out of line in their demands during the search or inspection.

Now, looking at the video that Isaac Dixon produced, I can only say that seeing the two attractive women, who look to be in their thirties, standing awkwardly by the front door inside the Morningland Dairy office in camouflage and combat boots has a surrealistic quality to it. "It was quite a surprise to us," recalled York. "It felt like they were trying to be bullies, an intimidation technique" — especially given that York and the Dixons had gone out of their way to be cooperative with the regulators to that point.

By the next day, the FDA agents had changed into more traditional khaki uniforms, and pretty soon into white sanitized suits with blue booties to take sponge swabs of hoses, floors, sinks, and other spots around the cheese production facility where listeria tends to congregate. The two agents were joined by a third agent and spent three days testing. But the damage had been done. Probably more than any other single episode in the Morningland Dairy case, the appearance of the FDA agents in battle fatigues on the first day established a confrontational mentality on both sides, which continued for months.

In what should have been a big victory for Morningland, the FDA's tests showed no contamination in the dairy facilities. Since nearly all listeria contamination of raw milk cheese originates with contaminated facilities — contamination from cows producing listeria-contaminated milk is nearly unknown — the implication was that no systemic problem existed.

But that wasn't enough for the Missouri Milk Board. It expressed concern because a set of private tests Morningland commissioned on a small subset of cheese — and carried out by Morningland employees who had no experience preparing samples for testing — showed the presence of listeria in six pieces besides those found by the CDFA. Morningland asked the state to do a complete test of its cheese in inventory. The state refused, saying it had all the evidence it needed of serious contamination. Morningland offered to test any batches of cheese before shipping. The state refused.

Morningland was desperate to save the two hundred thousand dollars of inventory, which represented Joseph Dixon's retirement account. The Dixons might have considered disposing of the inventory if they knew they could resume production, but the Missouri Milk Board had, since the FDA inspection, come up with concerns about the cleanliness of Morningland's facilities — despite the clean bill of health from the FDA — and wanted thousands of dollars in dairy and production facility improvements before considering whether cheese making could resume.

The Dixons felt boxed into a corner. Their only options seemed to be to destroy their entire inventory, invest in assorted facilities improvements, and hope the Missouri Milk Board would allow production to resume. That approval was far from guaranteed.

After at first approving a late fall order to destroy the thirty thousand pounds of cheese, the Dixons changed their mind and refused the order. In their view, destroying the cheese was not only a financial catastrophe, but a symbol of humiliating injustice. The state immediately went to court. In early January, the Dixons would go on trial for refusing the order.

The imposing block-square gray building that houses the Circuit Court of Howell County is the largest building in West Plains, Missouri. About thirty miles from Morningland Dairy, it was rebuilt in the 1930s after an explosion, purportedly from a gas leak, at a nearby dance hall in 1928 had killed thirty-seven of sixty young people gathered for an evening of entertainment.

The town of twelve thousand, which is home to Missouri State University, has the kind of small-town feel you'd expect in the rural Midwest, with a number of small breakfast and lunch restaurants, a hardware store, and other retailers arrayed around the large courthouse building. It's a place where it's still possible to buy a sandwich and salad for lunch for less than five dollars.

The Missouri attorney general's office assigned two young lawyers— Laura Brown and Jessica Blome—to prosecute Denise and Joseph Dixon on behalf of the Missouri Milk Board. Brown, who looked to be in her late twenties or early thirties, slender with brown hair, made the state's opening statement: "This is about a very simple issue—whether the defendant violated the state's order to destroy the cheese," she said. "We ask the state to order the destruction of this unlawful product . . . or find that the defendant has interfered with the state . . . and enjoin the defendant to stop interfering with the state and comply with the law."

She quickly summarized the facts of the case: "The Missouri Milk Board was notified by the state of California's Department of Food and Agriculture that cheese sold in the state of California by the defendants . . . tested positive for the harmful bacteria listeria monocytogenes. . . . After consulting with many different sources, the Missouri Milk Board determined that the bacteria comprised a grave risk to the public health."

As if anticipating accusations that the state was engaged in a politically motivated vendetta against Morningland Dairy, Brown added:

> This is not about the state's goal to put this dairy out of business. This case is not a campaign against raw milk cheese or the raw milk movement. It is not about the defendant being subject to unfair laws. It is about protecting the health and lives of every Missourian and citizens across the nation. . . . This cheese can potentially kill those who consume it. . . . Our hard evidence will show there is very harmful bacteria in this cheese.

The state's first witness was Gene Wiseman, the head of the Missouri milk board, who recounted how he learned the news about contamination of Morningland Dairy cheese from the CDFA. Next was Don Falls, the milk board inspector. Falls was a balding and, like Wiseman, slightly paunchy man who looked to be in his fifties.

Blome, the young, bespectacled lead prosecutor, led Falls through notations on his inspection reports. Though the inspector had never issued any citations against Morningland Dairy for violations while the dairy was under the Dixons' ownership the previous two years, his testimony sounded as if he had plenty of reason to do so. There was reference to a need for a covered area for milk being brought to the bulk milk tank a covered area for cleaning the bulk tank ("to protect the tank from contamination when you are cleaning it"), the need to get rid of rusty areas at the bottom of certain stainless steel equipment, and the need to smooth some rough wooden surfaces "that can harbor dirt and bacteria." The cheese in the walk-in cooler was closer than the six inches above the ground allowed, and the cheeses were stored too tightly together.

Of course, Blome was seeking to create doubt about the cleanliness of Morningland's current owners — even if she was, by implication, criticizing Falls for giving Morningland passing grades for two years. But the most intriguing question to Falls had to do with Morningland's long-term safety record.

"How many times in your sixteen years has the Missouri Milk Board placed an embargo tag on a cooler?"

Twice, said Falls. The first time was during the summer of 1999. "We placed an embargo placard on the Morningland Dairy cooler because it had a positive reading for listeria monocytogenes." Apparently the FDA had taken some samples that were tested at a federal facility in Denver. "There was one sample that showed listeria monocytogenes. We placed a placard on the entire inventory."

What happened next? As Falls recalled it, "They initiated a voluntary recall, and additional testing didn't show any further pathogens. They destroyed the contaminated lot of cheese that tested positive and were allowed to sell cheese that had tested negative."

Blome seemed to relish the testimony, suggesting that Morningland had had a previous encounter with pathogens. "And the second incident?"

"The second incident," said Falls, "is the one we are talking about here — August 2010."

Not surprisingly, Blome failed to explore the vastly different official responses to the two similar events. The 1999 incident seemed to barely turn up any dust; Morningland recalled the cheese in question, destroyed inventory of just the questionable cheese, and then resumed production. Why did FDA inspectors in military fatigues descend on Morningland Dairy in 2010? Why did the state push back when the dairy was amenable to serious by-the-books testing of its inventory? Why did the FDA insist on a full product recall at a time when it thought only two varieties out of more than a dozen were contaminated? Why were two skilled lawyers from the Missouri attorney general's office preparing briefs and then running a full-court press in a small-town courtroom? Why was a small dairy being pushed to the edge of insolvency, with all the follow-on ramifications, including the loss of a half-dozen or more jobs in the midst of an ongoing recession — all in the absence of any illnesses?

In other words, what had changed in the eleven years between the two incidents? It turned out that a lot had changed in attitudes and approaches toward food safety.

More than a century ago, outbreaks of illness tied to everything from concoctions promoted by traveling snake oil salesmen to tainted raw milk led to passage of the Pure Food and Drug Act of 1906. It was strengthened by passage of the federal Food, Drug, and Cosmetic Act in 1938, and the FDA — charged with overseeing the labeling of food, inspecting food production facilities to promote sanitary practices, and determining which additives and coloring were safe for food — was on its way to becoming a government mainstay.

A combination of factors (including vaccinations, antibiotics, and a greater understanding of safe food-handling practices like refrigeration, worker hygiene, and plant sanitation) helped to eliminate or reduce a host of serious illnesses spread at least partly by food — diseases like typhoid, tuberculosis, and brucellosis. By the 1950s and 1960s, the threats from tainted food had receded considerably. Of course, there would always be cases of food poisoning — often from bad restaurant food, or food at picnics left out in the hot sun. But by the 1950s, the public health establishment was far more focused on handling large-scale outbreaks of dangerous childhood diseases like polio and measles — and eventually, in the late 1950s and 1960s, with disseminating the polio vaccine.

Two factors changed the food safety complexion in a big way. The first was the rise of concentrated animal feeding operations (CAFOs) during the

1970s and 1980s. Food producers found they could lower costs by packing cattle, pigs, and chickens into huge warehouse-like facilities and fattening them quickly on corn and soy. CAFOs were animal agriculture's equivalent of the manufacturing industry's factory-style mass production systems.

One problem with CAFOs is that cows evolved to eat grass, not corn, and the change in diet turned their digestive systems into breeding grounds for pathogens. Dangerous bacteria proliferate in the huge volumes of manure within crowded CAFOs or remain within animals' intestines, and they can be spread when manure gets into rivers and streams and carcasses are ground into hamburger and other products.

As a publication of Purdue University's Extension put it, "Livestock manure can . . . contain disease causing microorganisms; and if manure is improperly stored or mishandled, these pathogens could pose a health hazard if they come in contact with water or raw foods. As such, there are concerns that the manure generated by CAFOs could result in infectious disease outbreaks in surrounding communities."[19]

The discovery in 1982 of a particularly dangerous pathogen, *E. coli* O157:H7, provided further evidence that CAFOs pose a threat to food safety. A 1996 paper from the Johns Hopkins School of Hygiene and Public Health tried to assess why *E. coli* O157:H7 was showing up in outbreaks from tainted food: "The livestock and beef industries have changed dramatically during the past several decades. While no one change can be singled out as the 'major' contributing factor to emergence of this pathogen, it is possible that these changes, alone and together, have created a setting in which this organism has been able to spread more readily through and into animal and human populations.

"In particular, big may not always be better: Consolidation of the industry, widespread movement of cattle, and increased use of large production lots for products such as hamburger may all have played a role in the process — and may provide a setting in which other 'new' pathogens can rapidly move into human populations."[20]

The second factor was more specific — the rise of a young Seattle personal injury lawyer, Bill Marler, as a food safety specialist and advocate. Even though *E. coli* O157:H7 had been discovered more than ten years before he arrived on the legal scene, and had been identified as the cause of several significant food-borne outbreaks, the pathogen wasn't well known in the food industry or legal arena until a serious outbreak associated with the Jack in the Box hamburger chain occurred in the Seattle area in 1992 and 1993.

It might seem like a stretch to suggest that one individual could profoundly change perceptions about food safety, but Marler is an unusual person. Even though he was young and relatively inexperienced in food product liability — he barely knew what *E. coli* O157:H7 was when a six year-old Seattle girl died in late 1992 after eating a hamburger harboring the pathogen — he quickly sensed the legal and financial opportunity to compensate families for their hospitalizations and suffering when more children and adults fell seriously ill during the episode. He lobbied aggressively, and successfully, to convince parents whose children had died or been seriously injured to select him as their lawyer over other more experienced personal injury attorneys. By mid-1994, Marler had settled the first cases in the Jack in the Box outbreak for an eye-popping $23.6 million — a record at the time — and was on his way to carving out a lucrative practice in the new legal specialty of food safety.

"The Jack in the Box outbreak is considered the meat industry's 9/11," wrote author Jeff Benedict in his 2011 book about the Jack in the Box case, *Poisoned: The True Story of the Deadly E. Coli Outbreak That Changed the Way Americans Eat*. "As soon as hamburgers killed kids, everything changed. Congressional hearings were held. The national media put a spotlight on the industry. State and federal health codes were upgraded."

The publicity made Marler the go-to lawyer for food safety cases. Two years later, he became involved in a second high-profile case when dozens of children got sick after drinking unpasteurized Odwalla apple juice, apparently because the company used apples that had fallen to the ground — where they may have been contaminated by animal manure. Marler represented the families of several of the children who became the most seriously ill, and settled the cases for a reported $12 million.[21] In addition, Odwalla was indicted and pled guilty to sixteen criminal charges in connection with the case, paying a $1.6 million fine.[22] Food safety quickly turned into a high priority for corporations around the country.

Marler's rise in the new legal area of food safety coincided with the rise of the Internet. He was an aggressive promoter, and the Internet is the ultimate tool for promoting legal and medical expertise if used effectively. Marler seemed to have a nearly intuitive grasp of how to use it. In addition to his own blog chronicling his speaking engagements and charitable contributions — as well as publicizing food safety issues and research — Marler established individual blogs on *E. coli*, campylobacter, listeria, and food poisoning in general. By 2012 he had more than thirty blogs and other websites. He understood that when victims of serious food-borne illness are looking for a lawyer, they will likely search Google and contact the law firm displaying what appears to be the most credible information about their illnesses and the outbreaks that likely led to their illnesses. The law firm receiving that first e-mail or phone call inquiry is likeliest to capture what could be a multimillion-dollar case.

But rather than simply promoting his expertise and his legal wins, Marler — who bears an uncanny resemblance, in looks and voice, to former House Speaker Newt Gingrich — positioned himself as a champion of food safety. At several points, such as during a congressional debate over the Food Safety Modernization Act in 2009 and 2010, he advocated on its behalf with the tagline, "Put a trial lawyer out of business."[23] Of course, food safety legislation won't eliminate food-borne illnesses any more than new anticrime legislation will do away with crime; Marler likely understood that better than anyone.

The heightened visibility gave him ever more credibility, and influence, with government regulators. State public health officials nationwide have served as expert witnesses in his legal cases, helping his firm's credibility with opposing lawyers, judges, and insurance companies that must often approve legal settlements. Marler even has the distinction of being the only outside lawyer known to have helped the CDC create a website on food-borne illness — three video interviews of his clients are the main attractions of the CDC's recently constructed website warning about the dangers of raw milk.[24]

At times, Marler seemed to challenge legal convention, such as in 2008 and 2009, when he began posting Internet videos of clients who were sickened from raw milk and other foods — before the cases had gone to trial. The videos showed children and adults on life support and in physical therapy. Marler once explained his video approach to me as one part of his version of "shock and awe" (together with expert witness testimony and medical reports), and more often than not the videos had their desired effect — they resulted in out-of-court financial settlements from companies desperate to avoid having the videos shown to juries, which might hand out even larger damage awards than could be negotiated via settlements. He expanded his use of videos from raw milk cases to others involving individuals sickened by cantaloupes and ground beef.

By the time Benedict published *Poisoned* in 2011, Marler had settled $600 million in cases and was headed toward $1 billion.[25] Lawyers typically receive 25 to 33 percent of financial settlements or jury awards, meaning Marler's Seattle firm, Marler Clark, likely earned at least $150 million (and probably more).

As a white knight in shining armor protecting the public from big bad agribusiness "poisoning its customers," Marler became a media darling. He knew that reporters love a controversial quote, and he is by nature an affable charmer who can offer a sharp critique of seemingly negligent corporations. His law firm's website contains links to about one hundred articles that quoted or profiled Marler between 2008 and 2011.[26] One of those was a *New York Times* front-page profile of one of his clients, a professional dancer, who had been paralyzed from contaminated ground beef. The article won the reporter a Pulitzer Prize.

As a promoter, Marler knew instinctively how to keep his name in lights when a food-related cause emerged. For example, when his alma mater, Washington State University, canceled a speaking event with Michael Pollan, author of *The Omnivore's Dilemma* — ostensibly because of budgetary problems, but possibly because of political opposition to Pollan's anti-Big-Ag views — Marler advertised on his blog that he would pay the $40,000 that was thought to be required to keep the event. The story was tweeted widely, and the *New York Times* wrote a feature about Marler's largesse under the heading, "For Personal-Injury Lawyer, Michael Pollan's Book Is Worth Fighting For."[27]

There is an unfortunate downside to Marler's shrewd promotion, in my judgment, and that is the cultivation of an ever-mounting — and at times unwarranted — climate of fear around food safety. Thanks to Marler's blogs, along with those of other product liability lawyers like Fred Pritzker, each case of potentially tainted food announced by the FDA or state public health and agriculture agencies — no matter how minor — becomes a major news story echoing around the blogosphere. The crisis atmosphere prevails even if there are no illnesses, often to the chagrin of the food producer blamed for the contamination. And the reverberations can continue nearly forever, since it is almost impossible to rid the Internet of such material.

Its appearance becomes a kind of "scarlet letter" each time someone uses Google to search information about a particular company.

It concerns me that Marler relies on sensational individual cases to call for more regulation of a problem that we don't have much understanding about — for instance, why a few people get sick from pathogens and the vast majority don't. Even more fundamentally, I'm concerned that we don't even know the true dimensions of our food safety problem.

Beginning in 1999, the CDC issued data showing that there were 76 million food-borne illnesses, 325,000 related hospitalizations, and 5,000 related deaths each year in the United States. The data were all estimates, primarily drawn from the period from 1993 to 1997, and some of the data the study drew on went as far back as 1947. Moreover, about half (38 million illnesses) were estimated to be from the norovirus, which transmits as commonly from people as from food.

Actually, to call the data "estimates" is being kind. They are more akin to wild extrapolations. In 2011, the CDC revised its data from 76 million to 48 million illnesses each year attributed to food-borne illness. The explanation for its extrapolations? For each of thirty-one pathogens, "we gathered data from surveillance systems and corrected for underreporting and under-diagnosis. We then multiplied the adjusted number by the proportion of illnesses that was acquired in the United States (that is, not during international travel) and the proportion transmitted by food to yield an estimated number of illnesses that are domestically acquired and foodborne. Then, we added the estimates for each of the pathogens to arrive at a total, and used an uncertainty model to generate a point estimate and 90% credible interval."[28] Got that?

And if you look closely at how the estimates break down, you find that 38 million of those 48 million are from "unknown agents" — not from the usual pathogens like listeria or campylobacter. Only about 5 million are estimated to come from those known pathogens carried by food. So instead of one in six Americans estimated to become ill from tainted food, it's really one in sixty from food containing a known pathogen.

Once you depart from estimates, the numbers change significantly. As I pointed out earlier in this chapter, the real numbers of reported food-borne illnesses from the CDC, which it gathers from local public health departments, are a fraction of those estimates.[29] The 23,152 reported in 2008 was actually 5 percent lower than the average between 2003 and 2007, according to WebMD.[30] And the reported numbers for 2009 and 2010 were down sharply from 2008. There is an underreporting factor, of course. Typically there are between 20 and 40 unreported illnesses for each reported illness. But even multiplying 23,000 by 40 yields fewer than 1 million illnesses.

Creating further doubt are the discrepancies over deaths from food-borne illnesses. The total number of reported deaths from food-borne illnesses in 2008 was 22, not even remotely close to the 3,000 estimated by the CDC. And deaths are easier to track than mild illnesses, especially given the wide publicity provided by food safety lawyers like Marler to each and every death identified by the CDC and state agencies.

Raising those kinds of inconsistencies with Marler frequently put the two of us at loggerheads between 2009 and 2011. He came to accuse me of failing to acknowledge that raw dairy products can be contaminated and cause illnesses. "Raw Milk Outbreaks do happen despite what the Weston A. Price Foundation and The Complete Patient (a.k.a. David Gumpert) say," he headlined one of his personal blog posts.[31] This despite the fact that I had stated in *The Raw Milk Revolution* and in any number of media interviews after the book's publication that not only can raw dairy cause illnesses, but raw dairy is likely more risky than pasteurized dairy.

Marler seemed to develop a particular antipathy toward raw dairy, and the people who produce and consume it. According to *Poisoned*, in 2010 Marler successfully lobbied Wisconsin's governor to veto legislation passed overwhelmingly by both houses of the state legislature that would have legalized raw milk sales from state dairy farms on a limited basis. He also successfully lobbied Whole Foods to discontinue stocking raw milk in states where retail sales are legal.[32]

Over time, I'd say Marler and I gradually developed something of a respect for each other's viewpoints. In 2010, we actually engaged in a "debate" on a popular food blog on the subject of raw milk.[33] I pointed out that raw milk's popularity was growing because consumers didn't take FDA and CDC warnings about raw milk seriously, and he expressed his concern that certain groups like children and pregnant moms were especially vulnerable to getting sick from raw milk. Even though there was disagreement, at least there was discussion — unlike with the FDA and CDC, which assiduously avoid debate.

In the echo chamber that is the Internet's fearmongering about food-borne illnesses, however, the Morningland Dairy case reverberated as loudly as any other on three of the Marler blogs, even though there were no illnesses associated with the Missouri dairy. Marler's *Food Poison Journal* announced the initial embargo on August 26th.[34] The Marler *Listeria Blog* announced it a day later.[35] Then Marler's own personal blog announced that the Missouri attorney general was seeking destruction of all Morningland Dairy's cheese in inventory.[36]

The competition among food safety lawyers to be first out with an online posting about every imaginable food safety illness, recall, or legislative proposal inevitably made regulators like those at the Missouri Milk Board and the CDFA gun-shy about seeming to be soft on food safety. So between the first discovery of listeria in Morningland Dairy's cheese in 1999 and the second one in 2010, there had been a huge change in atmosphere. The atmosphere was one in which food companies felt so intimidated that they rarely fought back against the regulators.

Morningland Dairy was unusual in fighting back, a Missouri public health worker would testify at the trial. Mary Glassburner, a food safety supervisor with the Missouri Department of Health and Senior Services, suggested during her testimony that Morningland Dairy was the exception among businesses she regulated, because it had resisted a state order to destroy possibly contaminated product. In her experience, food producers accepted the state's word that a product was dangerous. "They aren't in business to make people sick . . . so they are usually very cooperative in taking care of that product" once a destruction order is imposed. The message: Morningland Dairy cared less about its customers than other companies she dealt with.

Beyond recalls and destruction orders, the changing atmosphere around food safety reverberated in all kinds of other ways, prompting supermarkets and other food purveyors to exhibit more caution about their food offerings. That way, if they were ever sued, they could show they had put thorough policies into effect. But those policies also increasingly had the effect of freezing out small food producers that, careful as they are, don't operate with all kinds of checklists and official policies and procedures on safety.

I got a good taste of how large corporations have buckled under when I attended the national conference of a Jewish food organization, Hazon, back in late 2009. It was held at a spectacularly beautiful spot on the Pacific Ocean, near Monterey, California, at a state park known as Asilomar. In a two-page memo within the program guide passed out to each of the six hundred attendees, conference organizers felt it necessary to explain that the good old delicious days of 2006 and 2007 had been replaced by the fear-oriented food safety days of the present:

> Those of you who were at the first or second Hazon Food Con-
> ferences, in 2006 and 2007 [at an East Coast retreat center], got
> to experience the extraordinary food we were able to serve. . . .
> In 2007 on Friday night we ate kosher meat from goats that were
> raised [at the retreat center] and that we schechted [slaughtered]
> that morning. It was an appropriately intense experience for
> those who were there, and entirely consonant with our desire
> to provide transparency and education in the food that we eat.[37]

The food was similarly outstanding at the 2008 conference in California, but alas, by 2009, things had changed drastically, reported the organizers, and there were "some specific challenges" new to the conference. "Asilomar is located within a California State Park, and the conference center is managed for the state by a private contractor. Between last year's Food Conference and this year's, the management contract changed hands, and in September a company called ARAMARK took over the management of Asilomar. In 2008, ARAMARK had sales of $13.5 billion and profits in excess of $1 billion. That's a lot of food. And a company that size naturally has systems and procedures about how it sources the food that it serves."[38]

The program guide memo noted that ARAMARK claims to be committed to serving locally grown, sustainably produced food. But the Hazon organizers encountered "a series of problems in the period leading up to the Food Conference." The first such problem concerned chicken. "We intended to source and serve local pasture-raised chickens from Green Oaks Creek Farm in Pescadero, about 80 miles north of Asilomar. Some of us had already visited the chickens that we would have served this Friday night, and were thus able to attest at first hand that they were well-tended chickens. They were to be schechted by . . . a young kosher slaughterer, under the supervision of [a rabbi] and plucked and kashered by conference participants . . . as we did last year. This year, ARAMARK's regulations prevented us from doing that."

Then there were difficulties associated with ARAMARK's "documented safety standards — standards that smaller farms often don't have the infrastructure to provide. Nine small farm suppliers were prevented from donating 500 pounds of apples, 500 pounds of cabbage, 25 dozen eggs, 230 pounds of squash, and 325 pounds of trout, among other items," according to the Hazon explanation, for lack of hazard analysis critical control points (HACCP) plans and formal trace-back procedures. "Last year our volunteers picked up donated food and delivered it directly to Asilomar. That way they were a living connection in the journey from farm to table. This year . . . that food will have to go via distributors."

The Hazon organizers were clearly upset with ARAMARK. "You could argue that these are small issues, and in some ways they are. And if these policies were not in place, and someone at our food conference got salmonella — for instance — ARAMARK as the operator would potentially expose themselves to liability by not having appropriate procedures in place. . . . But Blue Greenberg, one of the leading orthodox Jewish feminists, once said, 'where there's a rabbinic will, there's a halachic way.' What she meant is that Jewish tradition is rooted in halacha, Jewish law, and people often think of it as unchangeable; but if and when the rabbis wanted to change the law, they very often found a way to do so. We think that's a good analogy for the food sourcing procedures at Asilomar — and, by implication, in thousands of other ARAMARK facilities around the country."

Because ARAMARK did not bend, the food turned out to be embarrassingly mediocre for a conference with high standards and expectations. ARAMARK ran out of main courses at the first dinner (an uninspired mix of tofu and green beans); latecomers (I among them) wound up with an even less inspired plate of barley and canned mushrooms. Similarly, a breakfast of lox and bagels was missing the bagels — many attendees were clearly unhappy with the rice crackers that were substituted — and the lox ran out after about 20 percent of the guests had been served; the rest had to settle for a fairly ordinary smoked trout.

For Morningland Dairy, there would be no bending, either by state officials or by the state judge overseeing the case. A few months after the two-day trial ended, he wrote a decision siding with the state, speculating that listeria had gotten into the Morningland cheese via milk from diseased cows at the dairy, and declaring that the condemned cheese needed to be destroyed.

CHAPTER 8

FOOD RIGHTS
AND THE BUZZ SAW
OF LAW ENFORCEMENT

In 1969, seven anti–Vietnam War activists — Abbie Hoffman, Jerry Rubin, David Dellinger, and Tom Hayden among them — were put on trial in U.S. federal court on charges they helped incite riots outside the 1968 Democratic National Convention in Chicago, when police beat demonstrators protesting the war.

In the politically charged atmosphere of the late 1960s, the trial of the Chicago Seven, as they came to be known, turned into a political carnival. It stretched for months, with celebrities testifying — singers Judy Collins and Arlo Guthrie, writers Norman Mailer and Allen Ginsberg, and activists Timothy Leary and Reverend Jesse Jackson. Demonstrators marched frequently outside the courthouse. Hoffman and Rubin, in particular, had an eye for the sensational — and one day arrived in court dressed in judicial robes. They complied when the judge ordered them to remove the robes, and compounded the joke by having Chicago police uniforms underneath. Hoffman blew kisses at the jury.

Five of the defendants were found guilty; they were sentenced to five years in jail and fined five thousand dollars. (At the sentencing, Jerry Rubin offered the judge LSD.) The guilty verdict was eventually overturned on appeal, and the U.S. Justice Department decided not to retry the activists.[1]

It's doubtful such a trial could occur today. The 1960s were a time when the American justice system was seen as giving too many rights to the accused — "coddling criminals" as some critics put it at the time. The U.S.

Supreme Court had, just three years earlier in the Miranda case, ruled that police must, upon arrest, warn suspects of their Fifth Amendment right to remain silent and to have a lawyer present when they are questioned. At the time, many law enforcement professionals viewed the decision as potentially a major handicap to law enforcement, since evidence could be thrown out if suspects were questioned without a warning of their Miranda rights.

Prosecutors and politicians learned important lessons from the Chicago Seven trial about how activists can use the legal system to leverage political causes. They also learned how to adapt to the Miranda decision, especially as crime increased during the 1970s and 1980s. Toughening punishment for lawbreakers even became a major issue in a presidential race; in 1988, George H. W. Bush ran television ads accusing his Democratic rival, Michael Dukakis, of failing to effectively punish serious offenders because Massachusetts had allowed a convicted murderer, Willie Horton, to participate in a weekend furlough program while Dukakis was governor (Horton committed a robbery and rape while out on furlough). The matter put Dukakis on the defensive and was an important factor in helping Bush defeat him.

The American legal system was toughened via thousands of new laws and mandatory sentencing for certain drug and violent crime offenses. By the first decade of the new century, the United States, with 5 percent of the world's population, had nearly 25 percent of its prisoners — more total prisoners by far than any other country, including China. Whereas the United States had forty thousand people imprisoned for drug offenses in 1980, twenty-five years later the number had soared to nearly half a million.[2]

"Criminologists and legal scholars in other industrialized nations say they are mystified and appalled by the number and length of American prison sentences," said a *New York Times* report on the ballooning number of prisoners.[3] Four years after the *New York Times* report, the international finance magazine *The Economist* painted an even harsher picture: "Both political parties have driven America's criminal-justice policy in one regrettable direction: towards locking up more people for more crimes for more time. A combination of over-criminalisation, mandatory-minimum sentences, tough drug laws and excessive prosecutorial power have stuffed America's prisons to bursting. As of 2010 roughly 2.3 million Americans were imprisoned, and 7.1 million were under some form of correctional control (prison, probation or parole)."[4]

Kentucky senator Rand Paul was moved to observe in a spring 2012 Senate speech in support of an amendment to reduce the FDA's police powers: "Criminal law seems to be increasing [and] increasingly is using a tool of our government bureaucracy to punish and control honest businessmen for simply attempting to make a living. Historically the criminal law was intended to punish only the most horrible offenses that everyone agreed were inherently wrong or evil, offenses like rape, murder, theft, arson — but now we've basically federalized thousands of activities and called them crimes."[5] In September of 2012, Rand Paul and his father, Ron, published a book, *Government Bullies: How Everyday Americans Are Being Harassed, Abused, and Imprisoned by the Feds*, which included tales of ordinary people caught in the buzz saw of regulatory enforcement.

Prosecutors had learned to use the threat of long prison sentences to discourage defendants from seeking jury trials and instead accept plea bargains, typically with reduced charges and more lenient sentences than a judge might hand out with a jury conviction. Everyone seemed to get something in such an arrangement — prosecutors won more convictions and defendants gained a sense of leniency. Plus, defendants didn't have to wait many months, either out on bail or in jail, for a trial — or pay as much for lawyers to defend them. The main problem came with defendants who were innocent or had a strong case to make that particular laws were being unfairly enforced. The system pushed them to settle, no matter what the circumstances, to avoid legal expense and the consequences of a toughened system.

It was in this climate of tougher enforcement, with private food choice under attack, that the FDA and its state allies launched a number of harsh initiatives — nearly all of them against food producers who had signed lease agreements with the California nutritionist Aajonus Vonderplanitz. In most of these cases, the targeted individuals had little idea about this harsh evolution of criminal justice.

How do farmers who've never had any encounters with the legal system fight back against the might of the U.S. Justice Department, or a state attorney general's office, with their armies of Ivy League–educated and law-school-trained lawyers? More troubling, how do farmers whose religious precepts discourage hiring lawyers fight back?

Those questions became important in early 2011, when the U.S. Justice Department, on behalf of the FDA, filed a legal action in U.S. District Court for the Eastern District of Pennsylvania in Philadelphia against Daniel Allgyer, the Amish farmer who served the Grassfed on the Hill food club in the Washington DC area. The FDA sought a permanent injunction barring him from shipping milk across state lines to the food club. If successful, the action could put Allgyer out of the business he had built based on serving out-of-state food club members. "Unpasteurized milk and milk products contain a wide variety of harmful bacteria, including listeria monocytogenes, Escherichia coli, Salmonella, Campylobacter, Yersinia, and Brucella, all of which may cause illness and possibly death," the request stated in part. "Epidemiological studies have established a direct link between the consumption of unpasteurized milk and gastrointestinal illness."[6]

The FDA filed its action against Allgyer alone, ignoring the Grassfed on the Hill food club's members — whom it had been investigating intensively for more than a year via undercover purchases of raw milk. Allgyer may have been producing the raw milk, but members of Grassfed on the Hill were ordering it and drinking it, working with Allgyer to arrange for it to be brought across state lines.

The FDA may have decided to target only Allgyer knowing that the Amish are prohibited by their religious tradition from aggressively defending themselves in court proceedings. And the FDA may have decided to leave alone the DC-area food club leaders — Karine Bouis-Towe and Liz Reitzig — because the decision makers knew Bouis-Towe and Reitzig could (and likely would) challenge the charges, engage a tough lawyer, and refuse any kind of plea-bargain arrangement in favor of a highly publicized court hearing and appeals to higher courts if they lost. Sure enough, within weeks of the FDA's filing, the two food club leaders organized a rally, within sight of the U.S. Capitol, to support Allgyer.[7] They even arranged for a farmer to bring a milking cow to the event and handed out small cups of the cow's milk to participants.

Among the speakers at the rally was Jonathan Emord, a lawyer specializing in food and drug law who had prevailed against the FDA in several court actions.[8] Bouis-Towe and Reitzig hoped to hire Emord to defend Allgyer against the FDA action and possibly set an important precedent on behalf of private food rights in the process. They engaged him with an initial small retainer to provide advice, but he told me he required in excess of "several hundred thousand dollars" to fully pursue any case against the FDA.

Even more discouraging, Allgyer didn't attend the rally, which drew a couple hundred people on a sunny, warm Monday morning in May. The Amish don't like to be photographed for television or newspapers, or even to be at the center of attention at public demonstrations. If you ever see Amish farmers at a rally of any sort, they are way off to the side, in the background as much as possible. Unfortunately, it can be difficult to raise money for a defendant's legal defense even if he's a media darling — but if he's inaccessible, you can almost forget about it.

Allgyer himself was keeping with his Amish tradition and heading down a different legal path. The day the FDA announced its intention to seek a permanent injunction against Allgyer in federal court in Philadelphia — April 26, 2011 — happened to be the same day Aajonus Vonderplanitz was departing the United States for South Africa, where he was scheduled give a series of talks on raw food nutrition. Unfortunately, when Allgyer tried to phone him a few days after that, the Amish farmer couldn't make contact. Allgyer was upset. He had signed on with Vonderplanitz expecting him to be available and to take charge during a crisis such as this, with the government seeking to prevent Allgyer from supplying the Maryland food club. Now he couldn't even reach his protector.

When Allgyer checked around with other Amish farmers who had agreements with Vonderplanitz, he learned that the multiagency raid on Rawesome Foods the previous June 30th had opened festering problems between Vonderplanitz and his longtime friend and food club owner James Stewart. Vonderplanitz had long been unhappy with the quality of food provided by the single-mom farmer, Sharon Palmer — especially the eggs. He felt they might well have been outsourced, rather than coming from her farm; he also suspected the meat Palmer sold was not organic and not soy-free. Stewart stood by Palmer, expressing confidence in the quality of her food, and continued to offer her eggs and chicken — as well as raw goat milk via a herdshare arrangement between Rawesome and Palmer's farm (until the late summer of 2010, when Palmer discontinued the goat milk production in the hope it might end the regulator assaults on her farm). Stewart was upset with Vonderplanitz for similar reasons as Allgyer: when the raid at Rawesome occurred, Vonderplanitz was off traveling in Asia and couldn't help in defending the food club at the public health hearing or in interviews with the media.

In October 2010, the simmering dispute between the two men boiled over. That was when *The Colbert Report* television show decided to broadcast a comedy segment about the multiagency raid on Rawesome.[9] A video and production crew had interviewed Stewart and several of his close associates at the tiny space that comprised the buying club. The five-minute report aired October 6th, and as might be expected, it portrayed the events as laughable examples of an overbearing government: "Real Americans are standing up to the ruling elite."

Early on in the segment, James Stewart was asked to explain "the complex etymology behind the buying club's name."

"Awesome with an R in front of it," the tall, husky manager deadpanned.

"Why did the government thugs raid Rawesome?" the announcer asked ominously. A pause . . . "To seize their raw milk."

A smiling blond, Lela Buttery, one of Rawesome's young volunteer operators, intoned, "Here at Rawesome, we have a choice of cow, goat, sheep, and most recently . . . camel milk." Film clips of milk spurting from a goat or camel's teats followed.

When David Acheson, a former high-ranking safety official at the FDA, was shown in an interview describing in vivid terms the possible illnesses that could develop from tainted raw milk, which he said included bloody diarrhea, the announcer interrupted, "They're playing the bloody diarrhea card!"

"Clearly the government has declared war," the announcer concluded. On came representative Ron Paul with his one-liner: "It's pasteurization without representation."[10]

Little noticed at the time, one person not included in *The Colbert Report* segment on Rawesome was Vonderplanitz.

Vonderplanitz's charges alleging outsourcing by Palmer weren't a surprise to investigators in neighboring Ventura County and to the L.A. County District Attorney. While they had been investigating Palmer and Rawesome on and off since late 2008, the previous June (of 2010) one of Palmer's employees had contacted the Ventura County Sheriff "because of concerns he had with the manner in which suspect Palmer was operating her business, Healthy Family Farms."[11] The employee told Ventura County

Sheriff's Detective Raymond Dominguez and the L.A. County District Attorney agent Ken Ward of his concerns over alleged product source misrepresentation by Palmer.

According to Ward's interview notes, the employee "explained Palmer advertises that all her products are organic and farm raised. He had only seen at any one time five pigs on her farm. Yet, he delivered pork ribs to customers for 'weeks on end.' Even the customers were questioning the supply. . . . Obviously, all the pork products were not coming from her farm."[12] Another former employee countered that he collected eggs from chickens on the farm, and that he had seen Palmer take chickens to a slaughterhouse. Still another said he milked fifty-eight to sixty goats each day. Both, however, said they had never seen Palmer make cheese.

Palmer vehemently denied the accusations of outsourcing pork, chickens, eggs, and cheese. The employees suggesting outsourcing were people she had been forced to fire because of various infractions and were thus vengeful toward her, she said. She had bought conventional food — but not to sell, rather to donate to a charity she was involved with (as well as to partially compensate workers, she told me). Using food to compensate farm workers was a customary practice at small farms, she said.

Palmer eventually admitted that she provided eggs to Rawesome that came from an outside organic egg producer for about six months during 2008 and 2009, after a mountain lion decimated her chicken flock during an attack. Stewart said he visited the farm, and that it was "like a snowstorm" with chicken feathers everywhere. Stewart told me he understood Palmer would be providing outsourced eggs for about two weeks and was only vaguely aware that the arrangement extended much longer as Palmer rebuilt her egg-laying flock. He admitted that he should have placed a sign at Rawesome indicating the eggs during that period weren't from Palmer's own flock.

"It was three years ago," Stewart told me in October 2011. "It was not a big deal. Those were organic eggs. Did I make a mistake [in not putting up a sign]? Yes." Vonderplanitz wouldn't accept any explanation. He put up a website called Unhealthy Family Farm that detailed his charges. Then, in the fall of 2010, he paid a visit to investigators with the Ventura County District Attorney and explained his concerns. He wanted Palmer charged with fraud. The following January, Vonderplanitz and Larry Otting — the real estate executive who had extended credit to help Palmer acquire Healthy Family Farms — filed a lawsuit in California state court in Los Angeles against Stewart and Palmer alleging a number of crimes, including intentional misrepresentation and conspiracy to defraud. The suit requested about twenty million dollars in damages.

Prosecutors never filed formal charges against Palmer in connection with their investigation and Vonderplanitz's allegations about outsourcing. That wasn't the case with a number of other Rawesome-related activities.

As a result of the June 30, 2010, Rawesome raid, the FDA not only became involved in investigating Morningland Dairy in rural Missouri, but it honed in on Amos Miller. In April 2011, the same month Allgyer was hit with the request for a permanent injunction on his out-of-state shipments to Grassfed on the Hill, FDA investigators descended on Miller's farm. Two investigators, accompanied by a U.S. Marshal, showed up one afternoon with a search warrant and spent several hours carrying out a search and inspection of his farm — focusing primarily on the huge corrugated-steel shipping/storage/production building. Miller wasn't present when they arrived, so one of his associates argued with the investigators that the farm was involved in private food production and outside the FDA's authority. They ignored him. One investigator in a white coat hurried around taking samples from the bottling room and inspecting the freezer, cooler, and packaging, and storage areas. The other stationed himself at a desk containing order forms, snapping dozens of photos of current and past orders from food club members around the country.

The FDA investigators eventually sent Miller a report that pointed out several potential minor safety violations in terms of his equipment and sanitation measures, he told me, but there was no other indication as to where the official search might lead. For the amiable farmer, the search was another reminder of growing tensions around the Rawesome affair.

Even aside from the FDA's search, Miller had been feeling increasingly uncomfortable in his dealings with Rawesome Foods, as he heard more stories about the conflicts between Stewart and Vonderplanitz. As much loyalty as he felt toward Vonderplanitz for helping get the Amish farmer off the legal hook related to his Pennsylvania problems back in 2006, "James Stewart is the one who pays me for the orders. And he pays his bills on time." Miller decided he had to break his ties with Vonderplanitz.

⤸

The tenor of the voicemail messages the Amish farmers involved in producing raw dairy for food clubs were leaving for one another was shifting sharply. While the messages during the four years from 2006 to 2010 had mostly been to spread the word about Vonderplanitz's accomplishments, by late 2010 there were strong hints of worry — and a desire to shift allegiance. Increasingly, what the Amish farmers were telling one another was that there was a new legal outfit, one that also didn't rely on lawyers, known as ProAdvocate Group.[13]

Actually, James Stewart started the ball rolling with ProAdvocate. Shortly after the June 2010 raid on Rawesome, when his disputes with Vonderplanitz escalated, he began learning about ProAdvocate as a possible alternative to his friend's organization, Right to Choose Healthy Food — and telling Miller about the organization.

ProAdvocate is a legal advisory organization that, among other things, guides its clients on how to organize what it calls "private associations." It was the brainchild of Karl Dahlstrom, who put the organization together — operating out of a gleaming office park in Dallas — shortly after he was released from federal prison in 2003, following a five-and-a-half-year sentence for selling stock as an unregistered broker-dealer.

Prior to going to prison, Dahlstrom gave seminars on reducing and avoiding federal and state income taxes — and fighting tax audits. The Internal Revenue Service charged him in the late 1970s with income tax evasion; he was sentenced to five years in prison — and then successfully reversed the conviction on an appeal that went to the U.S. Supreme Court, he says. "The Texas Bar Association came after me four times" during the 1980s and 1990s for practicing law without being a lawyer, he told me. He successfully fended the lawyers off, a couple times in court — until the U.S. Securities and Exchange Commission caught up with him in the late 1990s for selling stock in a company involved in offshore oil production.

It's not clear what the Amish farmers knew about Dahlstrom's past, but enough voice messages were sent back and forth among the farmers that by early May 2011 a group of about ten Amish from the East and Midwest plugged into an unusual conference call. They wanted to hear Dahlstrom, who by then was a jowly man of seventy-two with slicked-back gray hair, make his case for something he called "First and Fourteenth Amendment private associations."

He didn't disappoint. Dahlstrom spent a half hour or so explaining his version of the legal principles that protect private associations. "You have a right to form one of these associations," he told them early on. Then he explained how ProAdvocate operates under the same auspices.

"I've been accused of practicing law without a license," he explained. "That's exactly what I am doing . . . I am doing it for my association. The fact that I'm doing it within a private association means it is legal. It is not only a right, but a protected right. The lawyers think it is competition. We're no competition."

Because the Amish have such an aversion to dealing with lawyers, Dahlstrom's statements rang especially true. Here was a way, in their view, to obtain legal assistance — and even protection — without having to deal with real lawyers. It sounded even more convincing when he added his sales pitch.

"In the ProAdvocate Group, you are number one. When you hire a lawyer, he has as his first priority the courts. Who is his second priority? It's the public. He has to put the public above you. His third priority is himself, as an officer of the court." He didn't have to say that the client is the lawyer's fourth priority, in this view. "We'll take your case to the U.S. Supreme Court at no extra cost, because you are number one to us."

When Dahlstrom opened the conference call to questions, a farmer asked whether he recommended notifying government agencies that the farmer has formed a private association. Absolutely, said Dahlstrom. But be prepared for negative feedback from the agencies, and from the farmer's accountant or lawyer.

"Your lawyers and CPAs don't want it to work. These lawyers send their kids to Harvard and buy them BMWs . . . because they collect judgments."

All that was a lead-in to the cost of joining ProAdvocate. "It's eighteen thousand dollars for a one-time lifetime membership fee," said Dahlstrom. "We defend you."

And what happens if Dahlstrom is no longer around, a farmer inquired. "I have a daughter, Carla," who is active in the business, Dahlstrom explained.

Amos Miller inquired, "Why did this association thing come into play?"

Going back in history, Dahlstrom said, "You didn't have all these agencies and rules. The U.S. Constitution doesn't mention freedom of association. It all evolved," and the U.S. Supreme Court has upheld the concept.

A farmer from Ohio asked, "What about if selling raw milk is a crime?"

Said Dahlstrom, "It's only a crime if you do it to the public. It's not a crime if you are in the private domain."

Amos Miller and Daniel Allgyer were sold. A few days later, Allgyer would answer the U.S. Justice Department's demand for a permanent injunction by suggesting that his arrangement with Vonderplanitz was flawed, and that he had since gotten religion — or at least, Karl Dahlstrom's version of religion. "This answer is intended to inform the Court and the FDA agency that any and all manufacturing and sale of our products to the public is hereby terminated. We now understand that the FDA agency has a mandate from Congress to protect the public. . . . Be it known that we will fully comply with FDA statutes, regulations and orders in the future. We are also aware that the FDA's jurisdiction and authority is limited to the public domain, except for clear and present dangers of substantive evil per U.S. Supreme Court decisions.

"We also apologize for the expense, time and effort that the FDA agency has expended thus far and hope they realize that we never had any intent to violate the law in the past or future. We acted upon information and understandings of our research and various other persons and organizations. Apparently, some of that research and information was incorrect which has caused some concern and an investigation on their part. Please inform us as to anything we can do to redeem and mitigate ourselves from any civil and/ or criminal sanctions by the FDA agency. We believe that our only fault was a good faith mistaken understanding of the law."

Vonderplanitz didn't take well to Allgyer's decision to shift Grassfed on the Hill to a private association formulated by ProAdvocate. He felt legally responsible for Allgyer, since the federal request for a permanent injunction against Allgyer happened while Grassfed on the Hill was part of Right to Choose Healthy Food. So he decided to file something in addition to what Allgyer filed — something called a "cross complaint in intervention." In July 2011, the judge in the case, Lawrence J. Stengel, denied Vonderplanitz's complaint — primarily because he wasn't a lawyer. In a memorandum, Judge Stengel concluded: "Although an individual may represent himself pro se, he is not entitled to act as an attorney for others in a federal court" under what the judge said were well-established precedents and rules.[14]

The memorandum wasn't a final decision in the case, but it offered insights into Judge Stengel's thinking. From the viewpoint of Allgyer and

Grassfed on the Hill members, the judge offered little hope for the possibility he might back private food rights: "The tangential issues raised in his [Vonderplanitz's] motion include: whether raw milk is a health risk to the public and whether raw milk has caused epidemics; whether Mr. Vonderplanitz and the entities he attempted to represent were within the jurisdiction of the United States, . . . whether pasteurized milk is dangerous and whether pasteurized milk has caused epidemics; whether FDA investigators committed perjury and fraud by stating the raw milk was sold even though they were aware of the contracts which provided the members owned the dairy; and whether the Government should be enjoined from 'continuing to propagandize the myth, unscientific rhetoric, that claims and declares that raw . . . milk and dairy are dangerous to health and life. . . .' The main issue in this case is whether Daniel Allgyer is in violation of federal law."[15]

A few days after ProAdvocate's Dahlstrom made his pitch to Amish farmers, on May 18, 2011, a handful of people waited on the sidewalk outside Rawesome Foods' corrugated metal door and wall fronting on Rose Avenue in Venice's commercial center. They wanted to be first in at the club's official opening time of noon on this Wednesday, the one weekday it welcomed members. (It was also open on Saturdays.)

Promptly at noon, one of the Rawesome workers—a man with short, brown, curly hair who looked to be about forty—opened the door. He was carrying a notepad, and as each person walked in he wrote down the individual member's name. Among those waiting was a woman who wasn't a member. She asked the man with the notepad if she could obtain a one-day pass to shop for a few items. The man told her to go inside and ask for "Cheryl." A woman who appeared to be in her late forties or early fifties, five feet six, and about 160 pounds, gave the would-be member a form for her to sign, which looked like a contract, and told the woman there would be a $1 charge for the one-day membership.

The now-temporary member proceeded to select a quart of whole milk (for $4.79), a quart of goat milk (for $9.25), and a pint of sheep milk (for $14.50) from a section in the trailer-cooler labeled with a large hand-printed sign AMISH. The woman brought the three items to the checkout counter, paid $28.54, and left. She then walked up the block to a spot where a man and another woman waited. The shopper handed the three items to the waiting woman, who placed them into a refrigerated cooler.

The woman with the cooler was Scarlett Treviso, the senior investigator for the California Department of Food and Agriculture (CDFA) — the investigator in charge of the Rawesome–Sharon Palmer investigation. The man with Treviso was Richard Ballou, a senior investigator with the L.A. County District Attorney's office. The identity and affiliation of the woman who did the shopping were crossed out in Ballou's official law enforcement report, from which I drew this information, so it's not clear if she was a government employee or a citizen recruited as an undercover agent for the shopping task. The three individuals had gathered on Rose Avenue in Venice, stated Ballou, "for the purpose of purchasing milk products and to verify if Rawesome Foods was conducting business."[16] The milk products would be tested to confirm that they were, indeed, unpasteurized.

There was an urgency for investigators to pick up on their investigation of Rawesome (and Sharon Palmer) from the previous year — and confirm that Rawesome was still serving members — because the one-year anniversary of the June 30, 2010, raid was rapidly approaching. California has a one-year statute of limitations for filing charges from evidence obtained via a search warrant, defense lawyers told me.

Of course, no one at Rawesome had any idea the investigators had returned. They remained focused on their internal disputes. As June 30, 2011, approached, the tensions of the previous year between those supporting James Stewart and those supporting Aajonus Vonderplanitz continued to poison the atmosphere at the Venice food club. For longtime regulars, it seemed nearly impossible to stand above the fray or to advocate peace. One of those who sought to avoid taking sides was Maurice Kaehler, a soft-spoken Los Angeles yoga teacher and organic food expert who worked as a consultant to food producers and vendors. "Just because I do not worship chemtrails, gold standard, upcoming Armaggedon, Zeitgeist, David Icke, pick your politician, nor have the appropriate hatred towards the imaginary Illuminati, Bilderberger, fill in your global conspiracy group, I am held with some sort of contempt, to where it has come to I have to go in, get my product and get the hell out," he explained at one point. "It's such a tangled web," another complained. "There is so much hearsay. . . . It's just such a divided movement." So poisonous was the atmosphere, she and other longtime members told me, they didn't want to be quoted by name as supporting one side or the other.

When June 30, 2011, came and went, some at Rawesome breathed a sigh of relief. Not that they were aware of the specifics of the statute of limitations, but it just seemed as if, despite all the internal squabbling, time was marching on at a good pace without any more outsider interference. The most notable regulatory encounter preceding the June 30, 2010, raid had happened five years previously. Was it possible Rawesome might have another four years of peace? "We always said James went through life with an angel flying overhead," one Rawesome volunteer worker told me.

As it turned out, Rawesome had barely four more weeks of peace. A huge government raiding party showed up at midmorning on Wednesday, August 3rd, just as Stewart and his staff were completing their stocking, readying the club for the noon opening time on a warm summer day.

While it might not have seemed possible in the aftermath of the raid on June 30, 2010, there were twice as many agencies represented this time versus the four that showed up fourteen months earlier. This time they included not only the FDA, the CDFA's Milk and Dairy Food Safety Branch, the L.A. County District Attorney's office, and the L.A. County Department of Public Health, but also new ones: the California Franchise Tax Board (the state tax collection agency), the L.A. Police Department, the L.A. Department of Building and Safety, and the CDFA's Division of Measurement Standards. Legal documents associated with the operation were filed on June 30, 2011 — the last day possible under the one-year requirement.

The dozens of officers and investigators, together with their cars and a flatbed truck they brought along, created a major ruckus on busy Rose Avenue; before too long, a few dozen Rawesome members had gathered around to video the proceedings.[17] A young couple hugged in sorrow as it became apparent what was going on.

One video showed police trying to close a gate to Rawesome's back entrance, while a woman intoned, "Welcome to America, where it's a crime to eat organic food."

Others asked the officers what "the crime" was.

"We have a search warrant," one of the officers replied.

Someone else asked about Stewart. "He's gone," an officer said.

"What's the charge?"

"You'll have to ask the Food and Drug Administration," said the officer.

Indeed, Stewart was gone.[18] Agents from the L.A. County District Attorney's office slapped handcuffs on Stewart, shoved him into a car, and took him the few blocks to his tiny, one-room, second-floor walk-up apartment to conduct a search.

"There were six agents in my apartment," he would recall later. "They could barely fit."

They took his computer and business papers, plus nearly $10,000 in cash he had on hand for paying suppliers and workers. Then he was driven to the Twin Towers Correctional Facility in Los Angeles — the largest jail in the world, with 1.5 million square feet of space. It's also one of the most notorious jails in the country, a place where gangs continue their street vendettas and the security is tight. The L.A. County District Attorney requested that bail for Stewart be set at a whopping $123,000.

At the same time Stewart was being hauled in, a second, even bigger surprise was unfolding about three miles from Rawesome, at the snug bungalow home of Victoria Bloch, the diminutive graphic designer who assisted Sharon Palmer at farmers markets on weekends.[19] As Bloch was pulling out of her driveway in western Los Angeles in her super-compact Mini Cooper, a male detective and uniformed female police officer approached.

"They asked me to get out of my car, and said I was under arrest. The woman said, 'I have to have your hands in back,' and she cuffed me." Bloch was placed in an unmarked car, and the threesome drove about forty-five minutes to a women's detention center in east Los Angeles. The L.A. County District Attorney requested $60,000 bail for Bloch.

And in Ventura County, sheriff's deputies went to Sharon Palmer's farmhouse to arrest her.[20] They were reasonably considerate, given their previous rough treatment of her — allowing her to get dressed and take a shower before handcuffing Palmer and taking her to the local jail. The L.A. County District Attorney requested bail of $121,000.

The charges? There were thirteen, including four counts of conspiracy, contained in a twenty-one-page criminal complaint.[21] The L.A. County District Attorney summarized them in its press announcement: Palmer, Stewart, and Bloch were arrested "on criminal conspiracy charges stemming from the alleged illegal production and sale of unpasteurized goat milk, goat cheese and other products." Stewart faced all thirteen counts,

Palmer and Healthy Family Farms were charged in nine, and Bloch in three conspiracy counts.

The press release neglected to mention anything about Count 13, which was only against Stewart, charging that three days after the raid on June 30, 2010, he "did willfully and unlawfully remove or fail to keep posted the notice of closure issued by the Los Angeles County Health Officer."[22] In other words, he was being charged for walking out of the July 1st hearing and reopening Rawesome on July 3rd.

What the press release also failed to report was that the raiding party didn't leave any receipts for food confiscated, as it did in the June 30, 2010, raid. That's because the search warrant this time made clear this wasn't just about getting food samples. "After representative samples have been obtained for laboratory analysis, the remaining products will be the responsibility of the Public Health Department, Food and Milk Program, California Department of Food and Agriculture, or the U.S. Food and Drug Administration. All dairy products or supplements manufactured unlawfully or from unapproved sources such that they can not legally be sold, will be seized or destroyed."[23]

The authorities didn't distinguish between dairy products and supplements and items like honey, beef, chicken, eggs, and so forth. They took everything — some $80,000 worth of food. All milk products were poured down Rawesome's sink drains. The rest was loaded onto the flatbed truck and transported to a local dump.

The arrests triggered varying reactions among food producers and Rawesome members — reactions that were emblematic of the stressful year-plus struggle on the part of individuals who cared deeply about their food community. Some individuals felt terribly let down by Stewart and Palmer. In their view, it was incumbent on the two — in the absence of official regulatory oversight — to demonstrate impeccable behavior to demonstrate the workability of the private food model. Instead, these Rawesome members felt as if Palmer's and Stewart's questionable behavior had attracted regulators, and the two deserved everything law enforcement might bring down on them — even if they weren't guilty of the specific charges.

Others opted for a big-picture view — that whatever errors or even crimes Stewart and Palmer might have been guilty of, the offenses were minor, and at most deserving of regulatory citations. The highly public heavy-handed arrests and felony charges, in this view, were indicative of the desire by local and federal officials to make an example of these individuals and sympathizers to demonstrate that private options for dairy, meat, and other nutrient-dense foods wouldn't be tolerated. Both sets of views were on vivid display in the aftermath of the shocking arrests.

Within hours of the L.A. County District Attorney's arrest announcement, Mark McAfee — the outspoken owner of Organic Pastures Dairy Company in Fresno — was on the phone with Rawesome workers and volunteers. He wanted to organize a protest outside the L.A. County Courthouse in downtown Los Angeles for the defendants — the Rawesome Three, as they quickly became known. To provide an ongoing source of outrage, he wanted Stewart and Bloch to remain in jail longer than they might otherwise have to if a bail hearing was held right away, so there would be a clear cause for people to protest. He was clearly in the camp of setting aside what he saw as petty personal disputes (such as the falling out he had had several years earlier with Stewart when he worked as McAfee's Los Angeles distributor) in the interests of the larger concern over private food rights.

The next day, about one hundred people gathered outside the tree-lined courthouse carrying signs as McAfee and several others pumped up the crowd about the injustice of what was occurring — jailings and criminal charges that could land the defendants in jail for up to eight years for what were (at most) licensing violations, in the crowd's view. The event was covered by various media, including the local NBC News affiliate in Los Angeles. Its report included Rawesome customers expressing disgust. "I want my freedom to choose," said one young woman demonstrator.

"It is simply unjust!" shouted McAfee for the camera. "I stand 100 percent behind James and Victoria and Sharon."[24]

But the arrests also triggered reactions from other people who had long been involved in the production of nutrient-dense food, and at least one saw the arrests as legitimate. Ron Garthwaite, the owner of Claravale Farm — a California raw milk producer and Stewart's former employer at the start of the new century — said in an e-mail, which he requested I post on my blog: "James Stewart was our distributor in Southern California early on when we first started selling in stores. He no longer distributes our milk and hasn't for years. It is our opinion that James Stewart deserves to be in jail. It's about time. I don't know anything about Sharon Palmer or her operation, but James Stewart is not the appropriate poster child for this movement."[25]

Mark McAfee was incensed by his competitor's reaction and encouraged the broader view: "I do not share the old negative James Stewart feelings that Ron Garthwaite shares. James has been a friend of California raw milk for 12 years. This must be remembered, acknowledged and recognized. We are all on one team. To wish jail on anyone besides a murderer or child molester . . . is a very sad comment. James is a great human being and holds very high moral and ethical beliefs. His error was actually attempting to exercise his rights as he thought them to be."[26]

Maurice Kaehler, the yoga teacher, was inclined to blame Rawesome for being as confrontational as it was: "If this movement continues to be adrenalin-fueled and war-based then it will just be pissing in the wind," he wrote on my blog. "And how much have these raids been brought on by those who operate these dairies, co-ops and buyers clubs themselves? By being contrary for the sake of being contrary. . . . We have met the enemy . . . and they are us!"[27]

Back and forth went the charges and countercharges. In my view, these were understandable emotional reactions. I felt it was healthy for all those who cared to air their opinions — indeed, the openness of people's reactions stood in sharp contrast to that of the regulators and lawmakers, who seemingly refused to engage in any open discussion about workable private food options.

Moreover, all emerging movements have had their questionable characters and their divisive debates. Under the laws in force at the time, the men who carried out the Boston Tea Party in 1773 were guilty of theft and destruction of private property and were at odds with other colonial residents who preferred a peaceful resolution of differences with the British rulers. The U.S. Constitution contains a section known as the Fugitive Slave Clause in Article Four that required slaves who had escaped to other states be returned to their home states; the clause was only overturned with passage of the Thirteenth Amendment in 1865.

People sometimes forget that Malcolm X, one of the best-known advocates of black nationalism during the 1950s and 1960s, was involved in gambling and drugs for many years in Boston, and in 1946 he was sentenced to ten years in jail for burglary; it was in jail that his views on black nationalism crystallized. Muhammad Ali, the heavyweight boxing champion who also became a symbol of black nationalism, was publicly vilified, stripped of his boxing championship, and convicted of draft evasion in 1967 for refusing to serve in the Vietnam War; he was eventually exonerated by the U.S. Supreme Court and resumed his boxing career after a four-year enforced layoff.

In the emotional postarrest atmosphere, Vonderplanitz remained outwardly supportive of Stewart but seemed to have become completely marginalized. In an e-mail to supporters, he described his experience attending the courthouse rally: "On August 4, 2011, I attended the rally and court proceedings. . . . It was a good turnout but no one knew how to organize it or knew what to do to take advantage of the press exposure. About 5 TV networks were there to cover the story. Approximately 25 people remained outside picketing and about 55 people inside. I offered the 4 network TV stations present my comments as President of Right To Choose Healthy Food, since I had built Rawesome. They began to move for taping but when I gave them my name, they refused to receive my comments. Who blacklisted me? Rawesome members or government-controlled media?"

Mark McAfee's idea that Stewart and Bloch remain in jail longer than they might otherwise have had to sounded good in theory, but it presented problems to the two defendants.

"It was tough in there," Stewart would tell me later. "You couldn't get out of line, or a guard would smash you. One guy walking behind me did something they didn't like and they pushed him up against a wall and he started bleeding." Then there was the food: "I couldn't eat," he said. "So I used the two days as a time to fast." Two bananas were all he consumed.

When Stewart finally appeared in the prisoners' holding area in an expansive L.A. County courtroom on Friday, two days after his arrest, Deputy District Attorney Kelly Sakir asked the presiding judge to set bail at the recommended $123,000. "He has shown he has no regard for the law," she intoned. The judge wasn't impressed with the government's arguments. After Stewart's lawyer explained the questionable nature of the charges and that Stewart wasn't a habitual lawbreaker, the judge lowered bail to $30,000. The bail terms stipulated that 8 percent had to be posted in cash. Stewart's son-in-law came up with $2,400 and James walked out free.

For Bloch, the experience was more sublime. "Being handcuffed is strange," she told me. "Especially not being able to scratch my nose when it itched." Being strip-searched was yet another kind of unwelcome experience. In the holding cell where she was first confined, the other women were curious about this obviously middle-class new prisoner. "Everyone was asking me, 'What did you do?' I had the highest bail request of anyone there. When I told them what I did, they couldn't believe it. They were in there for drug offenses, prostitution. They kept saying, 'You're in here for selling milk?'" Bloch says she tried to explain the government's crackdown on raw milk and other foods. "They couldn't understand. 'It's not OK to put what you want in your children's mouth?' one of them asked me." Bloch took to the jail food a little better than Stewart. "We were awakened at 3:30 and given a bran muffin and some bread." At lunch, there was a burrito of some sort. She ate at least some of what she was given. When she went into the prisoners' docket late Thursday, the judge quickly rejected the state's request for $60,000 bail and released her on her own recognizance.

For Sharon Palmer in Ventura County things moved at a slower pace, and it wasn't until Saturday that she was released on reduced bail.

Like most serious criminal matters, the Rawesome case seemed to drag on endlessly. Bail reduction hearings, certification of lawyers, setting a pretrial hearing at which evidence would be presented — after a time, all the judicial events became almost routine, with hearings appearing to be called simply to set a date for the next hearing.

Almost, but not quite. As Bloch put it to me in an e-mail following one of the hearings in 2012, "We were all nervous wrecks in the courtroom yesterday. I slept only a few hours. Sharon got as much done on the farm to get ready for the weekend as possible just in case. James was afraid he'd be going back to jail. This is clearly an effective tactic — I would have thought that the longer the case proceeded, the more it would become same old, same old; but I'm finding that psychologically, it's just the opposite and the more a sort of unpleasant low-level background-noise kind of dread is there far more often than I'd like."

The sense of dread she described wasn't wrongly placed. As one of these seemingly routine hearings for the Rawesome Three was ending in early March 2012 — the judge had just adjourned the proceedings, setting a pretrial hearing for two months later — the justice system reached out again in unexpected fashion. Before the Rawesome defendants could turn around to exit the trial area, three L.A. County Sheriff's Department deputies standing a few feet away ordered Stewart and Palmer to place their hands behind their backs so they could be handcuffed. They were then whisked out of the courthouse.[28]

They had been arrested under a warrant issued by neighboring Ventura County, where Palmer's Healthy Family Farms is located. Left alone in the L.A. courtroom was Bloch, who told me that not only was she in shock, but that the L.A. Country District Attorney's representative appeared just as surprised.

The new charges were emblematic of the new era of piling on charges and then seeking high bail because of the "seriousness" of the crime. Palmer was charged with thirty-eight felony counts and Stewart with thirty-seven felony counts — including grand theft, money laundering, and the illegal offering of securities. The felonies were alleged to have taken place between February 1, 2008, and April 1, 2009, when Palmer was borrowing money from Rawesome members and other sympathizers like Wayne Markel and Mary and Eric Hetherington to acquire the Healthy Family Farms property.

Larry Otting, the longtime Rawesome member and real-estate executive who put his credit behind a $1.1 million mortgage on the property, was charged with fourteen felony counts.[29] Because he was out of town the day of the arrests of Palmer and Stewart, he was allowed to turn himself in a few days later, spend about fourteen hours in jail, and post bail.

Palmer was held pending $2 million bail, and Stewart $1 million bail. By contrast, bail for the Pennsylvania State University coach eventually convicted on pedophile charges, Jerry Sandusky, was initially requested to be $500,000 in 2011; he was released on $100,000 bail.[30] Palmer had the felony conviction from 2001, which could have accounted for the higher bail. But still, she hadn't shown any inclination to flee the property and had remained in contact with the people she borrowed money from.

Eventually, after a week in jail for Stewart and three weeks for Palmer, bail was lowered for each of them — to $100,000 for Stewart and $500,000 for Palmer. This would occur at a bail hearing at which Ventura County prosecutor Chris Harman labeled Palmer "a wolf in sheep's clothing . . . a predator . . . in a community that distrusts government, which she used to her advantage."

Stewart was freed shortly after his bail was lowered when Mark McAfee, his old employer with whom he had quarreled, put up his Organic Pastures Dairy Company farm as collateral. Stewart would allege that he had been "tortured" while being kept for several days in holding areas of the L.A. County courts — left overnight in an unheated room with temperatures outside in the forties and not fed for many hours. "They never touched me, but it was torture all the same," he said. Palmer was eventually freed with help from friends and relatives.

The dragnet against farmers and food club managers with a connection to Aajonus Vonderplanitz wasn't over. There were two others on the government agenda, though these two pursuits wouldn't proceed quite as smoothly from the government's perspective. The first was David Hochstetler, the Indiana Amish farmer who had first signed on with Right to Choose Healthy Food in 2006 and reaffirmed his allegiance in the aftermath of failed negotiations with the FDA in 2010 about possibly ending his affiliation with food clubs in Michigan and Illinois.

In late October 2011, Hochstetler received a certified letter ordering him to appear before a federal grand jury in Detroit on the day before Thanksgiving. Among the documentation he was ordered to produce when he appeared was "any and all documents relating to or concerning the sale, purchase, delivery, receipt, production, packaging, transfer, disposal, marketing, promotion, furnishing, sharing, labeling, manufacturing, distribution, shipment, or transportation of milk during the Relevant Time Period."[31] And there was also a request for "any and all documents relating to, or reflecting communications with, Right to Choose Healthy Foods or Aajonus Vonderplanitz during the Relevant Time Period."[32] Richard Hebron, the Michigan farmer Hochstetler worked with in supplying food to his co-ops, was also subpoenaed.

Grand jury investigations are serious affairs, usually held in tight secrecy. While the U.S. Constitution's Fifth Amendment is generally identified with prohibiting self-incrimination and double jeopardy, it actually begins with something else: "No person shall be held to answer for a capital, or otherwise infamous crime, unless on a presentment or indictment of a Grand Jury." Moreover, witnesses called before such a jury of their peers have few of the rights that apply at a regular trial — including the right to be represented by a lawyer, or limits as to the kind of evidence that can be introduced. Additionally, grand juries rarely reject prosecutor requests for indictments. As a former assistant U.S. attorney told me, "We used to have a saying among ourselves, 'If a prosecutor asked a grand jury to indict a ham sandwich, it would indict the ham sandwich.'"

Vonderplanitz went to the aid of Hochstetler, asking the government to delay the proceeding until after Thanksgiving. That led to a testy exchange with a U.S. Justice Department lawyer, Ross Goldstein, who seemed well informed about Vonderplanitz's run-in with Judge Stengel on behalf of Daniel Allgyer. When Vonderplanitz sought to confirm via e-mail with the Justice Department attorney his understanding that the grand jury appearance had been rescheduled to two weeks later, Goldstein was abrupt and taunting: "As Judge Stengel explained in his order denying your motion for intervention in United States v. Allgyer, . . . 'Mr. Vonderplanitz is not an attorney and cannot represent others in federal court. . . . ' Although your email of this morning implies that you represent the legal interests of other individuals or entities, you may not lawfully do so. Accordingly, the substance of your communication . . . is of no moment and is being disregarded in toto. Moreover, I can see no reason why you should have any need to further discuss this matter with the United States at this juncture."[33]

Vonderplanitz wasn't about to be put off so easily and responded just as huffily: "You wrote with the authority of a judge yet you are a prosecutor. As a U.S. attorney, shouldn't you know more about law, especially the U.S. Constitution than you reveal? The decision by Judge Stengel in the Allgyer case does not set precedence in that case or any other case. I am simply waiting for the case to be resolved in Judge Stengel's court so that I can appeal the decision. . . . You will hear from me anytime you try to harass or stop a farmer with whom I have a PRIVATE club contract to produce healthy food for me and members of our private clubs. You have no legal jurisdiction over private clubs. Your jurisdiction is with the public."[34]

Despite Vonderplanitz's bluster, it seemed like another in a series of depressing setbacks for the food rights activist — except for a strange occurrence not long afterward.

A week or so after his appearance before the grand jury was rescheduled, Hochstetler decided to take the advice of friends who suggested he consult with his local sheriff. These law enforcement officers — there are more than three thousand of them nationally — are nearly all elected public officials. During 2009 and 2010, a small group of sheriffs had begun organizing something called the County Sheriff Project, committed to "enforcing the Bill of Rights and protecting the people's liberties," according to its website.[35]

The organization was the brainchild of a former Arizona sheriff, Richard Mack, and emerged out of growing frustration among sheriffs that the federal government was becoming ever less respectful of local authority in such areas as forestry management, gun control, and immigration issues — along with farm and food matters.

One of those involved in the County Sheriff Project was Brad Rogers of Elkhart County, Hochstetler's home county. Rogers had just a year earlier been elected sheriff of the Midwestern county after having served as an officer in the department for more than a decade. He campaigned as a Republican, emphasizing the need for closer attention to the U.S. Constitution, and its protection of local sheriff authority. He won in a competitive primary and then was elected with 73 percent of the vote.

When Hochstetler called and told the sheriff about his ongoing problems with FDA agents nosing around his farm, along with the grand jury subpoena, Rogers immediately drove to Hochstetler's farm. As Rogers would recall later, "I could see it was a clean operation." He tried to be honest with Hochstetler with regard to the requirement that he testify before the grand jury in Detroit. "I told him, 'I can't protect you in Detroit. But I can protect you here in Elkhart County.'"

His first step in emphasizing that latter point was to e-mail the U.S. Justice Department lawyer Ross Goldstein, warning the Justice Department not to conduct inspections of Hochstetler's farm without a warrant signed by a local judge. There had been "a number of inspections and attempted inspections on [Hochstetler's] farm," he stated. "Any further attempts to inspect this farm without a warrant signed by a local judge, based on probable cause, will result in Federal inspectors' removal or arrest for trespassing by my officers or I."[36]

That tough language prompted Goldstein to cite the U.S. Constitution's "supremacy clause," which he said "has been interpreted since the earliest days of this nation to mean that federal law trumps state law whenever the two conflict."[37] Goldstein argued further that the federal Food, Drug, and Cosmetic Act allowed federal agents "to enter Mr. Hochstetler's property . . . without a warrant at all — pursuant to a long line of federal cases." Moreover, he warned the sheriff, if push came to shove federal agents could arrest *him* — "that the 'refusal to permit entry or inspection as authorized by section 374' is in itself a federal criminal offense, which under certain circumstances is a felony punishable by imprisonment for up to three years."[38]

Rogers readied a three-page reply to Goldstein, explaining how he saw the U.S. Constitution limiting federal power: "When you assert that the federal law trumps state law, it is a distortion of the intent, content and extent of the supreme law of the land — the U.S. Constitution — seen through a myopic and misunderstood view of Article VI, section 2 (the Supremacy Clause)." He also included a reminder about the Fourth Amendment, which "guarantees that all citizens are 'to be secure in their persons, houses, papers, and effects, against unreasonable searches and seizures . . . ' and, as you know, requires Warrants." Rogers's conclusion: "Your 'cosmetic' regulations will never 'trump' those principles. The citizen in question is a good man and has committed no crime. He is an upstanding member of this community. He does not have to allow you access to his property for the FDA to conduct random inspections."

The letter was dated December 5th, and it still sat on Rogers's computer the next day when a certified letter from the U.S. Justice Department and attorney Goldstein arrived at Hochstetler's farm. Goldstein noted in the letter that Hochstetler had previously stated he wouldn't answer questions or produce documents based on his Fifth Amendment constitutional rights. "Based on your representation that Forest Grove Dairy is a sole proprietorship and that you refuse to produce any responsive documents based on the assertion of rights guaranteed by the Fifth Amendment of the U.S. Constitution against self incrimination, I write to advise you that you are released from the subpoena until further notice," Hochstetler read to me from the letter. For the time being, Hochstetler was off the hook. He had escaped the nearly-impossible-to-escape grand jury grilling.

Rogers became an instant Internet legend after I reported on my blog how he had helped the Amish farmer out of a tough fix. He estimates he received at least one thousand e-mails of congratulation, and the story went viral on other websites. Six weeks later, the straight-backed Rogers was a speaker at the first convention of the County Sheriff Project in Las Vegas. Standing in front of two hundred of his colleagues from around the country, he recounted the story of how he aided Hochstetler. "I sent an e-mail to the Justice Department trial attorney. . . . I said, 'If you come back to this farm without a search warrant signed by a trial judge, I will have you removed for trespassing.'" The audience interrupted Rogers with wild applause, and he continued. "Well, he didn't take to that too well. He said the federal government has precedence based on the supremacy clause. I told him the federal government is supreme if it has to do with the Constitution." When Rogers concluded by explaining how Hochstetler had been let off from testifying before the grand jury, the crowd interrupted him again, with even louder applause. "I want to protect citizens like Hochstetler," said Rogers. "That stuff is not going to happen in my county." Still, Rogers remained modest. "We'll never know if it was my letters that led to the withdrawal of the subpoena."

That evening in Las Vegas, Rogers attended a convention banquet for his new organization; at its first awards presentation after dinner, he was given a special plaque, one of only three awards handed out that evening. Inscribed under his name was this: CSPOA Interposer: For Meritorious Valor for Interposing Himself on Behalf of His Citizens. He had received the award because of his efforts to protect Hochstetler.

The days of 2011 ticked down toward a New Year, and past the year-and-a-half mark since Vernon Hershberger had triumphantly cut the seals placed on his food coolers by Wisconsin's Department of Agriculture, Trade, and Consumer Protection (DATCP) inspectors on June 3, 2010. The raw milk, yogurt, butter, eggs, and meats his small farm produced had once again become available to the nearly two hundred grateful members of his rural community buying club.

Since that dramatic moment, nothing had happened beyond a couple of searches immediately afterward. He and his club members anxiously awaited DATCP's response. Would Hershberger be arrested for his brazen act of defiance? Put on trial? As time marched on uneventfully the outlook for the pensive farmer appeared positive. Word had it that the local prosecutor was shying away from pursuing the case, having decided that going after a deeply religious local farmer with an Amish past who was supplying area residents with food wasn't a great strategy to win votes.

Hershberger also heard that the local sheriff's deputies who had accompanied DATCP inspectors in their searches and sealing of his coolers a year and a half earlier didn't want to repeat the experience. He told me that a local sheriff's deputy relayed to a good friend of Hershberger's: "If there was ever a time I didn't want to be in law enforcement, that [raid on Hershberger's farm to tape the coolers] was it. There isn't anything going to happen to that case, because there are too many people in law enforcement who feel the same way." That attitude was part of what helped discourage the local prosecutor from filing charges, Hershberger concluded.

But pressures to go after Hershberger were building outside his rural Sauk County. The ruling in August 2011 by a state judge, Patrick Fiedler, against two other Wisconsin farmers, Mark Zinniker and Wayne Craig, who sold raw milk and other products privately from their on-site stores didn't bode well. The judge had agreed with DATCP that such private arrangements as cowshares or leasing agreements weren't exempt from the agency's requirement that they register for retail licenses. Of course, there was no retail license that allowed the sale of raw milk, so the judge was essentially prohibiting raw milk distribution of any kind.

Might the FDA have been encouraging DATCP as well to go after Hershberger (and by extension, Vonderplanitz)? I don't have evidence linking the FDA, only speculation based on data obtained by food rights activist Max Kane via open records requests showing that FDA funding to DATCP was rising rapidly — from slightly over $200,000 in 2007 to more than $500,000 by 2009. USDA funding, which was at a much higher level, had leveled off during that period. All this at a time when Wisconsin, like many states, was facing highly public — and contentious — budgetary constraints. FDA funds for DATCP were more crucial than ever.

Whatever the exact drivers, DATCP prevailed on the state's attorney general to bypass the local Sauk County prosecutor and act as "Special Prosecutor for the County of Sauk" for the purposes of pursuing Hershberger. The state of Wisconsin filed four misdemeanor charges against Hershberger at virtually the same time as the Hochstetler grand jury struggle was taking place.[39] Indeed, it was announced the same week as Hochstetler was having his subpoena canceled in December 2011. The four counts accused Hershberger of operating without a retail license, dairy license, or dairy plant license — as well as of violating a "holding order" by breaking the DATCP seals on his coolers. The potential penalties? Two and a half years in jail plus $13,000 in fines.

As per the Amish tradition, Hershberger refrained from engaging a lawyer. He had left the Ohio Amish community to which he belonged in 2009. He felt "they are too much a tradition, basing their faith on tradition, and not basing their faith on Christ," he explained as we sat in his small farm office on a warm August day in 2011. "You might say they are more focused on traditions than religious principles."

As a result of his departure, Hershberger was excommunicated. Although he had other family members still living in Amish communities, he could well be treated harshly should he return. He told me how a formerly Amish woman went to her mother's funeral at an Amish community and was forced to sit in the back of the church. Other punishments can include not being able to shop in Amish stores or even being denied food.

But Hershberger held onto a number of Amish traditions, including staying as far outside the legal system as possible. "I just feel very strongly not to join in their game. That's what I call it. When they came here to close us down, they were trying to get me to join in their game. Get a lawyer. Try to release my products . . . I just didn't play. I just kept on selling. Once they get you in their game, they'll suck you dry." It's not as if he wouldn't take legal advice. He took it from Vonderplanitz, and he occasionally spoke with Pete Kennedy, the head of the Farm-to-Consumer Legal Defense Fund. "I've learned a lot about the law," Hershberger said. But one important lesson: "I've learned you can't depend on someone else."

So when he appeared at his arraignment on January 4, 2012, Hershberger was his own lawyer. (Vonderplanitz's name appeared on court filings as "Fiduciary . . . not a lawyer.") A couple days later, when I spoke to him, he sounded dejected. To be released on his personal recognizance, Hershberger had had to sign a statement in which he agreed to "no sale of food without a valid retail food establishment license" and no production or distribution of milk. There was to be "no impeding, obstruction . . . or interference with any DATCP inspection." Moreover, and this was the most troubling, "the defendant may not allow anyone else to operate his farm, or any room or building on his property in violation of any of these conditions."[40] So he couldn't designate one of his two older sons (seventeen and twenty years old) to operate the farm and provide members with food in his place.

"If I hadn't signed, they would have thrown me in jail, right there," he said. His wife was pregnant with their tenth child. He understandably felt as if he couldn't just leave her without his protection. But he also knew he had deviated from his path of civil disobedience and felt badly about it. He decided he had to do something to recant his agreement to the terms. Three weeks later, the opportunity arose, when Hershberger was back in court for a hearing on a motion he had filed, at Vonderplanitz's urging, to dismiss the case.

After the judge rejected the dismissal request, Hershberger asked if he could make a statement. The judge agreed, and Hershberger began: "I cannot in good conscience tell the hundred-plus families who own the food and depend on it to feed their families, that they can no longer get food to feed their families. The Almighty God has spoken and I cannot do otherwise."

He went on to quote from the New Testament, including this: "But whoso has this world's good, and seeth his brother have need, and shutteth up his bowels of compassion from him, how dwelleth the Love of God in him?" He then answered his own question. "Your honor, I have spent many sleepless hours since signing the bond due to my conscience being plagued by the thought of shutting up my bowels of compassion to my Brethren who are dependent on the food that is provided by and for them on our farm. To most of them it is not merely a matter of preference but much more a matter of life or death! If the owners of the food cannot eat their own food, aren't we living in a communist state? If our farm stopped feeding its owners' families, there will be literally hundreds of children who will suffer malnutrition and even starvation. Your honor, I would much rather spend the rest of my life behind bars or even die than to be found guilty of such a gross sin before the Almighty God."

The judge didn't respond, and Hershberger walked out of the court feeling relieved because, in his mind, he had unshackled himself from the bail agreement. Hershberger fought back on another important level as well. Although he came out of the Amish tradition and mind-set, Hershberger was decidedly non-Amish in one key respect — his willingness to use modern technology. He was in e-mail contact with Vonderplanitz and other supporters. He knew how to scan court documents so he could distribute them to media representatives. He had a cell phone on hand at all times. Perhaps most significant, he became adept at using video. So each time a regulator came around or he made a court appearance, he recorded what happened. Then, he and a son edited his material down to the ideal YouTube length of between three and six minutes — and presto, he was a movie producer.

When DATCP inspector Jackie Owens, a woman who looked to be in her forties, came to his farm accompanied by two colleagues a month after the arraignment, in early February, she was confronted by Hershberger's son wielding a video camera; Hershberger was out doing errands. She politely asked permission to inspect Hershberger's farm; the bail terms gave DATCP the right to inspect the farm any time they wanted. As the camera recorded, Owens spoke to Hershberger on his cell phone and asked him if he would grant permission for her to inspect the farm. No, he wouldn't, Hershberger responded. Owens and her entourage left the premises, and within three days Hershberger posted video of the encounter on YouTube, and from there it was posted on food and health blogs around the blogosphere.[41] Within two weeks of the encounter with the DATCP inspectors, Hershberger received notice that the judge in his case was being asked by the prosecution to act against him for violating his bail terms. He could be thrown into jail.

On March 2, 2012, as some seventy supporters filled the small Sauk County courthouse on a snowy afternoon, and another hundred crowded a basement conference room with a television feed of the proceedings, Hershberger again stood his ground. When sheriff's deputies told him he couldn't have his son, Andrew, video the proceedings, he refused to enter the courtroom. Finally, a compromise was negotiated: since I was sitting in the media section up front, I would handle the camera. Hershberger came into the courtroom, about fifteen minutes late.

Two prosecutors, Eric Defort and Phillip Ferris, of the Wisconsin Department of Justice's Office of the Attorney General, sat dressed in business suits at a table to the right of the judge. They had sent the judge a letter the previous week complaining that Hershberger was violating the bail terms by making raw milk and other farm products available to his food club members — and alleging, based on Inspector Owens's report, that he was running a retail store. According to Defort, Hershberger was guilty of "willful violation of the pretrial release conditions."[42]

Guy Reynolds, the thin, white-haired judge, acknowledged he had received a letter from the attorney general's office about Hershberger. But what he said next surprised everyone, including Hershberger, who expected the judge was about to have him taken from the courtroom and locked up.

"This court will not respond to letters," he told Defort. "This court responds to motions."

It wasn't a complete win. The judge warned Hershberger that he could be in trouble with the court if the attorney general's office filed a motion and the judge agreed with it. Violating bond conditions "could be a separate crime subject to separate punishment. I admonish you that you are to follow my bond conditions."

Hershberger, sitting alone at the defendant's table with his Bible in his hand, reminded the judge that he had previously disavowed the agreement he signed in early January as a condition of being released pending trial for four misdemeanors related to making raw milk available to his nearly two hundred club members. Many of them were among those in attendance, he said. "I do not have jurisdiction over that food," Hershberger told the judge. "It belongs to the members."

But the prosecutors never filed a motion, and Hershberger continued about the business of supplying his food club, as he declared he would. The entire case was scheduled to be decided at a trial the following January (of 2013) by a jury of Hershberger's peers. The farmers were beginning to get the hang of the American justice system.

CHAPTER 9

THE FLICKERING PROMISE OF FOOD SOVEREIGNTY

In 1831, during a tour of the United States, the French historian Alexis de Tocqueville marveled at how the rule of law seemed to be universally accepted in the New World, even if strangely applied. In his book *Democracy in America*, he wrote, "Nothing is more striking to an European traveller in the United States than the absence of what we term the Government, or the Administration. Written laws exist in America, and one sees that they are daily executed; but although everything is in motion, the hand which gives the impulse to the social machine can nowhere be discovered."[1] De Tocqueville added that a contradiction often existed between titles and appearances for regulators and other administrators — that "the office might be powerful and the officer insignificant, and that the community should be at once regulated and free. In no country in the world does the law hold so absolute a language as in America, and in no country is the right of applying it vested in so many hands."[2]

Even in today's more regulated United States, de Tocqueville's observations about the contradictions between appearances and reality are apt, especially with regard to food regulation. A big challenge facing many of the farmers I have written about in previous chapters has had to do with varying interpretations not only of the food laws and regulations, but of whether there is in fact a private sphere where individuals can make their own choices about which foods are safe and what sort of processing and other manipulation they are willing to accept or not accept for themselves and their families.

While de Tocqueville admired the way things seemed to "work," he likely didn't fully appreciate how difficult it could be for those charged with administering the laws (along with those being administered to) to make things work, given this country's decentralized political and government structure. Part of the difficulty in making sense of American food rules stems from the fact that there are fifty states — each with its own public health and agriculture laws and regulations — and countless counties, cities, and towns with separate public health departments charged with executing still more laws and regulations. Different states have different laws regarding the sale of food produced in home kitchens, for example. Sometimes the regulation isn't even in state hands, but in the control of individual towns and cities. And sometimes there is no law on the books — at either the state or local level. Meat that is slaughtered within a particular state and sold within that state is subject to different inspection requirements than meat produced for sale across state lines, where the USDA holds sway. Even food products that cross state lines are subject to confusing food safety oversight. The FDA, for example, regulates eggs — but the USDA is in charge of chickens and other meat.

Raw milk regulation is fairly typical of the confusing oversight. Essentially, each state has its own set of laws and regulations, which means there are fifty variations on the theme. Even in states that don't allow its sale, some may allow herdshares, while some ban them and some don't have any legal or regulatory reference to herdshares at all. That doesn't mean regulators back off; in Massachusetts, for example, the state's Department of Agricultural Resources told a dairy farmer with just two cows who formed a herdshare in 2010 that she needed to "cease and desist" because herdshares were illegal, even though there is no reference in the state's laws to herdshare arrangements. A similar problem came up with herdshares in California beginning in 2011, when local prosecutors — at the request of the California Department of Food and Agriculture — began sending out cease-and-desist notices to several dairies around the state that distributed milk via herdshare arrangements (once again, with no provision in state law either for or against). In states that allow raw milk sales, there may be differences in how often farms are inspected, what kinds of lab tests are required, and the frequency of testing. Some places require monthly tests, while others call for quarterly or annual testing.

Then there is the federal component — since 1987, there has been a ban on interstate shipment and sale of raw milk. The FDA complicated that situation further when, in 2011, it issued a statement, in response to protest demonstrations on behalf of Amish farmer Daniel Allgyer, stating that it "has never taken, nor does it intend to take, enforcement action against an individual who purchased and transported raw milk across state lines solely for his or her own personal consumption."[3]

And as de Tocqueville suggested, even within the variations in laws and regulations, there are differences in enforcement — the result, he implied, of a certain informality and resistance to authority that prevails among Americans. In dairy regulation, farmers and state dairy inspectors often get to know each other, learn from each other about effective safety measures, and develop mutual professional respect. In such an environment, inspectors may informally alert farmers to safety or sanitation problems in their facilities and give them time to make adjustments, rather than formally cite them for violations.

Or regulators may even come up with informal arrangements within the confines of existing law that allow some farmers to escape regulation entirely. For years, the state of Maine had just such an arrangement for dairies producing and selling raw milk. Then in 2009, an official effort ending the arrangement led to the establishment of a major new front in the battle over food rights.

Maine is one of the more permissive states vis-à-vis raw milk, one of just ten that allows retail sales. To qualify for a raw milk permit, farmers must meet certain requirements for the type of facility they have; for example, milk generally must be stored in a separate building meeting certain plumbing and structural requirements — a potentially large expense for a farmer with just a few cows who bottles milk in a home kitchen and sells it to a handful of neighbors.

For many years — no one is even sure exactly when or how it started — Maine regulators applied an informal two-tier regulatory approach to raw milk producers. Those that were large enough that they promoted their dairy products via ads in local papers or sold to retailers were subject to the standard regulations. But many dozens of small farms, usually with fewer than ten cows, which operated out of public view — in other words, they refrained from any kind of advertising or promotion — were excused from obtaining permits.

In late 2009, as the debate about raw milk and food rights swirled around the country, Maine regulators reexamined their two-tier policy on raw milk and turned it into a one-size-fits-all policy whereby each dairy that sold raw milk, whether it advertised or not, would be required to have a state permit. In late 2009, letters went out to all dairy farms, advising those that sold raw milk without permits to get them.

In the letter, Hal Prince, director of the Division of Quality Assurance and Regulation of the Maine Department of Agriculture, Food, and Rural Resources, observed that "there seems to be confusion among businesses and inspection staff alike as to whether or not a license and inspection is needed by those 'not pasteurized' [raw] milk processors who do not actively advertise the sale of 'not pasteurized' [raw] milk. In the rule, there is no exemption of any kind that allows the sale of milk or milk products without a valid license. As such we will begin immediately to identify those processors who are operating without a license and assist them into compliance through proper inspection and licensing."[4]

I was able to examine internal documents relating to Prince's edict involving Maine regulators as part of a cache of nearly seven hundred pages of material obtained under Maine's Freedom of Access Act by lawyers, including the Farm-to-Consumer Legal Defense Fund, who became involved in the Maine raw milk conflict. In these documents, the officials contradict each other about why a change was made.

At the time the letter was going out to dairy producers in late November 2009, Maine's chief veterinarian, Donald Hoenig, wrote in an e-mail to Prince, the department director, "My recollection is that when the determination was made to only license those folks who 'advertised', it was on the advice of our assistant AG. . . . I believe it was the AG's office who probably advised us that 'offer for sale' could be interpreted to mean 'advertise'. I'm sure there could be other interpretations also but what you're proposing is a significant change in policy which could impact dairy farmers who may just sell a few gallons out of their tank sporadically. We made the decision to not require those people to be licensed since the practice was widespread at the time. It's probably not as common now as most dairy farmers are scared of the liability and think it's just a pain in the neck."[5]

Hoenig said further in a 2011 e-mail answering an inquiry on this subject, "In talking with one of the dairy inspectors who has worked for the state for 30 years, I'm told that this policy (no need to be licensed if you did not advertise) was in place when this person began work in 1981. When oversight of the program switched from my division (Animal Health) to Quality Assurance in July 2009, a decision was made to take a new look at the enforcement of all the dairy rules and that's when the policy changed."[6]

Among the regulators themselves, the debate about the two-tier approach to regulating raw dairies continued after the Prince letter went out in November 2009, and the matter became the focus of statewide debate. In August 2010, a laboratory evaluation officer, Cathleen Cotton, sent an e-mail that seems to have gone to everyone in the department, stating, "There has been a misconception that if you didn't advertise, you didn't need to license. This is not true now, nor has it been. It was simply a problem of resources — with only 2 Dairy Inspectors it was impossible to check every place that may be selling milk without a license. Now the Dairy program is with Quality Assurance and Regulations and we have many more inspectors around the State to keep their eyes open for unlicensed sellers of milk or milk products."[7]

So to some, the state's attorney general had sanctioned the two-tier approach, while to others it was a matter of not having enough dairy inspectors. Whatever the real reason, the licensing practice was part of a long-standing tradition; one of those practices that, as de Tocqueville suggested, wasn't terribly clear-cut or etched in stone but seemed to work.

Why does this minutiae in Maine agricultural regulation matter to the world at large? Because a directly related issue, known as "food sovereignty," would become an important aspect in a highly charged political and legal dispute affecting the entire movement for food rights.

Had the late-2009 shift by the Maine Department of Agriculture, Food, and Rural Resources occurred as a result of some outbreak of illness attributable to raw milk, it might have made sense to farmers. But coming out of nowhere, as far as they were concerned — without any outbreaks from raw milk in at least five years and probably longer, according to departmental documents — the action seemed arbitrary. So one predictable result of the shift was a bunch of unhappy dairy farmers.

One such farmer was Heather Retberg, a woman with an engaging smile who, with her husband, runs a small farm in the scenic coastal community of Penobscot. Over several years, they had built up a nice little business raising chickens, slaughtering them at a neighbor's regulator-approved facility for producers of less than one thousand chickens annually, and then selling the chickens to people in the area who valued chickens raised on pasture and not cooped up in tight facilities.

But in early 2009, the Maine Department of Agriculture, Food, and Rural Resources changed the rules so that people with an approved facility to slaughter fewer than one thousand chickens needed an additional permit to slaughter chickens for a neighbor. Such farm facilities tended to only do the slaughtering for a few neighbors, so for most people it didn't make sense to invest in the facilities upgrade that would be required to qualify for the additional permit.

There was an outcry around the state, and eventually the legislature made changes to ease life for those slaughtering fewer than one thousand chickens, but the Maine Department of Agriculture kept key obstacles in effect for neighbors helping each other. Bottom line, Retberg was still prohibited from slaughtering the chickens at her neighbor's and told she needed to either construct her own thirty-thousand-dollar facility or else have the chickens slaughtered at an approved facility many miles from her farm — all prohibitively expensive, she told me. So she exited the chicken business, as did a number of other small chicken farmers and processors. A Maine Department of Agriculture survey in 2011 found that 40 of 165 processors who responded to a questionnaire it sent out on the subject had exited the business. The biggest reason, offered by one-third: "over-regulation."[8]

When Retberg exited the chicken business, she was determined to focus more on her farm's raw milk business, selling privately to a few neighbors and area residents, under the state's long-standing exemption from regulation for small farms that didn't advertise. When she received the agriculture department's raw milk notice in late 2009, warning her she would need a special Maine permit to sell raw milk from the farm under any circumstances, it seemed as if the agency was following her around — determined to sabotage her farming aspirations — since complying would require many additional thousands of dollars of facilities upgrades.

Rather than seek help from a legislature that in her view seemed beholden to Big Ag's interests, she joined forces with another farm owner — Deborah Evans — and several neighbors who were active in fighting the chicken slaughtering problems. They became determined to go local — much in the spirit of de Tocqueville. In addition to expressing admiration for America's approach to the "rule of law," de Tocqueville had been even more amazed by the town meeting system that prevailed in hundreds of New England towns. "In America, not only do municipal bodies exist, but they are kept alive and supported by public spirit," he wrote in *Democracy in America*. "The township of New England possesses two advantages which infallibly secure the attentive interest of mankind, namely, independence and authority. Its sphere is indeed small and limited, but within that sphere its action is unrestrained; and its independence gives to it a real importance which its extent and population may not always ensure."[9]

Retberg and her farm friends had been following the cases of Daniel Allgyer, Vernon Hershberger, and the Rawesome Three and were convinced there had to be a clearer way than food clubs to achieve a legally sanctioned means of buying and selling food privately. The state legislature? The farmers concluded that the legislature wouldn't help them. They had tried that tack with the chicken situation and come to the same conclusion that activists in other states came to: Many state legislatures with significant agriculture seem to have been co-opted by Big Ag via campaign contributions to key agriculture committee members. They have not only resisted efforts to help small farms but deferred on implementation of the laws to the regulators, giving them free rein to do as they see fit — even if that is to defer to FDA and USDA wishes.

Instead of going to the legislature, the Maine farmers decided to petition their individual towns to pass ordinances allowing local farms to sell their food privately, directly to individual buyers. The big advantage of going to the towns was that unlike the efforts to sell via private food clubs, as was happening elsewhere around the country, the Maine arrangements would actually have the force of law behind them. If they could get small towns to adopt ordinances that would legalize private sales outside of the state or federal regulatory structure, that would legitimize something that was mostly in legal limbo around the rest of the country.

They started with their own towns along Maine's rugged coast — Penobscot, Blue Hill, Sedgwick, and Brooksville, quaint old towns of just a few hundred or thousand people, with longtime streaks of independence. The key element in the proposed ordinances was protection of "direct farmer/

grower/processor-to-customer sales from unnecessary regulation." The first proposed ordinance stated: "So long as there is one willing seller and one willing buyer, the producer or processor of local foods is exempt from federal or state permitting, certification or licensure. The one-on-one private contract between the local farmer/processor and their local customer provides sufficient oversight through the customer's interest in and knowledge of how the food is raised, harvested, and prepared, and the farmer/processor's honesty and integrity."

There were other items in their proposal, including protection of bean suppers, bake sales, and traveling food fund-raisers (for example, a series of food-in-the-field events with profits going to charity) that had come under attack; expansion of agritourism; and a requirement that all producers who sell directly to consumers label their products, "including their name, address, ingredient list and the date the product was prepared" to "provide accountability, traceability and transparency."

During the spring and summer of 2010, the supporters began discussing within their communities, including with their selectmen (who determine town meeting agendas), the idea of introducing their proposals during the winter and spring town meeting season of 2011 — when small towns in New England traditionally take up new ordinance proposals. They found town officials receptive, with a number expressing disbelief that small-scale chicken slaughtering and bake sales had come under attack. Proponents even developed a "Declaration of Food Freedom" petition for town residents, stating in part that the petition signer believes "that my access to farm raised food should be unfettered and free of one-size-fits-all regulations formed at federal levels and enforced by the state."

While everything seemed to be moving in the direction envisioned by de Tocqueville — with town meeting debate and discussion about food sovereignty — there was one factor at work during 2010 and 2011 that the French historian didn't observe during his American visit of 1830: the increasing centralization of power, such that the food sovereignty proposals, making food regulation an entirely local affair, would seriously threaten state and federal government agencies and authority. (The term "food sovereignty" originated in a late–1900s peasant movement in underdeveloped countries on behalf of locally produced food.)

Word of the local organizing by Retberg, Evans, and others seemed to quickly get back to state agriculture officials in Augusta, Maine's capital. Retberg remembers that she and her friends did a little dramatic skit called "Food Rules," poking fun at the layers of rules for farmers, in front of a few farmers. "Four days later, in early August, a dairy inspector was in our driveway. . . . He came up with a form that said we can't sell milk unless we have a license." She came to conclude that an area farmer had become a turncoat, alerting the officials about the fledgling food sovereignty campaign and identifying the farmers involved.

The inspector's visit to Retberg's farm was just an initial step. Before long, Maine agriculture and public health officials were planning an unusual campaign to raise fears about raw milk. Their campaign was to associate illnesses from a condition known as cryptosporidium with raw milk. Cryptosporidium — or "crypto," as it's commonly known — is a nasty parasite that causes diarrhea and stomach upset. The CDC says that "while this parasite can be spread in several different ways, water (drinking water and recreational water) is the most common method of transmission. Cryptosporidium is one of the most frequent causes of waterborne disease among humans in the United States."[10]

One CDC report calculated 10,500 cases in 2008 and noted, "The seasonal peak in age-specific case reports coincides with the summer recreational water season and likely reflects increased use of communal swimming venues (e.g., lakes, rivers, swimming pools, and water parks) by young children."[11] Other means of transmission are pets like dogs and cats, young farm animals, and sexual contact with someone who is infected, according to the CDC. Not mentioned as a means of transmission in the CDC's literature: raw milk.[12]

But the Maine Department of Agriculture seemed to have become convinced that raw milk was the cause of a number of crypto cases that cropped up in the state during the spring and summer seasons between 2009 and 2012. So top agriculture and public health officials in 2010 began to collaborate on finding cases of illness from raw milk, according to the internal e-mails and other documents I reviewed.

Each case of crypto involving an individual who drank raw milk prompted a flurry of e-mails among Maine agricultural officials. And ironically, one case involved Heather Retberg and the Quill's End Farm she runs with her husband. In the summer of 2010, just as Retberg was helping lobby on behalf of food sovereignty, a case of crypto was reported from someone who drank raw milk from Retberg's farm.[13] That prompted a visit from the Maine state vet, Donald Hoenig, on August 13, 2010.

Hoenig recounted his visit in a memo to four colleagues, including Hal Prince, director of the Maine Department of Agriculture's Division of Quality Assurance and Regulation. He noted, "[I] walked through their pastures and I had a chance to look over all the animals they are raising — sheep, goats, pigs, chickens, ducks, geese and cattle. I took three fecal samples from the cows and also took milk samples from the only container of milk which they had in their refrigerator. They did not have any unopened containers of milk but since we're not doing a bacterial exam on the milk and only looking for crypto at this time, I think this milk sample will be acceptable. We had a long discussion about the consequences of a positive test either from the fecal samples or the milk. I told them a positive milk sample would be the most significant and that they would likely have another visit from me and someone from the Maine CDC if the milk was positive."[14]

He added in his memo, "I am of the opinion that a positive fecal sample, while revealing, would not be that significant as crypto is very common on farms."[15] He also noted that the farm would "certainly have a fair amount of work to do before meeting our licensing standards. They currently milk on rubber mats placed over the hard dirt barn floor and do not have a milk room. They milk by hand and the milk is bottled in the kitchen. Currently, they do not have a sign advertising milk at the farm entrance. I was at the farm for two hours."[16]

Hoenig sent the milk and fecal samples from Retberg's farm to a lab at Cornell University in New York. On August 31st, the state's chief vet reported back to his colleagues: "All three fecal samples and the milk samples were negative for crypto."[17] Hoenig concluded, "Taking into consideration what I observed on my farm visit and the other risk factors for the patient, I think there is a low probability that the milk was the mode of transmission."[18]

Retberg remembers the incident well. She says Hoenig told her the woman who got sick "had been vacationing in the area. She had been swimming in an area pond and had eaten unwashed veggies." She also said Hoenig expressed his fears about the FDA taking over state agriculture responsibilities, and making life even more difficult for farmers like Retberg.

It was a fear expressed on a few occasions by agriculture officials in justifying their clampdown on raw milk licensing. The implicit message to farmers was this: the devil you know is better than the one you don't know. Retberg says she and her husband considered refusing Hoenig's 2010 request to conduct his inspection and concluded "that was a stressful step" they didn't want to take. It might, for example, lead to the state coming in with a search warrant and a forced inspection, as had happened to farmers in other states.

The search for crypto cases continued with other victims and farmers and also came up empty. One case involved a one-year-old boy who had drunk raw milk. An epidemiologist from Maine's Department of Agriculture wrote in a 2010 e-mail: "Parents wanted 'organic'. Child's physician was aware of milk source and mother knew it was not recommended. Family cottage in Strong, Maine on Toddy Pond. Water for the cottage is pumped from the pond, bottled to drink but baby bathed in pond water which he swallowed."[19]

In May 2011, Kate Colby, a field epidemiologist, wrote to her colleagues that a "probable crypto case . . . is a 58 yo female who is hospitalized at Mid-Coast. . . . Her daughter also became ill with similar symptoms on the same day within hours of the case. . . . They purchased raw skim milk from a farm in Topsham (unknown purchase date) during the exposure period. They ran out of their normal pasteurized milk and purchased it while they were there to get meat. This was the first time they had done this. Other exposures include tomatoes, lettuce, and hamburger from Fat Boy's restaurant in Brunswick, oranges, 2 pet dogs, pet rats, and transplanting strawberry plants in the garden without gloves. Drinking water is from public water supply and bottled water, no travel, no recreational water. The raw milk appears to be the only common exposure between her and her daughter. Her daughter is not currently ill and was not tested."[20] Though it's tempting to be suspicious of the raw milk in this situation, the reality is that food safety is an inexact science, and miscalculations occur even when experts are mobilized nationally. A huge outbreak of illnesses, with twenty-six deaths, from *E. coli* O157:H7 in Europe in May 2011 was blamed at different times on cucumbers, tomatoes, and lettuce before being finally traced to bad bean sprouts from Germany. In this situation in Maine, nothing approaching a thorough investigation was carried out.

Then there was another crypto case, reported by epidemiologist Megan Kelley in March 2011, of a forty-two-year-old woman from Islesboro who had "consumed raw milk purchased at Nealey's in Northport and produced by [a farm] in Belfast." The report noted that "her 19-year-old son, who usually drinks rice milk, also used the product and was symptomatic for 2 days. He was not tested. Her other exposures include staying in a shack in the woods on Islesboro with no running water and eating moose meat. She does not eat fruits and vegetables. Eats mostly beef and moose. She has no water exposures, animals or farm contacts. She does not know of any other persons who are ill. Islesboro has not seen other diarrheal cases in the last few weeks."[21]

Living in the wild subsisting on moose meat and water from unknown sources sounded a little suspicious to me, but that didn't dissuade the Maine Department of Agriculture. A sample from the woman was sent to the Maine Center for Disease Control and Prevention, according to an e-mail from Amy Robbins, a subordinate of state vet Hoenig. She reported to him in March 2011, "So it will be awhile before we have results from them. The lab was going to stress the need for a quick turnaround time due to the raw milk exposure."[22] Raw milk cases obviously received expedited attention.

It's not clear what the Maine CDC came up with — though no warning was ever issued, as the state would have done had crypto been found in the milk — and state vet Hoenig expressed frustration about the Islesboro case, as he commented in an e-mail: "Hard to figure out why immune compromised people are drinking raw milk isn't it? You'd think their physicians would make certain recommendations on dietary restrictions, if they were under a physician's care. I wish we had a better test for crypto in milk."[23]

The organized effort to link raw milk to crypto and other "enteric pathogens" was a group decision within the Maine Department of Agriculture. Robbins wrote Hoenig at the same time in spring 2011 that she was pushing for quick Maine CDC turnaround because of raw milk: "It's been about a year since we all last met to discuss raw milk exposures and enteric pathogens. At that time we came up with the plan to send an email to the group to receive feedback from everyone regarding next steps. I can reconvene the group to look at this approach for the future if that would help."[24]

Hoenig asked for a delay. "I think getting together again to discuss raw milk exposures is a great idea but we'll probably have to wait until the legislature calms down a bit."[25] It's not clear when the follow-up meeting to plan further actions against raw dairies actually took place.

ℰℛℴ

On a Saturday morning in early March 2011, Sedgwick, Maine (population about 1,200) held its town meeting in the quaint white wooden town hall, as it has every year since 1794. The proposed food sovereignty ordinance was number forty-two in a list of seventy-eight proposals being considered. Although all the town's citizens are entitled to vote yea or nay on proposals to spend their tax money and, in this case, enact potentially far-reaching laws with national implications, on this day there were about 120 in attendance.

The proposal, "To see if the Town will vote to adopt an ordinance entitled 'Local Food and Community Self-Governance Ordinance,'" followed one on a "wind energy facilities ordinance" and came before another one about "constructing a road to the property owned jointly by the towns of Sedgwick and Brooksville on Walker Pond."[26] Citing America's Declaration of Independence and the Maine Constitution, the food sovereignty ordinance proposed that "Sedgwick citizens possess the right to produce, process, sell, purchase, and consume local foods of their choosing." These would include raw milk and other dairy products and locally slaughtered meats.

The ordinance wasn't simply a declaration of preference. It added this warning to regulators: "It shall be unlawful for any law or regulation adopted by the state or federal government to interfere with the rights recognized by this Ordinance." In other words, state licensing prohibitions on unlicensed farms selling dairy products or producing their own chickens for sale to other citizens in the town would not be recognized in Sedgwick.

What about legal liability and state or federal inspections? It was up to the seller and buyer to negotiate. "Patrons purchasing food for home consumption may enter into private agreements with those producers or processors of local foods to waive any liability for the consumption of that food. Producers or processors of local foods shall be exempt from licensure and inspection requirements for that food as long as those agreements are in effect." Imagine — buyer and seller could agree to cut out the lawyers. It seemed almost un-American in twenty-first-century America. And, then again, very American.

After it was read, the 120 citizens in attendance raised their hands in unanimous approval, and Sedgwick became the first town in the country to enact a law that explicitly sanctioned private food sales. Afterward, the originators of the food sovereignty concept, Retberg and Evans, put out a press release that stated in part:

> Local farmer Bob St. Peter noted the importance of this or-
> dinance for beginning farmers and cottage producers. "This
> ordinance creates favorable conditions for beginning farmers
> and cottage-scale food processors to try out new products, and
> to make the most of each season's bounty," said St. Peter. "My
> family is already working on some ideas we can do from home
> to help pay the bills and get our farm going."
>
> Mia Strong, Sedgwick resident and local farm patron, was
> overwhelmed by the support of her town. "Tears of joy welled in
> my eyes as my town voted to adopt this ordinance," said Strong.
> "I am so proud of my community. They made a stand for local
> food and our fundamental rights as citizens to choose that food."

Before the spring town meeting season was over, five other area towns — including Penobscot, Trenton, and Blue Hill — would follow Sedgwick's lead. The news about the Maine towns spread quickly, stimulating inquiries to Retberg and Evans from as far away as Texas and California. Santa Cruz adopted California's first version of the ordinance. The food sovereignty movement was gaining traction.

While the food sovereignty ordinances were passing fairly easily in the Maine towns where they were introduced — by the spring of 2012 eight towns had adopted them — in the state capital of Augusta, a battle was play-ing out over the elimination of the informal understanding allowing private sale of raw milk. Legislation was introduced to allow it.

That didn't sit well with the Maine Department of Agriculture, and it invited the FDA to provide data and testimony that could help beat back the initiative. Included in the FDA's testimony to the state agency was an eighteen-page condemnation of raw milk supplied by John Sheehan, the head of the FDA's dairy division (which I quoted from in chapter 3).[27]

In the meantime, the state's governor, Paul LePage, was hearing from dairy farmers who were upset by the agriculture agency's assault on private sales of raw milk. The governor didn't like what he was hearing, and in

September, he wrote a memo to the agency's commissioner, Walter Whitcomb, stating, "I am particularly concerned about over regulating the small farms with large capital investments and costly licensing. In recent weeks I have received letters, emails and constituent visits concerning regulations involving intrastate commerce."[28] Attached to the memo was the proposed bill in the Maine legislature "that a license is not required of any person who produces and sells milk only on the premises of the producer and seller."[29] Underneath the text of the proposed legislation was a note that appeared to be from the governor or an aide: "This statute sounds reasonable. Please advise the problem you see with it?"

Also attached was the text of a talk by a Maine farmer, John O'Donnell, who wanted to let the governor know what was behind the food sovereignty movement, and why the FDA was out to stamp out small dairies: "As you may know, several Maine towns passed food sovereignty resolutions last year. This was mainly driven by small farmers experiencing unfair regulations that are barriers to entry, and restraint of trade. Many of these farmers fought for the same Maine bills I did, and saw how the Subcommittee on Agriculture was mainly under the control of the large farm and dairy interests and would never let small farm bills out of committee favorably. We also saw how the Department of Agriculture testified in these hearings that there would be repercussions from the USDA or FDA if we relaxed the standards for selling poultry, milk, and other products in our local communities and state."[30] Under this paragraph was a handwritten note, presumably from the governor or an aide: "Why would this concern us, if the products are sold intrastate."

There is no record of Whitcomb responding to the governor, but there is evidence of his department's fears of the FDA interfering in Maine's food affairs. This became apparent in follow-up communication Heather Retberg had with officials at the department. They pressed her to obtain a raw dairy permit after the testing of her farm's milk for crypto.[31] In a written response, Retberg posed a what-if question to a Maine agriculture official: If she had an agriculture department permit, would the agency be able to protect her from possible enforcement action by the FDA? She attached information about an owner of Estrella Family Creamery, a Washington State raw milk cheese maker that was shut down by the FDA in 2010. Retberg said that owner Kelli Estrella was "a licensed, prize-winning cheese maker in Washington state who had worked well and favorably with her Department of Agriculture, but was left unprotected from FDA aggression and is still struggling through an awful ordeal and has ceased making cheese and may yet need to sell the farm."[32] (The FDA eventually filed suit in federal court against the Estrella creamery, based on findings of listeria in its cheese-storage areas, seeking to force it to agree to stringent and costly FDA inspections.) Steven Giguere, a Maine Department of Agriculture program manager, responded: "If FDA attempts to regulate in-state sales of raw milk and we can show results of high quality milk being produced by licensed distributors who meet the standards for quality set out in the PMO [pasteurized milk ordinance] we can make a very good case that Federal intervention is not necessary."[33]

Actual evidence feeding the state regulators' fears came up in a May 2011 memo from the CDC to state epidemiologists and public health veterinarians, which stated in part: "In 1987, the FDA prohibited the distribution of raw milk over state lines for direct sale to consumers. Despite the federal ban on sale of raw milk across state lines and broad use of pasteurization by the dairy industry, human illness and outbreaks associated with consumption of unpasteurized products continue to occur. Raw milk is still available for sale in many states, and CDC data shows that the rate of raw milk-associated outbreaks is higher in states in which the sale of raw milk is legal than in states where sale of raw milk is illegal. . . . To protect the health of the public, state regulators should continue to support pasteurization and consider further restricting or prohibiting the sale and distribution of raw milk and other unpasteurized dairy products in their states."[34] In other words, become even more restrictive, the CDC was saying to states like Maine.

So when Whitcomb responded via a form letter to all of the people who had written in, including farmer John O'Donnell, the tension between federal interference versus the governor's concerns about burdening farmers with excessive regulation seemed as though it was coming to a head. The letter acknowledged O'Donnell and everyone like him who "shared . . . thoughts with the Administration regarding local food sovereignty ordinances."[35] Then it defended his department's posture. The letter stated in part: "Local food sovereignty ordinances leave the false impression that residence in certain towns exempt[s] individuals from food licensure and inspection requirements. Because the ordinances conflict and would frustrate the purposes of state food licensing and inspection laws, these ordinances are preempted by state law . . . persons who fail to comply [with state laws] will be subject to the Department's statutory responsibility to enforce state law, including the removal from sale of products from unlicensed sources and/or the imposition of fines."[36]

The Maine Department of Agriculture thus seemed to cast its fate with a federal agency rather than with its own constitutional superior, the governor — but perhaps for good reason. Civil service employees know well that politicians come and go, while the employees remain — often having to try to survive in an atmosphere of draconian budget cutting. The Maine agricultural regulators may have decided, as recalled in chapter 4's description of how the FDA influences state employees to cooperate with the agency, that their best opportunities for future revenue growth were going to come from the FDA as a reward for their support of John Sheehan and the FDA.

De Tocqueville marveled in 1831 at the degree to which towns and states worked together. "In the township, as well as everywhere else, the people is the only source of power; but in no stage of government does the body of citizens exercise a more immediate influence," he wrote. "In America the people is a master whose exigencies demand obedience to the utmost limits of possibility."[37]

As the debate over food sovereignty exemplifies, things are quite different in America today. Government agencies guard their power, and seek to expand it where possible. When the town of Blue Hill passed its food sovereignty ordinance a month after Sedgwick, in April 2011, Whitcomb wrote to Blue Hill's town managers a short and emphatic letter similar to what he would later write to farmer John O'Donnell: "The ordinance purports to exempt local residents from certain food licensure and inspection requirements. . . . The ordinance is preempted by state law. . . . Town residents involved in food processing and sales activities which are subject to state licensing and inspection are not exempt from those requirements. . . . Persons who fail to comply will be subject to enforcement, including the removal from sale of products from unlicensed sources and/ or the imposition of fines."[38]

True to its word, the agency ordered its inspectors during the summer of 2011 to begin monitoring local farmers selling food to residents in the towns that had passed food sovereignty laws. They took special note of a tiny farm owned by Dan Brown, a Blue Hill farmer with a single cow, who sold raw milk, cottage cheese, pickles, and jam from a small farm stand near his house, as well as at a couple of farmers markets. An agriculture department agent made purchases. The state tested the milk and cottage cheese for pathogens as well as for conventional bacteria counts. Shortly after, a Maine agriculture official working on the case e-mailed a supervisor: "Sounds like we have our first test case."[39]

In November 2011, the state of Maine and agriculture commissioner Whitcomb filed suit in state court seeking an injunction against Brown and fines for violations of three state laws: selling milk without a permit, selling milk in bottles without the right labels, and selling pickles and jam without a food establishment license. The suit said the department "informed the Defendant of the health risks involved with the sale of these products. The Department demanded that the Defendant stop the sale of the products until he is properly licensed, and offered to work with him to expedite the process. The Department received no response from the Defendant."[40]

Brown, an amiable, large-bellied man with a goatee, had on several occasions told the inspectors verbally that he didn't think he needed to obtain a permit to sell raw dairy, especially after his town passed the food sovereignty ordinance. He responded publicly after the suit was filed — via a Facebook page[41] and a YouTube recording.[42] He said he had become involved in selling raw milk a couple years earlier, after unhappy experiences in the conventional dairy industry, where farmers get "pennies a pound" for their milk from processors. The economics of selling raw milk were much more favorable, he indicated, and everything had been working out until the Department of Agriculture "changed the rules." He concluded: "I didn't change anything I was doing, they changed the rules."[43]

Maine's suit against farmer Dan Brown — or "Farmer Brown," as he came to be known — moved forward with all the trappings of a major case. The Farm-to-Consumer Legal Defense Fund became involved on behalf of Brown. Witnesses, including Dan Brown, were deposed. By the summer of 2012, the two sides had amassed 170 pages of arguments. In an early action, fairly routine for a major case, each side moved for "summary judgment" — asking a judge to rule in its favor in advance of the case going to trial.[44] Even if the judge took the unlikely step of making such a clear-cut early ruling, the case would likely proceed via appeals.

The 170 pages provided revealing insights into a case that might, for the first time in American history, provide judicial guidance as to the rights of municipalities to assert food rights in contradiction of long-standing state and federal regulations. Lawyers for the Maine attorney general sparred with defense lawyers for Farmer Brown over whether the food sovereignty ordinances passed by Maine towns should be allowed to stand. Lawyers for Brown argued that the state effectively allowed the private sale of raw milk by small farms that didn't advertise for many years prior to 2009. That was the year it began targeting all raw dairies for licensing. The state responded that the no-advertising provision was just one of a number it used to determine whether dairies needed to be licensed.[45]

Central to the case was the power of local rule versus state and federal authority. The lawyers offered divergent interpretations of Maine's home rule provisions, which allow wide municipal independence. Brown's lawyers argued that the Maine constitution, and home rule laws growing out of it, provided clear precedence for Maine towns to enact laws independent of state regulations. The state argued, essentially, that the home rule provisions were never intended to be applied so as to interfere with the state's broad powers to regulate food, and especially dairy. Food, after all, is a special area in the state's judgment, since it is so dangerous.

Especially revealing was the state's supporting evidence for its assertion that allowing private sale of raw milk and other products would "have serious public health consequences."[46] The largest single chunk — about 15 percent of the paper volume — consisted of printouts from the CDC about all the ways people can get sick from pathogens, how dangerous raw milk supposedly is, and how people can "protect" themselves from food-borne illness. A big chunk of that included the now-familiar "estimates" about the amount of food-borne illness in the United States — that 48 million people get sick and 3,000 die each year from food-borne illness, and detailed breakdowns of these "estimates" by pathogen.

There was no hard data covering the localities in question — for example, how many people had become sick from tainted food in Blue Hill and other Maine towns since they enacted the food sovereignty ordinances, most of them well over a year earlier. How many illnesses had there been from raw milk in the state of Maine over the previous five years, what with many dairies having opted out of the state's supervision? That question was raised to

Maine officials by a reporter with *Food Safety News*. Amy Robbins, an epidemiologist at the Maine Center for Disease Control and Prevention, replied via e-mail in November 2011: "In the past five years no outbreaks related to raw (unpasteurized) milk products have been identified in Maine." But, she added hopefully, "outbreaks related to raw (unpasteurized) milk products have occurred in other states."[47]

By the fall of 2012, the issue continued to reverberate in state legislative races. In one legislative race in the area of Portland, Maine's largest city, a Republican candidate (Mike Wallace) said in a newspaper debate with his Democrat opponent: "I would work to ease regulations for local farms, to allow them to sell directly to neighbors. Items such as raw milk, artisan cheeses and fermented foods are community driven, and thrive on best practices. Family farms do not have the resources to be concerned with how Augusta or the FDA will step in with largely arbitrary regulations. I will be an advocate for them."

It was encouraging to see politicians positively raise the food rights issue. But how would judges and juries rule in the many cases that were accumulating around the country?

CHAPTER 10

THE SEARCH FOR A ROSA PARKS MOMENT

As actions against farms and food clubs increased between 2010 and 2012, many consumers around the country dependent on private food became outraged. They wanted to fight back. But how? The food sovereignty movement based in Maine offered one approach. Its main drawback was that it was relatively quiet and obscure. The small towns passing ordinances didn't get a lot of media attention, and the legal challenge mounted by the state of Maine (which might spread to other states) could well slow the pace of town adoptions — with the actual outcome, after appeals and legislative battles, uncertain. One encouraging note by the end of 2012 and the beginning of 2013: legislators in a handful of states, including Virginia, Iowa, Wyoming, Ohio, and even Maine, were in the midst of pushing laws that would have a similar effect as the small towns' ordinances, of making food sovereignty a statewide option. They had to make it past their legislatures, though, and that wasn't a given in any of the places.

A national protest movement replete with rallies and petitions was another option. The main challenge for an emerging food rights movement was that even though the number of people regularly accessing food on a private basis was growing quickly, the total was still relatively small — perhaps one million nationally, according to an estimate by John Moody, organizer of a Kentucky food club and author of a handbook on establishing a food club. It's difficult enough to engage people to support rallies and protest activities when they have direct experience with the issue, but you can forget about attracting a critical mass if people have little or no personal knowledge of the issue at stake. Certainly many people I knew, even though they were interested in food issues like GMOs and organic production, and shopped at farmers markets, hadn't yet explored private food clubs and had difficulty appreciating the intensity of the crackdown by state and federal regulators.

Most people know the civil rights movement exploded during the 1960s, but what tends to be overlooked is that it actually launched fifty years prior, with the founding of the National Association for the Advancement of Colored People (NAACP) in 1909. The push for racial equality directly affected millions of people — 20 percent of the population was black, after all — yet it sputtered for nearly half a century, with decades of ongoing official and unofficial segregation, voter discrimination, lynchings, and negative court rulings before Martin Luther King Jr.'s Southern Christian Leadership Conference began its large-scale demonstrations in the early 1960s.

Comparing the food rights movement to the civil rights movement might be a tad grandiose; a more comparable movement might be that for homeschooling that began in the early 1980s. At that point, homeschooling was banned in all fifty states. The movement began with small groups of parents insisting on the right to educate their children at home, rather than in public or private schools. Yet the homeschooling movement seemed not to have to confront the intensity of official resistance and harassment as the food rights movement was encountering. By the early 1990s, lobbying and court actions had eliminated many of the obstacles in various locales, like curriculum approval and student competency assessment — although legal battles over school credits and registering continued. By the first years of the new century, the bureaucratic inhibitions were even fewer, and a handful of states didn't even require homeschoolers to register.

So the perceived discrimination and tough state and federal resistance to food rights continue to prompt comparisons to the civil rights struggle. In the view of food rights advocates, there was one tactic the civil rights movement used to great effect: civil disobedience. It was civil disobedience — ignited when Rosa Parks refused to move to the back of a Montgomery, Alabama, bus in 1955 and eventually affirmed when the U.S. Supreme Court ruled that the bus company's segregation was illegal — that in retrospect was key to what followed. The power of one or just a few people to attract media attention and energize supporters turned the tentative civil rights movement into a full-fledged national issue in the 1960s.

The leadership that was taking hold around food rights began looking at civil disobedience as a potentially galvanizing tactic. Up until the 2010 raid on Rawesome Foods, the food rights leaders had been the raw milk proponents Aajonus Vonderplanitz and James Stewart. They were leaders more by default than because of their ability to organize and plan strategy. Their public and bitter falling out following the government raid of June 2010 undid any claim to national leadership they might have had, however. Into the lurch stepped several mothers of young children who had been members and organizers of two of the food clubs most directly affected by the government assaults — Grassfed on the Hill in Maryland and Rawesome in California. Liz Reitzig and Karine Bouis-Towe of Grassfed were joined by Laurie Cohen of Rawesome and became the de facto leaders, with help from food clubs and sympathetic organizations around the country, including the food sovereignty movement in Maine. They started the Farm Food Freedom Coalition, which aimed to bring farmers and consumers together for the cause of food rights — and out of that arose a new organization to use civil disobedience to challenge the FDA's prohibition on the interstate sale of raw milk, known as the Raw Milk Freedom Riders.

Reitzig, the mother of five young children she homeschooled, was the organized and disciplined leader. She felt that farmers were shouldering much more of the risk from government interference in private food than they should. It was up to consumers to step up to the plate — indeed, to form a shield around "the courageous farmers who are sacrificing everything for our food."

Reitzig insisted on regular conference calls involving local food rights leaders from around the country, especially in states that had experienced crackdowns like Wisconsin, Minnesota, and California. They received important backing from a sensitive and charismatic leader with important experience in civil disobedience — Michael Schmidt, the Canadian raw dairy farmer who had been raided three times by Canadian food authorities between 1993 and 2006 and then charged with multiple violations of the dairy laws of Ontario, where he lived. Through all the assaults against him, which cost him three-fourths of the land on his farm to pay off legal and other debts — as well as his first marriage — he preached nonviolence and negotiation to find common ground. He won a huge court victory against the Ontario government when a judge ruled in his favor in early 2009 on the dairy law violations, agreeing with Schmidt that private food organizations are entitled to operate apart from the publicly regulated food system. Unfortunately, Canada doesn't have as complete a prohibition against double jeopardy, as the United States does, so the government appealed his acquittal — and an appeals court reversed the ruling in late 2011. Schmidt then went on a thirty-seven-day hunger strike that attracted wide attention in Canada and the United States and ended only when the Ontario premier agreed to Schmidt's demand for a personal meeting. From a leadership perspective, Schmidt's only problem was a big one — that he was Canadian, and not American, and thus not fully familiar with the American political and judicial system, and also not a direct victim.

Reitzig delegated authority and organized demonstrations in support of Daniel Allgyer in Washington and Vernon Hershberger in Wisconsin. She encouraged local groups of food club members to do the grunt work. She was demanding — she became upset when participants said they had to skip a food rights event because of kids' soccer games or dance recitals — but full of effusive public praise for those who pitched in. Reitzig recognized early on that a successful civil disobedience campaign required two essential ingredients: victims who aroused sympathy and an incident that aroused indignation — of the Rosa Parks sort.

As for the victims who could potentially arouse sympathy, there were plenty: Daniel Allgyer, Vernon Hershberger, David Hochstetler, Michael Hartmann. Some aroused more sympathy than others. Though Michael Hartmann, the Minnesota farmer, had fiercely loyal customers, he had the shadows of a 2010 outbreak of illness linked to his raw milk hanging over him. One family had actually filed suit against him, alleging their young son had been hospitalized with hemolytic uremic syndrome (HUS), a dangerous side effect from infection with *E. coli* O157:H7, supposedly from the Hartmann milk.[1]

But not only did the farmer and food club organizer victims need to arouse sympathy, they needed to be resilient to stay the course — and their families needed to stay tough as well. As it turned out, that was a lot to ask. While these four farmers were all outraged by the government attacks, they were also inexperienced standing up against the pressures of intensified law enforcement. They were, after all, mostly law-abiding citizens before running up against the Food Police.

Law enforcement professionals, on the other hand, specialize in bringing pressure to bear on accused lawbreakers. Police know how to mount an intimidating show of force, play potential defendants off against each other, and scare defendants into ratting on each other or pleading guilty to accusations so as to try for judicial leniency. A number of the farmers and food club managers failed to appreciate the intensity of and assorted tactics in the regulator and prosecutor bags of tricks.

Take Daniel Allgyer. The lanky Amish farmer had expressed his commitment on a number of occasions to continuing to produce food for the Grassfed on the Hill food club regardless of what the federal judge in the case, Lawrence Stengel, ruled. The expectation was that he would issue a ruling backing the U.S. Justice Department. Everything in the months since the agency had filed for the injunction in early 2011 had favored the government—including acceding to its requests to hold all hearings and conferences by phone and via written filings, so that there would be no court appearances where supporters of Allgyer might congregate and make their views known. And, indeed, when Judge Stengel did finally issue his ruling on the FDA's request for a permanent injunction, in early February 2012, the result was pretty much as expected. He went along with the agency's request to block Allgyer from supplying the Maryland food club with milk for at least five years, but he did so in harsher terms than Allgyer supporters might have hoped.

Judge Stengel gave no credence to the private contractual arrangement between Allgyer, Grassfed on the Hill, and Right to Choose Healthy Food (RTCHF). At the time the injunction was requested, RTCHF had leased Allgyer's cows, and the members of Grassfed on the Hill were members of RTCHF—having signed individual agreements and paid annual dues. In footnotes accompanying the decision, the judge mistakenly labeled the leasing arrangement "a cow share," an error that may have been a reflection of his disdain toward private food arrangements—almost as if to say, "cow share, herd share, leasing, whatever the hell you call it, it's all the same BS to me, just verbiage to avoid following the law."

Judge Stengel wrote: "The contract between Mr. Allgyer and persons entering into a cow share agreement is merely a subterfuge to create a transaction disguised as a sale of raw milk to consumers. The practical result of the arrangement is that consumers pay money to Mr. Allgyer and receive raw milk, which is transported across state lines and left at a 'drop point.' As such, despite any artful language, the agreement involves the transfer of raw milk for consideration, which constitutes a sale and is lawfully regulated by the FDA."[2]

In fact, given other statements from the judge, it seems doubtful he would have approved of the milk moving from Pennsylvania to Maryland even if it only happened to be in someone's pudding or cereal. He suggested in a footnote that individuals who traveled to Allgyer's farm to pick up their milk and bring it back to Maryland would be in violation of federal law as well. He said that "the purchase of raw milk by one who traveled between states to obtain it, or traveled between states before consuming it or sharing it with friends or family members, implicates 'commerce between any State.'" He noted that courts have interpreted the purpose behind the interstate commerce provision of the federal Food, Drug, and Cosmetic Act to be to "safeguard the consumer from the time the food is introduced into the channels of interstate commerce to the point that it is delivered to the ultimate consumer."[3]

Judge Stengel appeared to be interpreting the ban on interstate raw milk shipments even more stringently than the FDA, which had said it wouldn't enforce the prohibition for individuals bringing it across state lines for their own use. In other words, Judge Stengel was implying, the agency should be listening to the National Milk Producers Federation, which had warned the FDA in November 2011 to "stand firm" and "hold fast" against raw milk advocates, who were advocating weakening or eliminating the ban on interstate raw milk shipments.[4]

The only potential good news in the judge's decision was that it did not affect Allgyer making milk available in Pennsylvania, where it is legal to sell raw milk, nor did it prohibit him from supplying food other than raw milk to the Maryland club. But the club members most of all wanted their milk, and they were located in Maryland, not Pennsylvania. Raw milk can't be legally sold, or even made available via a cowshare, by Maryland farms.

The main hopes put forth by the judge for lifting of the order were if Congress were to pass a law rescinding the interstate ban on raw milk or a federal judge were to rule against the FDA in a suit challenging the ban — such as that brought by the Farm-to-Consumer Legal Defense Fund in early 2010. "If the FDCA [Food, Drug, and Cosmetic Act] is amended or modified to allow the interstate sale of raw milk or raw milk products," then Allgyer could resume shipments to Maryland, the judge said.[5]

Unfortunately, a few months after Judge Stengel wrote those words, a federal judge in Iowa dismissed the Farm-to-Consumer Legal Defense Fund suit challenging the FDA and its ban on interstate shipments of raw milk, saying the Farm-to-Consumer Legal Defense Fund hadn't shown injury to any of the plaintiffs.[6] Representative Ron Paul had introduced legislation to lift the federal ban, but it had only a few committed supporters by 2012.

The only other potentially encouraging news for Allgyer was that the judge refused to grant the FDA its request for open-ended inspections of his farm — and to be able to charge Allgyer expensive hourly fees that could total thousands of dollars per inspection. The judge cited a 2009 case involving Organic Pastures Dairy Company, in which a California federal judge denied a similar wide-ranging request from the FDA after Mark McAfee's dairy pleaded guilty to selling raw milk across state lines. It was as if the judge saw himself standing up for the Amish farmer by refusing to grant the FDA *everything* it sought, and maybe helping the poor guy stay in business by throwing him a few crumbs. "Like Organic Pastures Dairy Co., I find that the proposed injunction submitted by the government in this case is overly broad."[7]

What about appealing the case? That would be difficult in any event, and nearly impossible without a lawyer — but the question turned out to be moot. A few days after Judge Stengel issued his order, Allgyer shocked Reitzig and Bouis-Towe, telling them that not only would there be no appeal, but that there would be no more food. He was opting out of farming completely. He and his family had had enough of the stress of dealing with government authorities. He and his wife, Rachel, wouldn't risk the safety of their eight children with gun-toting agents visiting the farm to check on their activities. He was planning to sell his animals and equipment and do something else, perhaps returning to carpentry.

In a statement to members of Grassfed on the Hill, Bouis-Towe said: "Dan and Rachel Allgyer have determined that they will discontinue service to our group and close down the farm. Dan has served many of us for more than six years and he is very saddened to have to make this decision but the stress and strain that his family has been under for the past few years due to the case and now the decision has given them no other choice."

Club members reacted with understandable anguish to having their supply of good healthy food yanked out from under them.

"NO! NO! NO!" exclaimed one on the club's listserv. "I am deeply anguished. I truly wish that those wicked people whose combined efforts led to this horrible outcome could have a share in our suffering."

Said a second member: "This made me cry as I do drink the milk for medical reasons. If anyone finds another source please call me at the number below. Thank you."

And a third: "Dan has to shut down the farm to stop the unrelenting war on his family, the very serious danger to his wife and children, from federal officers supported by your taxes. . . . It is easy and safe to attack the Amish, since they are well known to be pacifists. The federal officials supported by your taxes are not brave."

But Tim Wightman, a farmer-turned-dairy-consultant and head of the Farm-to-Consumer Foundation (an offshoot of the Farm-to-Consumer Legal Defense Fund), probably captured the difficulties confronting Allgyer better than anyone. His observations were based on Wightman's own difficulties dealing with Wisconsin authorities a decade earlier, when an outbreak of illnesses was tied to raw milk from his dairy. When Allgyer announced he was discontinuing farming, Wightman wrote that food club members couldn't appreciate the tension that existed in the persecuted farmer's family dynamics. They "don't know the ill feeling one gets of cars that slowly drive by the end of the lane. . . . You hate the mistrust within that greets every new face and you worry when you let it drop if it was the conversation that just did you in. These things cannot be balanced with the natural flow of the land or families, no matter how many families are involved in our current arrangements, it is still the one farm family that is asked to bear the brunt of the issue, deal with each choking aspect of worry, which makes the very food you produce stick in your throat."[8] Once the decision is made to move on, "you hope this will begin the process, the dreams of anguish will fade and the smiles will return to the table of your loved ones and that food can be enjoyed once again. You pray for the strength for the scars to be healed."[9]

For the Rawesome Three, the situation was more tangled. There wasn't just a farmer (Sharon Palmer) legally ensnared, but a food club manager

(James Stewart) and a consumer who helped the farmer at farmers markets (Victoria Bloch, a graphics designer). After the arrest of Stewart and Palmer on additional charges in Ventura County in March 2012, they had two sets of charges against them — the original Los Angeles County charges related to selling unpasteurized milk without a license and the new charges concerned with loans to Palmer from Rawesome members and sympathizers for acquiring her Healthy Family Farms — which together could lead to up to forty years in jail for the duo.

Stewart was completely outraged about the new charges against him. "It's all lies," he told me. While he said he might have signed some legal paperwork at the request of Rawesome members who made loans to Palmer, "I had nothing to do with any of those loans." Eventually, at a four-day preliminary hearing in May at which some of the lenders testified, no one seemed able to link Stewart directly to either promotion of the loans or handling or signing documents in connection with the loans. Still, a judge concluded there was enough evidence for the case against both Palmer and Stewart to move to trial.

Stewart began seeking out advice from nonlawyer legal advisers similar to ProAdvocate. By mid-July 2012, he had missed a couple of court hearing dates — one in Los Angeles County on the original Rawesome charges and another in Ventura County on the new charges. Mark McAfee learned about the missed court dates and became concerned that the hundred thousand dollars he had pledged via the deed on his dairy as bail for Stewart might be forfeited.

In another bizarre twist to this already bizarre tale, McAfee engaged bail bond security agents, who have police powers to arrest individuals charged with skipping bail; they took Stewart into custody by luring him outside his Venice apartment, dazing him with pepper spray, and handcuffing him before whisking him away to jail. By October 2012, three months later, he remained jailed in Ventura County while awaiting trial. He had lost weight and rediscovered yoga, prompting other inmates to nickname him "Stretch."

Eventually, friends of Stewart would mount an online petition campaign to free him as well as to get charges against Palmer dropped.[10] They alleged a variety of misconducts on the part of the Ventura County District Attorney's office, including the filing of charges even after they knew Palmer was pushing hard to repay the lenders from a legal settlement she had received. By the summer of 2012, Palmer had indeed repaid seven lenders a total of $750,000. This included $60,000 to Mary and Eric Hetherington, according to Mary.

The pressures in the Rawesome case not only got to Stewart, but they got to the third member of the triumvirate, Victoria Bloch, who was only charged in the original L.A. County case. Like Daniel Allgyer, she had pledged to fight the charges accusing her of handling raw milk distribution at farmers markets on behalf of Palmer and her community-supported agriculture establishment, and thus violating prohibitions on selling raw milk and improperly labeled products. The charges were less onerous than those against Palmer and Stewart but could still land her in jail for more than two years.

Eventually, Bloch's enthusiasm for fighting the charges flagged. More than a year after the original charges had been filed, in September 2012 — just as a long-awaited preliminary hearing was about to get under way at which the state would finally have to present its key evidence in the case — Bloch, together with Palmer, took a deal from the prosecutor. Bloch pleaded guilty to one misdemeanor — selling improperly labeled milk — paid a one-hundred-dollar fine, and would be on probation for a year. Palmer pleaded guilty to a single misdemeanor of selling raw milk produced in unsanitary conditions, paid a five-hundred-dollar fine, and would be on probation for three years. (Because Stewart was jailed in Ventura County and had a court date there that conflicted with the L.A. County preliminary hearing, his proceedings in L.A. County were delayed; he didn't get a plea-bargain offer at that time.)

Perhaps the saddest case of opting out involved Rae Lynn Sandvig, the sociable and gregarious Minnesota mom I described in chapter 4, whose home was forcibly searched for raw milk and beef by agents from the Minnesota Department of Agriculture (MDA), local police, and public health authorities in 2010 in the aftermath of an outbreak of illnesses from raw milk. Later that year, Sandvig was summoned to an administrative hearing at the MDA, where she brought a lawyer and protested that she wasn't re-selling milk or meat, but rather just allowing her garage to be used as a drop site. The MDA eventually decided not to seek criminal charges against her and instead wrote her a letter of warning saying that if she didn't discontinue her activities, she could face criminal charges. Sandvig's inclination was to continue her activities as a drop site for the farmer, Michael Hartmann, and challenge the MDA to bring criminal charges against her. But by 2012 she had backed away. She told me her husband had insisted she dispense with offering their garage as a drop site, and her mental state had suffered to such an extent she wasn't about to fight him.

"I had always been a very outgoing person. I always used to pick up the phone. I don't now. I screen all my calls. We got drapes in the living room. We got a new lock for the front door. My husband watches who's driving on the street. . . . I saw two Jehovah's Witnesses coming up my walkway. I hid in that corner." She pointed to a corner of her spacious modern kitchen, tears welling up in her eyes. She wondered if she was showing symptoms of post-traumatic stress disorder.

To continue getting raw milk and meat from Hartmann, she picked it up from a friend who volunteered her garage as a drop site instead. That woman, along with at least eight other families, received warning letters from the MDA during the spring of 2012 saying that they could be subject to criminal charges for their activities.

All these events — the legal sanctioning of farmers like Daniel Allgyer, the complexity of charges and court proceedings that wore down and confused individuals like Victoria Bloch, and the intimidation that people like Rae Lynn Sandvig experienced — made it difficult for food rights organizers to come up with an incident of civil disobedience, or as some referred to it, "a Rosa Parks moment."

How would this special moment work? In the fantasies of food rights activists, it might well be an expanded version of an incident that occurred at John Moody's Kentucky food club. On a Friday afternoon preceding Memorial Day weekend in 2011, as a worker at the food club was setting out raw milk and other food for pickup by members, an inspector for the Louisville Metro Department of Health and Wellness appeared at the church basement storage site. He presented two pieces of paper: a cease-and-desist order (from the Louisville Metro Department of Health and Wellness) and a quarantine order (from the Kentucky Department for Public Health). And he placed "quarantine" notices on each of several coolers containing seventy-six half gallons of milk.

By the time members arrived later in the day, a new piece of paper had been placed on the coolers, Moody told me, which stated:

I, the undersigned, hereby declare that I have taken my milk that comes from cows I own via private contract under the protection of the KY constitution (articles 1, 2, 4, 6, 10, 16, 26), and if the county health department would like to speak with me about this matter, I can be reached at the number given below.

Before the afternoon was out, about forty members of the buying club had signed the statement and taken their quarantined milk. "A large number of my members pulled in and ignored the cease-and-desist and quarantine orders," Moody told me. In other words, these buying club members openly defied the Louisville public health authorities. In so doing, they became the first consumers to participate in such an act of group resistance in the name of food. That weekend, Moody and other members called state legislators at home to protest the regulators' move. Within a couple weeks, the public health authorities had backed off. The quarantine was over, and the food club had scored a big victory.

Unfortunately, it was inherently difficult to plan for such a moment, since one never knows when or how the authorities might pounce. If they conducted a raid to seize food, would food club members insist on taking possession of their food — especially if the enforcement agents were armed and possibly shouting orders to back off and threatening serious penalties?

Reitzig certainly would — she had read widely on various applications of civil disobedience through history and she organized "rights workshops" in Minnesota, Wisconsin, and Washington DC at which she and other food rights supporters advised local food rights organizers about how to challenge enforcement authorities. So while many were scared off by the events in Pennsylvania, California, and Minnesota, Reitzig convinced others to join her in a plan: Let's create a Rosa Parks moment. Have consumers publicly and openly transport raw milk across state lines and thereby challenge the FDA to make arrests and file charges.

The newly established Raw Milk Freedom Riders organized car caravans transporting raw milk across state lines and ending with demonstrations. In November 2011, they planned a seven-car caravan to transport raw milk from Pennsylvania to Maryland, where they planned a demonstration in front of FDA headquarters. The task of alerting the FDA was left to Max Kane, the brash young Wisconsin food club owner and raw milk activist, who attempted to telephone FDA dairy chief John Sheehan with the news a couple weeks in advance. He recorded his effort to inform the FDA of "a crime . . . a big illegal shipment of raw milk" in a thirteen-minute video he posted on YouTube. Not surprisingly, he never got beyond Sheehan's voicemail.[11]

A second caravan a few months later went from Wisconsin to Illinois, ending with a rally at a park in Chicago. Both events attracted a few hundred supporters and garnered a fair amount of media attention, but the FDA stayed away. In August 2012, the Raw Milk Freedom Riders teamed up with an organization protesting against the public health crackdown on lemonade stands. The two groups held a joint protest near the Capitol in Washington DC, at which they sold both raw milk and lemonade. One purpose of the protest was to attract the attention of the U.S. Capitol Police, who would hopefully arrest some of the one-hundred-plus participants for selling raw milk, lemonade, and other items without a permit. But the police kept their distance and avoided the entire affair.

The FDA and other enforcers appeared careful not to encourage more media coverage by arresting participants. Could a Rosa Parks moment possibly occur in court, perhaps by turning the trial of a farmer into a political event with lots of supporters, whose presence would help convince a jury to acquit — a kind of mini–Chicago Seven affair?

In May 2012, the Raw Milk Freedom Riders gathered a protest of more than two hundred people at the Hennepin County courthouse in downtown Minneapolis to support farmer Alvin Schlangen as he was due to go on trial. Authorities had, within a one-year period beginning in June 2010, raided his farm (two hours outside Minneapolis) and then his delivery van and a warehouse storage area in St. Paul and Minneapolis. The raids were followed by misdemeanor charges in 2012 of illegally selling unpasteurized milk off the farm on more than an "occasional" basis (as limited by law), selling unlabeled products, selling food without a retail license, and selling "adulterated" food products — which could lead to more than two years in jail.

But the effort to support Schlangen by showing up in large numbers at his court proceedings ran into another government tactic — delay. As dozens of protesters sat out in the hallway and in the courtroom with Schlangen, the prosecutor successfully maneuvered to have the proceedings delayed until September. You could almost hear the air come out of the collective group. It was a vivid lesson on the difficulties of providing organized national support to local court cases. They could easily be delayed, and the protest effectively disrupted. When Schlangen finally went on trial the following September, there were only about thirty or so people in the gallery instead of more than one hundred.

The authorities seemed to be outstrategizing their opponents. They also seemed to have the judges completely on their side. The federal judge in the Allgyer case agreed with the government's view that there was no such thing as private food rights. So did the Wisconsin judge who ruled against two farmers running private food clubs there (see chapter 4). In Missouri, the state judge had ruled against Morningland Dairy in its effort to stop the state from forcing it to dispose of more than two hundred thousand dollars of cheese. By 2012, a three-judge appeals panel had confirmed the first judge's ruling, agreeing that the cheese had to be disposed of.[12] How could Alvin Schlangen reasonably hope for anything different when he went on trial in September 2012?

It was late on a Wednesday evening, September 19, 2012. Alvin Schlangen was dead tired. He had just completed his third day on trial in a Minneapolis court, facing three misdemeanor charges alleging he sold raw milk and other foods without proper licensing and labeling (one of the original four charges had been dropped). The case had late in the afternoon gone to the six-person jury hearing the case, but after an hour and a half of initial deliberation, the three men and three women had ended their day without reaching a verdict and gone home.

Schlangen, a slender, soft-spoken man who with his closely cropped white hair looked quite fit for age fifty-five, joined about thirty members of the Freedom Farms Co-op he ran — mostly moms and their young children who had attended the trial proceedings — for a potluck dinner at one member's home. Then he hit the road for the two-hour drive back to his five-acre farm in Freeport. He would have loved to have stayed over in Minneapolis to avoid not only the trip home that evening but a return trip at seven the next morning, but he dared not leave his wife, Alice, alone.

Alice had been completely stressed by the events of the previous twenty-seven months leading up to the trial, beginning with the search of the couple's property on June 23, 2010, by agents from the Minnesota Department of Agriculture (MDA) accompanied by police. The targeting of Schlangen had nothing to do with any complaints from consumers or suggestions that his food made people sick. Rather, it was part of a crackdown (growing out of illnesses traced to the farm of another farmer, Michael Hartmann, the previous month) by the MDA on farmers and food clubs.

Coincidentally, the raid on his farm occurred just as Schlangen was in the process of partnering with another man to organize the food club. He had just a month earlier put three thousand dollars into setting up the arrangement. It was all part of a huge transition, begun in 2000, when he exited the conventional egg production business with some eighty thousand laying hens and began an organic egg production business that in 2010 morphed into the food club, which he served with just eighty hens at his farm. He also had lease agreements, modeled on Aajonus Vonderplanitz's arrangement, with nearby Amish farmers to supply unpasteurized milk and other food for his 140 food club members.

The details of the state's offensive against her husband didn't especially matter to Alice Schlangen, who was the family's breadwinner as a hospital coding expert — the person who figures out how to code the endless patient procedures carried out at hospitals for reimbursement by insurance companies. All she knew was that she and her husband seemed to have just lost three thousand dollars, on top of many thousands before that in the transition to organic and private food sales — losses that had them in serious debt to credit card companies. Now he was in trouble with the law.

"She thought it was a disaster financially, and the idea that her husband was a criminal was more than she could handle," Schlangen told me. Alice Schlangen moved out shortly after the MDA's search in June 2010. Members of Alvin Schlangen's own large family — he was one of eleven children — distanced themselves as well. "My siblings were embarrassed," Schlangen explained. One of them had served in Vietnam during the war there in the 1960s and 1970s and had trouble with Alvin's idea of protest.

Within a year of the MDA search of his farm in June 2010, there was more trouble from the MDA. On March 9, 2011, as he was delivering eggs and milk to members in the St. Paul area, Schlangen was stopped by MDA agents. They emptied his van of five thousand dollars worth of food. Later that day, they confiscated yet more food he stored at a Minneapolis warehouse. That second series of government raids was a low point for Schlangen. He felt very much alone.

Things seemed to begin getting better a few months later, when he rec-
onciled with Alice. "She had had time to understand it was our government
that was doing this, not the people of Minnesota."

At the start of the September 2012 trial, the Hennepin County judge,
Robert Small, had encouraged Schlangen to accept a prosecution offer to
plead guilty to one misdemeanor and walk out of the court a free man,
responsible only for two hundred dollars in court costs. At least Schlangen
thought that was the deal: "I didn't really understand the details of what the
judge was saying. I have a significant hearing loss from working in a machine
shop for ten years in my younger years. But I didn't need to hear the details.
If he didn't make the charges go away, I wasn't going to take any deal."

It didn't matter to Schlangen either when the judge warned that he
wouldn't feel bound to the terms of the prosecution deal proposal in the
event that Schlangen was convicted. In other words, the judge reserved the
right to impose harsher punishment on Schlangen, up to the maximum of
ninety days in jail and a thousand-dollar fine on each count, or a total of
nine months in jail and a three-thousand-dollar fine. Moreover, if he were
convicted in Hennepin County, the chances were good he'd be convicted
on similar charges in Stearns County (where there were actually six misdemeanor counts, including added ones associated with his alleged failure to
keep his eggs at prescribed temperatures, selling custom-slaughtered beef
and chicken, and removing embargoed food). Another eighteen months
there plus six thousand dollars in fines and he could be looking at more
than two years of jail time, plus nearly ten thousand dollars in fines. So the
stakes were high when he rejected the prosecution deal and plowed ahead
with a trial. And in the initial courtroom proceedings, it didn't necessarily
look like a smart decision.

The prosecutor, Minneapolis assistant city attorney Michelle Doffing-
Baynes, looked to be in her late thirties, with long brown hair and grown-
out highlights. She wore a black suit, and she played the fear card in her
opening statement. "This case is about a man," she said. "A man who chose
his business over public safety."

One of the state's key witnesses, twenty-eight-year-veteran MDA inspector James Roettger, testified that the reason Minnesota's law on raw milk
limited sales to the farm was so that buyers could "get it on the farm that
day and consume it that day." Each day after production, bacteria in the milk

quickly multiply so that after a "week's period of time [bacterial growth] may be ten, fifteen, maybe twenty times higher than what pasteurized milk was."

Roettger, a solidly built gray-haired man who appeared to be in his sixties, had achieved some measure of notoriety in the food rights community in December 2010 when he was caught on video confiscating raw milk being delivered to a Minneapolis suburb by a brother of farmer Michael Hartmann.[13] He was wearing a department beret and was dubbed "Beret Boy" by some food rights supporters. In his testimony, he claimed the "danger" was that "raw unpasteurized milk contains organisms like campylobacter, listeria, salmonella. All those things are food-borne illness organisms that could make someone very, very sick or could kill them."

Roettger's statements were an exaggeration because the naturally occurring "good" bacteria that multiply after production don't affect the milk's safety. And raw milk rarely contains pathogens, so whether milk is consumed the day it is produced or a week or two later is irrelevant. But Schlangen's lawyer, Nathan Hansen — a pleasant, goateed man engaged by the Farm-to-Consumer Legal Defense Fund, who was also a member of Schlangen's food club — didn't challenge Roettger on those assertions.

A second MDA official, compliance officer Levi J. Muhl, described the conditions at the warehouse where Schlangen stored food as being unkempt, with "potential vermin harborage." Produce he examined "was severely molded" and had a "very putrid" odor. Eggs, he said, "were held at room temperature, which is another violation of food code." He was much younger than Roettger, dark haired and fit, and had been with the MDA for eight and a half years. He described in ominous terms some kefir in Schlangen's storage area he had come across, describing it as "kind of a liquid yogurt type; I've never had it."

The state also pushed hard to make the case that Schlangen's private food club was nothing more than a food business like any other, geared toward maximizing sales and profits. Roettger, the MDA inspector, introduced about eighty exhibits — photos of food in Schlangen's van and in coolers, "invoices," "drop tickets," and product and price lists — all designed to communicate that Schlangen was taking and filling orders much like a retail business would. The prosecutor had Roettger read off the contents of members' orders, to emphasize her point that people were simply ordering food. Ann Walters, a middle-aged blonde woman and an MDA compliance officer for eleven years, pointed to exhibit #26, which she said was a photo of green beans, strawberries, and probably blueberries. She said there might be sausage or bratwurst in the photo as well. No matter — they were all things for which it would be necessary to have a retail food license to sell in the state of Minnesota.

The effort to stir up fear and distrust of the food provider was beginning to sound a lot like the Morningland Dairy case in Missouri nearly two years earlier, except there was one critical difference between the two court cases. The decision making on the Morningland case was entirely in the hands of a judge, but the decision making for Alvin Schlangen was in the hands of a six-person jury, three men and three women. In fact, Schlangen's was the first food rights case to come before a jury. All the others up until then had been heard by judges, and since the 2006 Ohio herdshare case decided in favor of dairy farmer Carol Schmitmeyer, none had exonerated a farmer or food producer.

There was no reason to think that the Schlangen case would turn out any differently except for the possibility that a jury of his peers might have a different perspective on the case than a judge would. That is, ordinary citizens might be more receptive to the notion that the state's regulations were unclear and arbitrarily enforced. They might more readily accept the idea of people obtaining their food outside the public food system, within a private realm not subject to the same bevy of rules.

Schlangen's lawyer initially attempted in his cross-examination of the MDA inspectors to demonstrate the vagueness of Minnesota's raw milk law, which limits sales to farms on an "occasional" basis. How often, he asked James Roettger, was "occasional"? If a consumer purchased from a dairy once a month? Twice a month? Three times a month? "I would think at that point in time [three times in a month] you're starting to get to the point where it's more than occasional and I would investigate it, yes," Roettger stated. When the defense lawyer asked the same question of Levi J. Muhl, he thought half a dozen purchases a month would be more than occasional. (The prosecution and defense witnesses weren't allowed to hear each other's testimony.)

The key defense witnesses were two members of Alvin Schlangen's Freedom Farms Co-op. One of them was Kathryn Niflis Johnson, a holistic health counselor who had trained as a registered nurse. As Hansen led her through her rationale for consuming raw milk and joining a food club, a much different picture than that provided by the prosecution began to emerge.

Hansen inquired as to why Johnson drank unpasteurized milk.

"I believe in the health benefits," the intense brown-haired woman said. "I believe that pasteurized milk is a processed food."

"And how do you obtain this product?"

"Through a private buying club of which I am a member."

"Who assists with that, the administration of that buying club?"

"Alvin Schlangen."

"Could you explain the process for obtaining this product?"

"Well, it's my understanding that as a member we lease or own these animals, and so we have a right to whatever they produce. And so what we do is we place an order and food amount, and you know, I'm using the term order because this is like the way I look at it, this is a whole new model of relationship. . . . We place an order and then the food products are delivered by Alvin. And we pay our amount that goes toward overhead and labor it takes to produce that food."

"Is it your understanding that obtaining unpasteurized milk in Minnesota is legal?"

"Oh it's absolutely legal to obtain it, yes. Inconvenient maybe, but legal, yes. And that was the purpose of setting up this new model, because farms that you want to purchase the milk from are not close anymore. As they may have been in 1945 or whenever the statute was written."

"Do you know the farm and the farmer where your unpasteurized milk comes from?"

"Yes, I do."

"It doesn't come from more than one farm?"

"No, it doesn't."

"Have you had the opportunity to visit the farm where your cows are leased and where the milk comes from?"

"Yes, I have. And so has my fourteen-year-old daughter, who is accompanying me today."

"Have you ever received rotten or spoiled food that made you sick from your private buying club?"

"No, and I've been drinking — my family has been drinking raw milk for over ten years and it's never made us sick. And as a matter of fact, it has made us healthy."

"How often do you consume unpasteurized milk?"

"On a daily basis. I may not have some every day. On a regular basis certainly. I just had some for lunch!"

"Is it your intention when you obtain this product to be in violation of Minnesota law?"

"No, it's totally the opposite. The people who belong to this club, I would say . . . [each of us] wishes to be a law-abiding citizen. But it's really difficult to find a way to comply with the law that can be interpreted in so many ways. And so this was one way to find a way to be, to obtain this product legally. Another way is that, you know, two years ago there was a bill introduced to the legislature in both the House and the Senate to change the law, to clarify and change the law so it would be easier to be in compliance."

"How long would it take you to drive to get your unpasteurized milk?"

"Two and a half hours in one direction. So I could be spending five hours if I wanted fresh milk weekly."

"How much would that cost you gasoline-wise?"

"I haven't estimated, because I don't intend to do that. I want there to be a legal way for that to happen, and I believe there is."

As expected, the cross-examination by the prosecutor, Michelle Doffing-Baynes, was more challenging.

"Ms. Johnson, you said that you bought other products other than unpasteurized milk from Mr. Schlangen — is that right?"

"Well, you know, I'm not sure if we should use the term 'bought,' but yes, I have obtained other products from him."

When she said she obtained mostly milk and eggs, the prosecutor inquired if the milk came from Schlangen's farm or another farm. Johnson explained that while eggs came from his farm, the milk came from another farm, which she had also visited.

"Have you been to his Minneapolis warehouse?" Doffing-Baynes asked Johnson.

"I have been to the warehouse in Minneapolis . . . I don't really consider it 'his' warehouse. It was my understanding that he just leased a small portion of the warehouse. And I was even concerned that the description of the coolers, which by the way aren't like camping coolers, they're mechanical coolers, they're refrigerators."

Doffing-Baynes then asked if Johnson had seen a promotion for a winter market at the nearby Traditional Foods Minnesota club that had been shut down, or whether she had seen Schlangen's website promoting the special market. Johnson said she didn't recall having seen the flyer or having been at the winter market, but that it didn't surprise her that Schlangen's website was included. "The people who go to all the trouble to research this food are a community and we all work together. And so if somebody's, you know, holding an event, then somebody else might help promote it and might take part in it. So this doesn't mean that it was his, you know, winter market necessarily. But, obviously, he was involved in it in some way."

Doffing-Baynes wondered if Johnson was aware if Schlangen's food was inspected.

"I guess I can't really speak to that," she said.

"Do you know whether or not he has a license to handle food in the state of Minnesota?" the prosecutor asked.

To which Johnson responded, "I am under the understanding that with this model that we're operating under, that's not necessary. And actually, I don't think you can obtain a license to handle or distribute raw milk, so it's kind of a catch-22."

"But the food, you can obtain a license to handle food, right? Like a grocery store or a food truck?"

"I suppose you could. But it's my understanding that, you know, we are under private contract and, you know, we probably discuss our food and know more about it than most people who eat."

"OK, so you don't think he has a license, right? Is that your testimony?"

"I don't know."

Finally, near the end of the second day of the trial, it was Schlangen's turn to testify. He had decided to testify, even though the U.S. Constitution's prohibition against self-incrimination meant he didn't have to, and that it wouldn't be held against him by the jury. But if he decided to testify, he would be subject to cross-examination.

There was no question in Schlangen's mind that he was going to testify, just as there was no question he wasn't going to take a plea deal. Schlangen is a sincere man, but given to roundabout explanations to simple questions. So easy questions from his lawyer about how he started the club or how he exercised care in transporting food at optimal temperatures elicited lengthy explanations about how slow-cooking meat with lots of fat is healthy for people, and about the inner workings of thermostats and how he arranged jars of cream in his coolers and alternated jumbo and extra-super-jumbo eggs in the cartons rather than separating eggs by size, like in the supermarket. Were the jurors tuning out?

Schlangen departed from the typical criminal defendant garb of dark conservative suit, white shirt, and tie and on the first day of the trial donned a Farm-to-Consumer Legal Defense Fund T-shirt, which had this affirmation on the back: WE'VE GOT YOUR FARMER'S BACK. On the day he was testifying he wore a light blue and green polo shirt. Would jurors be more sensitive to the political overtones of this case or turned off by the possibility he was a wacko, and his supporters in the gallery a bunch of wacko supporters?

The prosecutor tried to make similar points to those she had tried with Kathryn Niflis Johnson.

"You talked about raw milk. And you testified that you believed it is safe to drink; is that true?"

"I didn't make a general statement of raw milk safety."

"OK. So sometimes it's unsafe to drink raw milk; isn't that right?"

"I didn't say that and I won't."

"Have you heard of people getting sick from drinking raw milk?"

"Have I heard — I have never heard from an individual that they got sick from raw milk."

"You've heard it in the news, right?"

"I've heard it in the media, yes."

"You don't possess a license to sell food in the state of Minnesota, do you?"

"I don't have one."

"And you understand that grocery stores get inspected, right? In the state of Minnesota?"

"I don't know anything about what happens in a grocery store."

"But you're not inspected, are you?"

"Not by the Department of Ag, no."

The prosecutor then shifted to a photo of a sign on Schlangen's delivery van that said the van was private property, warning government agents to stay away, and asked the farmer to describe what he saw.

"It's the sign that identifies our space as being private."

"And not open to the public, right?"

"Right."

"Not open to the government, right?"

"The government is public to me, yes."

"OK. So it's fair to say that you're antigovernment, is that right?"

"That's not accurate."

"Just for your business?"

"I am antioverregulation."

"Your website says it's organic eggs. Is that right?"

"Right."

"But you're not an organic egg farmer, are you?"

"Are you kidding me?"

"Are you an organic egg farmer?"

"Our farm is not certified as organic."

"You're not?"

"Nobody owns that word."

"Because the government owns that word. Is that right?"

"I said nobody owns that word."

"But it's a government designation for food products, isn't it?"

"Certified organic is a designation of a food product."

"Do you think it's misleading that your website is called organic eggs?"

"The word organic is not owned by anyone. This is freedom of speech. If it's an organic — do you know what that word means?"

"I think I'm doing the questioning here, Mr. Schlangen, not you."

"OK."

"So the question is, are you a certified organic egg farmer? And the question could be answered by a yes or no."

"We are not certified organic at this time."

There was a fair amount of discussion about whether the Freedom Farms Co-op was really a conventional business in disguise as a cooperative volunteer effort. The prosecutor expressed confusion about the way his bills were paid, between Schlangen's personal credit card, farm checking account, and co-op checking account.

Schlangen explained how it made sense. "The food club is based on twenty different farms for a collective resource for 140 families. Our farm is just one of those potentially. And it [Schlangen's farm] is a business, it's supposed to be profitable, I'm not saying that it is." He added that "the

Freedom Farms Co-op account is used to pay for fuel, used for delivery . . . to pay for all the food that comes into the club."

Doffing-Baynes then concluded with questions about the price of eggs and milk.

"Mr. Schlangen, what are the prices on some of these products? For instance, you're an egg farmer. How much does an average carton of eggs cost at the grocery store?"

"I don't shop at the grocery store."

"How much do your eggs cost on this document?"

"We have values for our food."

"Are they four dollars per dozen? Is that right?"

"That would be the established value for that."

"And your milk is seven dollars per gallon, is that right?"

"A gallon of raw milk from our club is valued at seven dollars."

"Is it fair to say that your products cost more than the products in the grocery store?"

"I don't shop at the grocery store."

As he ended his testimony and returned to the defense table, Schlangen noticed that a number of the jurors were smiling. "I thought one of them was going to stand up and shake my hand," he said. Of course, it's difficult in such situations to know what people are thinking — whether the smiles were smiles of approval, or of sympathy for someone in trouble.

There had been another potentially encouraging development on the second day of the trial. Judge Small commended the half-dozen or so young children in the gallery section with their moms, saying he had never seen such "unfidgety" children before.

"It's the raw milk," one of the moms intoned.

"I didn't hear that," the judge responded. But, of course, the judge did hear it — and, more important, the jurors heard it.

But then, the same rule applies to judges — they can be nice to the defendants and defendant's supporters, even if they are convinced the defendant is guilty.

In her concluding remarks, the prosecutor summarized each witness's allegations. For example, one MDA employee "testified that Mr. Schlangen does not possess a food handler's license in the state of Minnesota. The state is requesting a verdict of guilty on all counts."

In his concluding remarks, Hansen, the defense lawyer, reminded the jury, "Raw milk is legal in the state of Minnesota, that's not disputed. The question is what the law says and how it is interpreted." According to the state's witnesses, he said, "every single person has to drive to the farm and get it for themselves. It is a cynical view or interpretation of the law as it is written. . . . There is no support as it is written for the things they read into it."

He described that in the case of Freedom Farms Co-op, "A voluntary group of people sends one person" to obtain the milk. He said there was no report of anyone receiving adulterated food. "There has been no testimony of anyone getting sick. And you know there would be if it had happened." On top of that, the food "was the property of the food club and not Mr. Schlangen." He concluded: "The Department of Agriculture's interpretation of these laws is ridiculous and I ask that you return a verdict of not guilty on all counts."

Prosecutor Doffing-Baynes was allowed to present a brief rebuttal argument. "A person in the United States can go into any grocery store in the United States and purchase an apple, have no concerns. A person can go into a store in a foreign country, buy an apple, and they may have concerns. Why? Food safety laws."

Shortly after the jury began its deliberations, it sent out a question to the judge: Were cowshare arrangements legal in Minnesota? The judge responded that the jury "has all the laws they need in front of them," and that they should continue their deliberations on that basis. But the fact that they knew about cowshare and herdshare arrangements suggested an unexpected sophistication about the matter of private food.

By 4:30 p.m., after an hour and a half of deliberations without having reached a verdict, the judge sent the jurors home. Schlangen had dinner with his supporters, then made his way to his farm, his fate still very much up in the air. There were all kinds of possible outcomes. While he could be found guilty of all three counts, Schlangen could also be found guilty of only one or two counts, and acquitted of one or two counts. Would a partial acquittal be a victory? It was also possible the jury could deadlock, with most in favor of acquittal or conviction, but one person holding out for the opposite outcome. In that event, the judge could declare a mistrial, and another trial might be held.

The possibility of being convicted was very much on Schlangen's mind that Wednesday night at his farm, so, tired as he was, he wrote an e-mail to the 140 members of his Freedom Farms Co-op:

> This note is to thank all of our FFC family that has prayed and otherwise projected helpful energy toward our goal of food freedom. . . . I tried to connect with (hug) every one of you as I recognized that you were there. This court experience was actually very much overdue for me. Although I do not look forward to being in this position again, I am much convinced that it will benefit me in the future. At this point, I am prepared (and explained to Alice) for the possibility that this jury may not know that they have the power to ignore a bad law and dismiss this case entirely. WE ARE PREPARED FOR THIS POSSIBLE OUTCOME! I've mentioned to some, that our food freedom movement might actually benefit from the shock of a trial having this outcome and that might be a reason for our creator to allow it to happen . . .

He reaffirmed his lawyer's contention about the inherent injustice of forcing people to travel hours to a farm for certain foods and concluded by considering the practical realities were he found guilty: "If this jury is confused about their power to do the right thing in this case, the thought of doing some jail time does not affect my determination to continue to volunteer for services to my food community. I've been told that in a misdemeanor case (such as this) it is common to take a few days to process and set an appeal bond to allow for a managed amount of cruelty (like putting a hen in a cage) based on the seriousness (or lack of) in the verdict. Thanks to all of you for being part of my (our) community! I've been hesitant to ask, but is there a member of our FFC coop family that would consider holding this volunteer position on a temporary basis?"

The next morning, about twenty-five of his supporters were in the Minneapolis court hallway, joining hands in an "energy prayer circle." By lunchtime, before anyone could volunteer to take over Schlangen's duties should he be jailed, the jury returned with a verdict. The clerk read out the verdicts:

Count 1: "Limitation on sale, milk pasteurization . . . not guilty."

Count 2: "Adulterated or misbranded food . . . not guilty."

Count 3: "License required for a food business . . . not guilty."

Schlangen remained stone-faced for several seconds, seemingly disbelieving what he had just heard — until he turned around. Behind him, in the spectator area, there were hugs and kisses and crying among the thirty or forty members of his food club and other supporters who had gathered in anticipation of the verdict. As Schlangen and his supporters prepared to leave the courtroom, someone asked in a hushed voice about that day's milk/food delivery, which had been postponed until the following day. Someone else piped up: "Hey! We can talk about it out loud now, can't we?" The Minneapolis *Star Tribune*'s front-page story the following day: "Minnesota Farmer Cleared in Milk Case."

The regulators were not conciliatory, however. There was no talk of potential cooperation with food club members, no mention of respecting the law. Within hours of the jury's verdict, the MDA issued a defiant statement that "we strongly disagree with this ruling." It added that "the fact that the jurors deliberated for as long as they did shows that they found the decision a difficult one to make."[14]

In point of fact, the jurors had little difficulty coming to agreement on their decision. After the verdict was issued, I made contact with the jury's foreman, Eric Hemingway, the square-jawed thirty-seven-year-old owner of his own investment advisory service. He said the reason the jury took nearly an entire day (spread over parts of two days) was because the judge had provided highly detailed instructions for determining guilt "beyond a reasonable doubt, and we tried to be very methodical in going through his instructions."

In the end, there were two key factors in the decision to acquit, Hemingway told me. First, the fact that no one became sick from Schlangen's food was very important. One of the three misdemeanor charges accused Schlangen of providing "adulterated or misbranded" food, and the absence of illnesses suggested no adulteration. As Hemingway put it, "No one was injured. . . . If anyone had gotten sick, that would have weighed on me." A second important factor was the notion that Schlangen wasn't selling but rather distributing food he obtained on behalf of members. "He was just connecting up people who wanted this food through his club," according to Hemingway. "People went in with their eyes wide open." Likewise, Schlangen "was a very credible witness," as were Kathryn Niflis Johnson and a second food club member who testified for the defense.

Hemingway indicated that there never was a lot of disagreement among the six-person jury. "Different people had different ways of explaining things to the others. Some played devil's advocate, some did what-ifs." In the end, though, there wasn't a situation where one or two jurors dissented and had to be convinced by the others, he said.

Hemingway told me that he knew little about the struggle over food rights before he was assigned to the jury, and that food choices aren't a huge deal in his family. He knew vaguely that more people were drinking raw milk, "but I've never had raw milk, I didn't grow up on a farm." He said when it comes to food in his family, "My wife does the shopping and I go to the refrigerator." Nor were other jurors raw milk drinkers. They were a diverse group, including a mechanic, a molecular genetic scientist, a corporate district manager, a marketing consultant, and a technical solutions architect — along with Hemingway, the investment adviser.

Hemingway added that his focus was on "being impartial. We were very deliberate and thorough." In the end, though, "the state failed to make its case. . . . You have to look at the law. You can't look at your own beliefs of what the law should be. . . . [Schlangen] was not in violation of the law." The law wasn't very clear in a number of areas, he noted. For example, the state charge that Schlangen was selling food without a retail license fell short in part because the law isn't specific in requiring food licenses for distributing food privately. The message from the six jurors — people without a vested interest in the outcome — seemed to be that so long as private food distribution wasn't making people sick, the government should back off.

And Hemingway's view may have been more detached than that of other jurors. I was also able to speak afterward with the mother of one juror, who had spoken with her daughter about the case. She didn't want to be identified nor did she want her daughter identified, but she told me that her daughter, the juror, said Schlangen "was a courier for the milk. . . . These people should have the right to drink what they want." She added that her daughter was moved after the verdict was announced. "It hit her heart that these people [Schlangen supporters] were so thankful. She felt real good about the decision she made."

If the jurors felt good, Schlangen felt even better. He recommitted himself to the fight for food rights — not only for himself, but for farmers around Minnesota and the rest of the country, even though he still faced similar criminal misdemeanor charges in another Minnesota court (along with MDA administrative charges in an administrative court). "Because of all of the energy in this community, I am able to become the man I truly want to be," he said in a follow-up e-mail to his supporters.

The full impact of the Schlangen decision won't be known for some time. But it sent an important message to regulators: prosecutors will likely be less inclined to accede to regulator demands to bring criminal charges against farmers and food clubs for distributing food privately. Prosecutors, after all, want to bring cases that will result in convictions, not acquittals.

"The fog has lifted," Schlangen told me.

The nascent food rights movement may well have experienced its Rosa Parks moment, but ironically, it didn't stem from civil disobedience. It came about because one man insisted on the right, guaranteed by the Sixth Amendment of the U.S. Constitution, that "in all criminal prosecutions, the accused shall enjoy the right to a speedy and public trial, by an impartial jury of the State and district wherein the crime shall have been committed . . ."

EPILOGUE

It would be nice to say this book has a happy ending, and that it's time to move on to the next issue, but life is rarely so tidy. The struggle over food rights will very likely be an ongoing one, certainly for many of the individuals and organizations featured in this book. Here is an update on some of them:

Grassfed on the Hill resurrected itself after the FDA's undercover investigation. Under the leadership of Liz Reitzig and Karine Bouis-Towe, it once again has hundreds of members in the Washington DC area. The food club now keeps information about its relationships with farmers highly confidential.

Rawesome Foods disappeared from its site in Venice, California—but members created at least three new food clubs, each of them smaller than the original Rawesome, and each with no permanent location. Their operations are also highly confidential.

James Stewart was released from jail in November 2012, after spending four months in custody. He had lost nearly 40 pounds, going from about 205 pounds down to just under 170 pounds. He says he lost much of his weight during the last five days after he was transferred from the Ventura County jail, where he says he was treated decently, to the Twin Towers Correctional Facility in Los Angeles, where he says he was shackled hand and foot and placed in the toughest part of the massive facility because there was a notation in his record that he had "attacked guards." "I have never attacked anyone," he told me. His lawyer was able to get him released on his own recognizance, and he emerged to a mountain of legal problems. He was able to quickly negotiate a plea bargain on the original Rawesome raw milk charges (like his two codefendants, Sharon Palmer and Victoria Bloch), pleading guilty to two misdemeanors and paying a small fine. He still faced the Ventura County charges, which were due to come to trial in early 2013, but eventually were delayed until at least the spring. According to one of his lawyers, Ajna Sharma-Wilson, in addition to the legal issues described in this book Stewart faced additional felony charges associated with income tax evasion on allegedly unreported revenues from Rawesome Foods. He also lost his one-third holding of the land where Rawesome was built when L.A. County sued him, and the other owners sold the property and used the proceeds to pay legal fees. While he spoke frequently in the days immediately after Rawesome was shuttered in August 2011 about resurrecting the food club, after he was released from jail in late 2012 he said he planned to "go in a new direction" and distribute premium olive oil. He said he had no regrets about having established and grown Rawesome and still can't understand why the legal system came down so hard on him: "I never hurt anyone, never made anyone sick."

Sharon Palmer was expected to go on trial in Ventura County in early 2013 on the charges in connection with the loans she secured to obtain her farm, though as noted, the case was delayed until at least the spring. She continued operating Healthy Family Farms and selling at farmers markets.

The owners of Missouri cheese maker Morningland Dairy, Denise and Joseph Dixon, shut down their cheese-making operations. As of the end of 2012, the thirty thousand pounds of cheese the state sought to have destroyed still sat in a cooler at the Missouri facility; in January 2013, with at least half the cheese rotten, the Dixons agreed to have the state cart it away and assembled a small group of friends to ceremonially mark the end of their resistance. The Farm-to-Consumer Legal Defense Fund appealed their case to the Missouri Supreme Court.

In Maine, a judge ordered the state and dairy farmer Dan Brown to attempt to negotiate a settlement of the state's suit of the farmer for failing to obtain a raw milk dairy license and a food retail license. By early 2013, the sides were reported to still be significantly apart. Presumably if they failed to come to a compromise, the case would go to trial.

The outcome of Alvin Schlangen's criminal trial, rather than discouraging or tempering the Minnesota Department of Agriculture, actually seemed to energize the agency to pursue him ever more aggressively. The MDA pushed ahead on an administrative case, seeking to have Schlangen declared in violation of state dairy and retail food laws. If the administrative judge issued such a declaration, and Schlangen didn't obey, he could once again be charged criminally. Plus, he still faced misdemeanor charges in his home county (Steans County) similar to those he was acquitted of in Hennepin County, and the prosecutor there moved forward aggressively toward a trial; he opposed a move by Schlangen's lawyer to dismiss three of the six charges, which were nearly the same as those he was acquitted of in Hennepin County, and in February 2013 a judge agreed with the prosecutor, ruling Schlangen could be tried on all six charges. The trial was scheduled for late spring 2013.

Wisconsin dairy farmer Vernon Hershberger was due to go on trial for criminal misdemeanor charges in early January 2013. The road to that trial turned out to be rocky, though. In advance of a pretrial hearing in late fall 2012, Hershberger received a plea deal offer: plead guilty to two misdemeanors, pay a fine, and agree to never again distribute food without a license. He told me he explained to his lawyer "that I would consider taking their offer if they can find me an injured party in this case. If they cannot find an injured party I would have to decline their offer because the Bible instructs me to help the poor and the needy and to share this world's goods with other people." Then, just a few weeks in advance of the scheduled trial, disputes broke out between the prosecution and defense over a variety of procedural issues, including jury instructions and which witnesses would be allowed to testify. The judge finally decided to delay the trial until at least spring of 2013, to review briefs by the two sides to resolve some of the disputes.

Daniel Allgyer was reported by friends to have shifted from farming to doing carpentry.

Aajonus Vonderplanitz's civil suit (together with Larry Otting) against Sharon Palmer and James Stewart seeking millions in damages for alleged slander and libel was reported to have been dismissed. Sharon Palmer continued to pursue a counter-suit against Vonderplanitz and Otting, in which she was seeking at least $4 million in damages for defamation and breach of contract.

Vonderplanitz continued the lease arrangements he had negotiated with a number of farmers via his Right to Choose Healthy Food organization, and he was never prosecuted in connection with Rawesome or any of the other farms and food clubs he was associated with.

California Department of Food and Agriculture investigator Scarlett Treviso was reported by the CDFA in early 2012 to "have taken another job."

ACKNOWLEDGMENTS

When you get lost in the details of writing a book over a period of many months, certain things become clear only in retrospect. Now, more than two years after I first decided to write a book about the struggle for food rights in America, it is clear to me that I had little sense of the enormity of the task that lay before me.

The big problem was explaining and documenting the scope of the issue. To most people, there is no obvious food rights problem. They go into a supermarket, and the bins and shelves are overflowing. How could there possibly be government-imposed limitations among scenes of such plenty?

Moreover, our government never declared itself in opposition to private food rights, at least at the time in 2010 when I first contemplated this book. That has changed — under the pressure of legal challenges from those experiencing the impingements on food rights, regulators and judges have declared limitations on our rights to access the foods of our choice, even if mostly on a private direct-from-the-farm basis.

Perhaps more significant, the government bodies have never revealed any kind of organized enforcement campaign against food rights — a declared war on private food akin to the wars on drugs and terrorists. Certainly there was evidence to the contrary, in the form of assorted enforcement actions, but these were always portrayed as discrete actions (usually undertaken on a local level) unrelated to one another.

So a much bigger challenge than I expected was simply documenting the extent of the unofficial campaign against food rights, connecting the dots (as it were) to make the case that much of the crackdown, via increased enforcement activity, is related — part of an organized campaign directed from Washington DC.

Regardless of how compelling you and others judge I made the case, I can say without hesitation that I couldn't have made the case nearly as well as I have without the selfless input of many individuals.

It's been my good fortune to have had many wonderful people supply me with or guide me toward important information, including thousands of pages of documentation necessary to describe the sometimes nearly unbelievable events that are the basis of this book. Certainly much of the information was of a sensitive nature, intended by government officials and investigators to be kept out of public view. Some of the individuals who provided information did so at personal risk, after deciding that it was in the interests of public education and debate to make the data available.

First and foremost, I want to thank the brave farmers who have been targeted for potentially serious criminal prosecution for the simple act of privately distributing food to individual consumers. Though going public heightens their legal risks, they have without exception trusted me to share their stories. These farmers include Daniel Allgyer, Amos Miller, David Hochstetler, Vernon Hershberger, Alvin Schlangen, Mark Nolt, Dan Brown, Michael Schmidt, Richard Hebron, and Denise and Joseph Dixon and son Isaac.

I also owe a debt of gratitude to many individuals in the budding food rights movement for their endless ideas, guidance, support . . . and patience. Putting together all the pieces of the jigsaw puzzle that is this book took longer than many of them expected, and it would have been natural for some to have given up on it, wondering if it would ever appear. But like the farmers, these individuals have stood by me — Liz Reitzig, Karine Bouis-Towe, Victoria Bloch, Doreen Hannes, Natasha Simeon, Melinda Olson, Sea J. Jones, Mark McAfee, John Moody, Max Kane, Deborah Evans, Heather Retberg, Laurie Cohen, Angela Doss, James Hopkins, Ajna Sharma-Wilson, Gayle Loiselle, Mike Adams (Natural News), Maurice Kaehler, Judith McGeary, Abby Rockefeller, Joseph Heckman, Yannick Phillips, Kristin Canty, Cyndy Gray, and Brigitte Ruthman. (There were so many that I fear having left some out; if I did, my apologies.)

I don't want to suggest that everyone in the food rights movement who supported my research was always in agreement with my interpretation of events — or with each other. The stresses that arose as government enforcement efforts intensified involved three especially controversial food rights activists who are a part of this book — Aajonus Vonderplanitz, James

Stewart, and Sharon Palmer. As terribly as they may have tangled among themselves, and sometimes even with me, each remained respectful and helpful in my work to complete this book.

Then there are the dedicated folks at the Farm-to-Consumer Legal Defense Fund — especially the organization's chief lawyers, Pete Kennedy and Gary Cox, together with board members Elizabeth Rich and Steve Bemis, and conference organizer/fund-raiser Cathy Raymond. They have been on the front lines of the legal struggle described in this book, and endless in their patience explaining various cases and subtleties of law to me. Of course, the FTCLDF wouldn't be able to do its noble work without backing from Sally Fallon and the Weston A. Price Foundation.

I was fortunate as well to recruit two very capable students at Suffolk University Law School in Boston — Chris Consoletti and Nimisha Parikh — to assist me in my research, thanks to references from a professor, Gabe Teninbaum. I was pleasantly surprised to discover they were mature and knowledgeable beyond their years about the investigative task at hand to verify events and issues in this book. Chris on the legal side and Nimisha on the policy side helped me gain access to important documentation that I wouldn't otherwise have known about. A physician friend, Leonard Finn, was an important sounding board about matters around pathogens and illness.

Then there were people on the government side who, even though they didn't necessarily agree with my views about food rights, went out of their way to help me obtain accurate information. There was Los Angeles County prosecutor George Castello and Ventura County prosecutor Chris Harman, who each took my calls and helped me track down documents and understand sometimes complicated legal issues. I had the same experience with Heidi Kassenborg, a dairy regulator with the Minnesota Department of Agriculture; Donna Gilson of the Wisconsin Department of Agriculture, Trade, and Consumer Protection; Annette Whiteford, California's state veterinarian; and Jessica Blome, a prosecutor with the Missouri Attorney General. Two former federal prosecutors — Tom Roche and John Fleder — also shared important insights and information, as did former FBI agent John Gamel. And Hugh Kaufman, long of the Environmental Protection Agency, provided important guidance on accessing relevant information.

I must also acknowledge essential support from the editorial side. Indexer Shana Milkie was selfless in helping me at a crucial time organize the book's voluminous endnotes, and thus give substance to this essential documentation. Jennifer Sharpe, a Los Angeles freelance radio reporter and writer, was exceptionally generous in sharing time and expertise. Brianne Goodspeed, a senior editor at Chelsea Green, and Margo Baldwin, its publisher, have also been extremely supportive with their criticisms and guidance in helping me get a handle on the endless complexities of this book's narrative and then in helping improve its readability via old-fashioned line editing, pointed questions, and assorted specific suggestions. My agent, Jennifer Unter of the Unter Agency, has been a patient and objective critic of my various ideas and drafts.

Virginia farmer Joel Salatin has been a supporter of this project from the beginning, providing me with ideas and encouragement all along my reporting and writing journey. I am honored that he wanted to author the book's foreword (the second time he has taken on this role — the first being for my previous book, <i>The Raw Milk Revolution</i>).

Last but not least, I must profusely thank my wife, Jean, for her endless patience and support as this book's research and writing extended well beyond what I originally expected, and thus intruded ever more into our lives.

DECLARATION OF FOOD INDEPENDENCE

MARCH 2012

In a spirit of humility, and with respect for both the just law of the land and the laws of nature, there are certain fundamentals in life which cornerstone the ideals of human dignity, and which a just society should hold untouchable from the opinions of the majority.

We hold that the right of the individual to exercise their personal judgment for the purpose of qualifying the food they eat is such a fundamental. We hold this right is given by God to all people.

In the spirit of natural human cooperation, we hold that consenting individuals are endowed by their creator with the right to procure the foods of their choice from a willing producer. We affirm the right of the People to peaceably assemble for the purpose of feeding themselves.

We affirm the right of the People to secure their preferred food through peaceful, private contractual trade without permission from the majority. The undersigned respectfully submit that we will reject, via peaceful noncompliance, laws and regulations that infringe on our rights to obtain and eat the foods of our choice.

We would rather be struck by the hand of the oppressor than comply with laws and regulations that compromise our dignity and demoralize the very essence of what it means to be a free person.

For the support of this declaration, with a firm reliance on the protection of God, we mutually pledge to each other our commitment to secure this end for ourselves, our fellow citizens, and our mutual posterity.

(Written and edited by organizers of the Raw Milk Freedom Riders during early 2012 and unfurled as a six-foot-high document at several food rights demonstrations in 2012.)

NOTES

INTRODUCTION

1. Farm-to-Consumer Legal Defense Fund, Grassway Organics Farm Store LLC et al. v. Wisconsin Department of Agriculture, Trade and Consumer Protection, Case No. 09-CV-6313, Dane County Circuit Court Branch 8, Wisconsin, Decision and Order, September 9, 2011, 4, http://www.thecompletepatient.com/sites/default/files/WIorder-clarification9-11.pdf.
2. Bill Ganzel, "The Cost of Living during the Cold War," Wessels Living History Farm, http://www.livinghistoryfarm.org/farminginthe50s/money_01.html (accessed October 29, 2012).
3. "Typical American Family Expenses & Annualized Expenditures," eHow.com, http://www.ehow.com/info_7811523_typical-family-expenses-annualized-expenditures.html (accessed November 1, 2012).
4. "How Safe Is That Chicken?" *Consumer Reports*, January 2010, http://www.consumerreports.org/cro/magazine-archive/2010/january/food/chicken-safety/overview/chicken-safety-ov.htm.

CHAPTER ONE

1. Grassfed on the Hill cooperative, member information package, written and edited by Karine Bouis-Towe and Liz Reitzig, 2007–2008 (obtained from court documents in case United States of America vs. Daniel L. Allgyer, in U.S. District Court, Case No. 11-02651).

CHAPTER TWO

1. "FDA Raids Amish Farmer Dan Allyger," National Independent Consumers and Farmers Association, http://www.nicfa.us/newandupdates.html (accessed October 29, 2012).
2. Ibid.
3. Establishment Inspection Report, Rainbow Acres Farm, Kinzers, PA 17535-9766, FEI (establishment identifier number): 3007402882, EI Start: 04/20/2010, EI End: 04/20/2010, page 3.
4. Joshua C. Schafer and David L. Pearce, U.S. Food and Drug Administration, notice of inspection conducted at Rainbow Acres Farm, April 20, 2010, photos attached as exhibit 24. Obtained from court documents in case United States of America vs. Daniel L. Allgyer, in U.S. District Court, Case No. 11-02651.
5. Aman Singh, "Choice at the Supermarket: Is Our Food System the Perfect Oligoply?" *Forbes Corporate Social Responsibility Blog*, August 6, 2012, http://www.forbes.com/sites/csr/2012/08/06/choice-at-the-supermarket-is-our-food-system-the-perfect-oligopoly/.
6. "Armed Authorities Raid Family Farm: Ohio Department of Agriculture Traumatizes Women and Small Children," Farm-to-Consumer Legal Defense Fund press release, December 15, 2008, http://www.farmtoconsumer.org/press/press-15dec2008.htm.
7. Jacqueline Stowers et al. v. Ohio Department of Agriculture, Case No. 08CV159968, Lorain County Court of Common Pleas, Ohio, Complaint for Declaratory and Injunctive Relief, Motion for Preliminary Injunction, and Writ of Mandamus, December 17, 2008, http://www.farmtoconsumer.org/docs/complaint_final.pdf.
8. Iso Rabins, San Francisco Underground Market, "Underground Market Shutdown: An Update," http://us1.campaign-archive2.com/?u=5bb29e249d33f56d1f219edeb&id=20ea4e0156&e=191bba18a9 (accessed October 29, 2012).

9. Laura Bledsoe, "Farm-to-Fork Dinner Fiasco," Farm-to-Consumer Legal Defense Fund, October 24, 2011, http://farmtoconsumer.org/quail-hollow-farm-dinner.htm.

10. "Why Lemonade Freedom?" Lemonade Freedom, http://www.lemonadefreedom.com/what-is -lemonade-freedom-day/ (accessed October 29, 2012).

11. David K. Shipler, *The Rights of the People: How Our Search for Safety Invades Our Liberties* (New York: Alfred A. Knopf, 2011), 7, 9.

12. Ibid.

13. Jimmy Carter, "A Cruel and Unusual Record," *New York Times*, June 24, 2012, http://www .nytimes.com/2012/06/25/opinion/americas-shameful-human-rights-record.html?_r=1 &adxnnl=1&ref=todayspaper&adxnnlx=1340637051-fSgZaPPaw3EBo1zI6i2m3g.

14. U.S. Food and Drug Administration, "Food Security Guidance: Availability," *Federal Register*, January 9, 2002, https://www.federalregister.gov/articles/2002/01/09/02-542/food-security-guidance-availability.

15. Amanda Kondolojy, "Food Network Delivers Best Quarter in History," TV by the Numbers, March 26, 2012, http://tvbythenumbers.zap2it.com/2012/03/26/food-network-delivers-best -quarter-in-history/126036/.

16. *Obama Foodorama: The Blog of Record about White House Food Initiatives, from Policy to Pie*, http://www.obamafoodorama.com.

17. "More Than 1,000 New Farmers Markets Recorded across Country as USDA Directory Reveals 17 Percent Growth," U.S. Department of Agriculture press release, August 5, 2011, http://www.ams.usda .gov/AMSv1.0/ams.fetchTemplateData.do?template=TemplateU&navID=&page=Newsroom&result Type=Details&dDocName=STELPRDC5092527&dID=153449&wf=false&description=More +than+1%2C000+New+Farmers+Markets+Recorded+Across+Country+as+USDA+Directory +Reveals+17+Percent+Growth&topNav=Newsroom&leftNav=&rightNav1=&rightNav2=.

18. "Winter Farmers Markets Expand: Now More Than 1,200 Locations for Fresh Local Foods," U.S. Department of Agriculture press release, December 15, 2011, http://www.usda.gov/wps/portal /usda/usdahome?contentid=2011/12/0516.xml&contentidonly=true.

19. State of New York, Department of Agriculture and Markets, Hearing Officer Report in the Matter of Considering the Issuance of an Order to Meadowsweet Dairy, LLC/Barbara and Stephen Smith, May 16, 2008, http://www.thecompletepatient.com/sites/default/files/MeadowsweetHearingDec.pdf, 18.

20. Maryn McKenna, "How Your Chicken Dinner Is Creating a Drug-Resistant Superbug," *The Atlantic*, July 11, 2012, http://www.theatlantic.com/health/archive/2012/07/how-your-chicken -dinner-is-creating-a-drug-resistant-superbug/259700/.

21. "Commerce Clause," Legal Information Institute, http://www.law.cornell.edu/wex/commerce _clause (accessed October 30, 2012).

22. Syllabus for *Wickard v. Filburn*, a U.S. Supreme Court decision (317 U.S. 111) from 1942, available via the Legal Information Institute of Cornell University Law Schools, http://www.law.cornell .edu/supct/html/historics/USSC_CR_0317_0111_ZS.html.

23. "Club Membership Agreement, Right to Choose Healthy Foods," RA Healthy Foods Club, http:// www.rahealthyfoods.com/assets/membership_agt.pdf (accessed October 30, 2012).

24. Farm-to-Consumer Legal Defense Fund et al. v. Kathleen Sebelius et al., Brief in Support of United States' Motion to Dismiss Plaintiffs' Amended Complaint at 25, April 26, 2010, http:// www.farmtoconsumer.org/litigation/ey100426--ds_mtd_memo_in_support.pdf.

25. Ibid., 26.

26. Ibid.

27. Farm-to-Consumer Legal Defense Fund, Grassway Organics Farm Store LLC, et al. v. Wisconsin Department of Agriculture, Trade and Consumer Protection, Case No. 09-CV-6313, Dane County Circuit Court Branch 8, Wisconsin, Decision and Order at 4, September 9, 2011, http:// www.thecompletepatient.com/sites/default/files/WIorder-clarification9-11.pdf.

28. Ibid.
29. U.S. Food and Drug Administration, Warning Letter to Daniel Allgyer/Rainbow Acres Farm, April 20, 2010, http://www.fda.gov/iceci/enforcementactions/warningletters/2010/ucm209276.htm.
30. Daniel Allyger, letter to customers, April 26, 2010.
31. Ibid.
32. Ibid.

CHAPTER 3

1. Department of Health & Human Services, Public Health Service, Centers for Disease Control and Prevention (CDC), Memorandum to State and Territorial Epidemiologists, State Public Health Veterinarians, May 3, 2011; obtained from public records disclosure in 2012 by Maine Department of Agriculture, Food, and Rural Resources.
2. Robert Hartley, *An Historical, Scientific, and Practical Essay on Milk as an Article of Human Sustenance* (Manchester, New Hampshire: Ayer Publishing, 1977), http://books.google.com/books?id=i1p3WSCex0EC&pg=PA132&lpg=PA132&dq=Robert+Hartley,+distillery+dairies&source=bl&ots=0CRTmdjcw0&sig=8zzBeAxsvXT09OmyldvAPvpezk&hl=en&ei=DjOxSZfoENLjtgf8tKzCBw&sa=X&oi=book_result&resnum=7&ct=result#PPA139,M1 (accessed October 31, 2012).
3. Ibid.
4. Patrice Debré, *Louis Pasteur* (Baltimore, Maryland: Johns Hopkins University Press, 1998), 235–38.
5. Moira Davidson Reynolds, *How Pasteur Changed History: The Story of Louis Pasteur and the Pasteur Institute* (Sarasota, Florida: McGuinn & McGuire Publishing, 1994), 36.
6. Ibid., 41–42.
7. Ron Schmid, *The Untold Story of Milk* (Winona Lake, Indiana: New Trends Publishing, 2003), 54–55.
8. Debré, *Louis Pasteur,* 359.
9. Ibid.
10. "Élie Metchnikoff," *Wikipedia,* http://en.wikipedia.org/wiki/Metchnikoff (accessed October 31, 2012).
11. J. R. Crewe, "Real Milk Cures Many Diseases," *Certified Milk Magazine,* January 1929, available on the website of the Weston A. Price Foundation Campaign for Real Milk, http://www.realmilk.com/milk-cure.html.
12. Alan Czaplicki, "Pure Milk Is Better Than Purified Milk," *Social Science History* 31, no. 3 (2007): 411–33, doi: 10.1215/01455532-2007-004.
13. Robert V. Tauxe, "Food Safety and Irradiation: Protecting the Public from Foodborne Infections," *Emerging Infectious Diseases* 7, no. 3, supplement (2001): 516–21, http://wwwnc.cdc.gov/eid/article/7/7/01-7706_article.htm.
14. "Real Raw Milk Facts: Hot Topics," Real Raw Milk Facts Working Group, http://www.realrawmilkfacts.com/raw-milk-hot-topics (accessed October 31, 2012).
15. U.S. Centers for Disease Control and Prevention, "Salmonella Dublin and Raw Milk Consumption: California," *Morbidity and Mortality Weekly Report* 33, no. 14 (1984): 196–98, http://www.cdc.gov/mmwr/preview/mmwrhtml/00000318.htm.
16. Stephen Barrett, "Why Raw Milk Should Be Avoided," Quackwatch, December 22, 2003, http://www.quackwatch.com/01QuackeryRelatedTopics/rawmilk.html (accessed October 31, 2012).
17. Ibid.
18. Aajonus Vonderplanitz, letter to City of Los Angeles, Office of Finance, CDU Tax Discovery Unit, December 30, 2007.
19. Ibid.
20. Centers for Disease Control and Prevention (CDC), *Foodborne Active Surveillance Network (FoodNet) Population Survey Atlas of Exposures* (Atlanta, Georgia: U.S. Department of Health and Human Services, Centers for Disease Control and Prevention, 2006–2007), 13, http://www.cdc.gov/foodnet/surveys/FoodNetExposureAtlas0607_508.pdf.

21. M. Waser et al., "Inverse Association of Farm Milk Consumption with Asthma and Allergy in Rural and Suburban Populations across Europe," *Clinical and Experimental Allergy* 5 (2007): 661–70, doi: 10.1111/j.1365-2222.2006.02640.x.

22. Georg Loss et al., "The Protective Effect of Farm Milk Consumption on Childhood Asthma and Atopy: The GABRIELA Study," *Journal of Allergy and Clinical Immunology* 4 (2011): 766–73, http://www.jacionline.org/article/S0091-6749%2811%2901234-6/abstract.

23. Ibid.

24. Testimony of John F. Sheehan, Director, Division of Plant and Dairy Food Safety, Office of Food Safety, Center for Food Safety and Applied Nutrition, U.S. Food and Drug Administration, Before the Joint Standing Committee on Agriculture, Conservation and Forestry, State of Maine Legislature, March 21, 2011, page 15 (obtained from public records disclosure in 2012 by Maine Department of Agriculture, Food, and Rural Resources).

25. Mark Holbreich et al., "Amish Children Living in Northern Indiana Have a Very Low Prevalence of Allergic Sensitization," *Journal of Allergy and Clinical Immunology* 129, no. 6 (2012): 1671, http://download.journals.elsevierhealth.com/pdfs/journals/0091-6749/PIIS0091674912005192.pdf.

26. Anna Petherick, "The Evidence Around Raw Milk," International Milk Genomics Consortium, http://milkgenomics.org/newsletter/the-evidence-around-raw-milk (accessed November 13, 2012).

27. Ibid.

28. Ibid.

29. Chris Masterjohn, "The 2010 USDA/HHS Guidelines: A Rather Bizarre Definition of 'Nutrient Dense,'" blog post on the website of the Weston A. Price Foundation, February 21, 2011, http://www.westonaprice.org/blogs/2011/02/21/the-2010-usdahhs-guidelines-a-rather-bizarre-definition-of-nutrient-dense/.

30. U.S. Food and Drug Administration, Warning Letter to Daniel Allgyer/Rainbow Acres Farm, April 20, 2010, http://www.fda.gov/iceci/enforcementactions/warningletters/2010/ucm209276.htm.

CHAPTER 4

1. Carl Zimmer, "How Microbes Defend and Define Us," *New York Times,* July 12, 2010, http://www.nytimes.com/2010/07/13/science/13micro.html?pagewanted=1&adxnnlx=1341883063-Vw8NDd5A5VH5%204pFE97hlw.

2. "Microbes Maketh Man," editorial, *The Economist,* August 18, 2012, 9, http://www.economist.com/node/21560559.

3. Carl Zimmer, "Bacterial Ecosystems Divide People into 3 Groups, Scientists Say," *New York Times,* April 20, 2011, http://www.nytimes.com/2011/04/21/science/21gut.html?_r=2&src=me&ref=general.

4. "'Friendly' Bacteria Protect Against Type 1 Diabetes, Yale Researchers Find," *YaleNews,* September 21, 2008, http://news.yale.edu/2008/09/21/friendly-bacteria-protect-against-type-1-diabetes-yale-researchers-find.

5. "Do Germs Protect Kids from Chronic Disease?" *Fars News,* June 4, 2012, http://english.farsnews.com/newstext.php?nn=9103080844.

6. Erin Millar, "Clean Freak," *Readers Digest Canada,* October 2012, 88.

7. Mary Ellen Sanders, "How FDA's Actions Are Guaranteeing Research on Probiotic Foods Is Not Conducted in the USA," California Dairy Research Foundation, October 13, 2012, http://cdrf.org/2012/10/13/how-fdas-actions-are-guaranteeing-research-on-probiotic-foods-is-not-conducted-in-the-usa/.

8. James M. MacDonald et al., "Changes in the Size and Location of U.S. Dairy Farms," in *Profits, Costs, and the Changing Structure of Dairy Farming,* Economic Research Report no. 47 (U.S. Department of Agriculture Economic Research Service, September 2007), http://www.ers.usda.gov/media/430528/err47b_1_.pdf.

9. Jerry Hirsch, "Dairy Farmers in Desperate Straits," *Los Angeles Times,* May 29, 2009, http://articles.latimes.com/2009/may/29/business/fi-milk-crisis29.

10. "N.Y. Dairy Farmer Kills 51 Cows, Commits Suicide," FoxNews.com, January 22, 2010, http://www.foxnews.com/story/0,2933,583703,00.html.
11. "Dairy Farmers Are Struggling for Survival Right Now — Why?" Farm Aid, February 2009, http://www.farmaid.org/site/apps/nlnet/content2.aspx?c=qlI5IhNVJsE&b=2723877&ct=6794923.
12. "Raw Milk Permits: The C.A.R.E. Perspective," Community Alliance for Responsible Eco-farming (CARE), http://www.pasafarming.org/files/CAREstatement.pdf/at_download/file (accessed November 3, 2012).
13. "C.A.R.E.: Community Alliance for Responsible Eco-Farming," *Spoon and Fork DC* blog, November 3, 2010, http://www.spoonandforkdc.com/2010/11/care-community-alliance-for-responsible.html.
14. David Gumpert, "Organic Valley Lays Down the Law on Raw Milk," Grist, May 26, 2010, http://grist.org/article/organic-valley-confronts-its-most-serious-crisis-ever-over-raw-milk/.
15. Robert G. Ehlenfeldt, administrator, Wisconsin Department of Agriculture, Trade & Consumer Protection (DATCP) Division of Animal Health, e-mail message to C. Thomas Leitzke, DATCP, Steven C. Ingham, DATCP, and Jacqueline C. Owens, DATCP, December 19, 2008, subject: Re: Brucellosis.
16. C. Thomas Leitzke, DATCP, e-mail message to Steven C. Ingham, DATCP, Robert G. Ehlenfeldt, DATCP, Cathy S. Anderson, DATCP, and Jacqueline C. Owens, DATCP, February 18, 2009, subject: FDA Raw Milk Conference Call.
17. Farm-to-Consumer Legal Defense Fund, Laurie Donnelly, et al. v. Kathleen Sebelius et al., Case No. C 10-4018-MWB, Iowa Northern District Court, Western Division, Plaintiffs' Complaint for Declaratory, Preliminary and Other Injunctive Relief, February 18, 2010, http://www.farmtoconsumer.org/docs/fda-suit--complaint-final-as-filed-02-20-10.pdf.
18. Farm-to-Consumer Legal Defense Fund et al. v. Kathleen Sebelius et al., Reply in Support of United States' Motion to Dismiss Plaintiffs' Amended Complaint, June 21, 2010, 5, http://www.farmtoconsumer.org/docs/ey100621--ds_mtd_reply.pdf.
19. Eric Wagoner, "Athens, GA Raw Milk Seizure, Part One," YouTube video posted October 22, 2009, http://www.youtube.com/watch?v=EMfQXxVAPgk.
20. Farm-to-Consumer Legal Defense Fund et al. v. Kathleen Sebelius et al., Defendants' Statement of Additional Material Facts, July 1, 2011, http://www.thecompletepatient.com/sites/default/files/FTCLDF-FDA-GAaccount.pdf.
21. Eric Wagoner, comment on "Finally, We Get the Real Story of the FDA's Role in the 2009 GA Raw Milk Pour-out: Let Your Imagination Go," *The Complete Patient* blog, July 13, 2011, http://www.thecompletepatient.com/article/2011/july/12/finally-we-get-real-story-fdas-role-2009-ga-raw-milk-pour-out-let-your.
22. State of Minnesota, County of Hennepin, Application for a Search Warrant and Supporting Affidavit, June 9, 2010, signed by Officer Chris Yates and Judge Robert A. Blaeser.
23. Michael Schommer, "FDA Awards $1 Million Rapid-Response Grant to Minnesota Department of Agriculture," Minnesota Department of Agriculture press release, October 4, 2011, http://www.mda.state.mn.us/en/news/releases/2011/~/media/Files/news/2011releases/nr-2011-10-04-foodsafety.ashx.
24. "MDA Receives New Grants to Bolster Food Safety," *Brainerd Dispatch*, September 14, 2012, http://brainerddispatch.com/news/2012-09-14/mda-receives-new-grants-bolster-food-safety.
25. U.S. Food and Drug Administration, *Food and Drug Administration FY 2011 Congressional Budget Request*, http://www.fda.gov/downloads/AboutFDA/ReportsManualsForms/Reports/BudgetReports/UCM207333.pdf.
26. U.S. Food and Drug Administration, *FDA Division of Federal–State Relations Year in Review: January–December 2010*, http://www.fda.gov/downloads/ForFederalStateandLocalOfficials/Meetings/UCM244055.pdf.
27. U.S. Food and Drug Administration, *FY 2011 Congressional Budget Request*.

28. U.S. Food and Drug Administration, *FDA Division of Federal–State Relations Year in Review: January–December 2010*, http://www.fda.gov/downloads/ForFederalStateandLocalOfficials/Meetings/UCM244055.pdf.
29. John Sheehan, e-mail message to Roberta Wagner, Director, CFSAN Office of Compliance and Lloyd A. Kinzel, Regional Milk Specialist, CSFAN, August 24, 2009, subject: FW: Additional Raw Milk Info.
30. Karyn M. Campbell, Director of Investigations Branch, Philadelphia Office, FDA, e-mail message to Mathew M. Henciak, Assistant to the Director of Investigations Branch, cc: Christine M. Smith, Director of Investigations Branch, Baltimore Office, FDA, October 15, 2009, subject: FW: Additional Raw Milk Info.
31. Karyn M. Campbell, e-mail message to Mathew M. Henciak, Christine M. Smith, Randy Pack, Anne Aberdeen, Stephanie Shapley, Lori S. Lawless, Kirk Sooter, Steven L. Carter, Richard C. Cherry, Calvin W. Edwards, and Michael D. O'Meara, October 15, 2009, subject: RE: Sample analysis confirms raw milk.
32. U.S. Food and Drug Administration, "Food and Drug Administration Office of Regulatory Affairs, Collection Report for Sample Number: 570827," March 1, 2010, 3.
33. Ibid.
34. Ibid., for sample number 570826, February 26, 2010, 3.
35. Ibid., supporting document #3, 1.
36. Ibid., supporting document #7.
37. Ibid., summary report, December 23, 2009.

CHAPTER FIVE

1. David Gumpert, "An Amish Entrepreneur's Old-Fashioned Approach," *BusinessWeek*, January 5, 2010, http://www.businessweek.com/smallbiz/content/jan2010/sb2010014_284280.htm.
2. U.S. Department of Agriculture, Office of Small Farms Coordination, "Small Farms Success Stories: USDA Small Farms and Beginning Farmers and Ranchers Coordinators' Collections, 2006–2008," September 2009, 4, http://www.csrees.usda.gov/nea/ag_systems/pdfs/small_farm_success_stories.pdf.
3. "About," Food for Maine's Future, http://savingseeds.wordpress.com/about/ (accessed November 4, 2012).
4. "Former Broker Gets Prison for Swindling Woman Out of Home," *Los Angeles Times*, June 18, 2002, http://articles.latimes.com/2002/jun/18/local/me-broker18.
5. James Stewart, memorandum to Rawesome members, December 30, 2008.
6. Ike's Pump & Drilling, Inc. v. Sharon Palmer, Case No. MS180146, Ventura, California, March 3, 2005, http://www.ventura.courts.ca.gov/via/CaseInformationSummary.aspx?CaseNo=MS180146.
7. FarmTek v. Judith Bliszcz et al., Case No. 56-2007-00307446-CL-CL-VTA, Ventura, California, November 14, 2007, http://www.ventura.courts.ca.gov/via/CaseInformationSummary.aspx?CaseNo=56-2007-00307446-CL-CL-VTA.
8. Danny Miles v. Sharon A. Palmer, Case No. 56-2008-00333883-CL-CL-VTA, Ventura, California, December 23, 2008, http://www.ventura.courts.ca.gov/via/CaseInformationSummary.aspx?CaseNo=56-2008-00333883-CL-CL-VTA.

CHAPTER 6

1. "Learn More: Cow and Goat-Shares," Farm-to-Consumer Legal Defense Fund, http://www.farmtoconsumer.org/cow-shares.html (accessed November 4, 2012).
2. Declaration of Amos Miller, Motion to Quash or Dismiss, Docket No. NT-0000305-06, Citation Number P2356246-4, District Court, County of Lancaster, Commonwealth of Pennsylvania, August 2006.
3. Docket for Commonwealth of Pennsylvania v. Amos B. Miller, Docket Number: MJ-02302-NT-0000305-2006, Commonwealth of Pennsylvania, June 2, 2006.

4. David J. Hochstetler and Aajonus Vonderplanitz, letter to U.S. Food and Drug Administration Investigator William G. Nelson, November 21, 2006.

5. U.S. Food and Drug Administration, Warning Letter to David J. Hochstetler/Forest Grove Dairy, February 8, 2007, http://www.fda.gov/ICECI/EnforcementActions/WarningLetters/2006/ucm076271.htm.

6. Michigan Department of Community Health, Summary Report of the March 2010 *Campylobacter* Outbreak Involving Consumption of Raw Milk, 8.

7. Carol Schmitmeyer v. Ohio Department of Agriculture, Case No. 06-CV-63277, Darke County, Ohio, Decision and Judgment Entry, December 29, 2006, 6–9, http://www.davidgumpert.com /files/12_29_06_decisi.pdf.

8. Regina v. Michael Schmidt, 2010 ONCJ 9 (CanLII), Ontario Court of Justice, Provincial Offences Court (Newmarket), Judgment, January 21, 2010, http://www.canlii.org/eliisa/highlight.do?text =raw+milk+british&language=en&searchTitle=Search+all+CanLII+Databases&path=/en/on /oncj/doc/2010/2010oncj9/2010oncj9.html.

9. RMAC Updates, "Case Statement for Amending Raw Milk Statute," Raw Milk Association of Colorado, May 10, 2010, http://www.rawmilkcolorado.org/rmac_updates.php.

10. Meadowsweet Dairy LLC, Steven Smith and Barbara Smith v. Patrick Hooker, Commissioner, Department of Agriculture and Markets of the State of New York, and Will Francis, Director of Division of Milk Control and Dairy Services, RJI No. 01-08-092475, County of Albany, State of New York Supreme Court, Decision and Order, November 18, 2008, http://www.thecomplete patient.com/sites/default/files/NYsmithdec.pdf.

11. Scarlett Treviso, Statement for Probable Cause, attached to Search Warrant and Affidavit, June 29, 2010, State of California, County of Los Angeles, signed by Judge Ronald R. Combest, 4–8 (investigation page ID no. 00196–00200).

12. Ibid.

13. Ken Ward, Los Angeles County Bureau of Investigation, Supplemental Report, Narrative, Case 2010-G-1523, July 22, 2010, investigation page ID no. 00170–00171.

14. Ibid.

15. Ibid.

16. Ibid.

17. Ibid., investigation page ID no. 00151–00152.

18. Ibid., investigation page ID no. 00159–00161.

19. District Attorney's Office, County of Los Angeles, Search Warrant Location Schematic, Case 2010-G-1523, June 30, 2010, investigation page ID no. 00382.

20. Ted Holst, Los Angeles County Bureau of Investigation, Supplemental Report, Narrative, Case 2010-G-1523, August 19, 2010, investigation page ID no. 0038–0040.

21. "Armed Police Raid Private Organic Co-Op Rawesome Foods, Security Camera Footage," YouTube video posted August 1, 2010, http://www.youtube.com/watch?v=G5zPhhNUakc.

22. Holst, Supplemental Report.

23. Ibid.

24. Ibid.

25. Rawesome Investigation, Environmental Health Hearing Sheet, Post Hearing Fact Sheet, EHMIS-TAR601, hearing date July 1, 2010, report date August 18, 2010, investigation page ID no. 0088.

26. Ibid.

27. Ibid.

28. Kunle Adesina, Complaint Report, County of Los Angeles Department of Health Services, Preventive Health Services, Environmental Management, July 1, 2010, investigation ID no. 0089.

29. P. J. Huffstutter, "Raw-food Raid Highlights a Hunger," *Los Angeles Times*, July 25, 2010, http:// articles.latimes.com/2010/jul/25/business/la-fi-raw-food-raid-20100725.

30. "(Rawesome Raid): The Story — The Police Raid, Part 1 06/30/10," YouTube video posted June 3, 2011, http://www.youtube.com/watch?v=cZnQYLMDQ3w.

31. Tommy Rosen, "What's the FBI Doing in My Milk?" Huffington Post, July 2, 2010, http://www.huffingtonpost.com/tommy-rosen/whats-the-fbi-doing-in-my_b_633344.html.

32. Ibid.

33. "Rawesome Food Club Raided by Local, Federal and Canadian Agents," Laguna Natural Health eNews and Tips, July 3, 2010, http://lagunanaturalhealth.blogspot.com/2010/07/rawsome-food-club-raided-by-local.html.

34. Adesina, Complaint Report.

35. Affidavit of Ken Ward attached to Order Sealing Search Warrant Documents, in the matter of Search Warrant 60637, County of Los Angeles, State of California, signed by Judge Michael D. Abzug, July 7, 2010, investigation page ID no. 00259–00261.

36. Ibid.

37. Ibid.

38. Affidavit of Ken Ward attached to Order Sealing Search Warrant Documents, in the matter of Search Warrant 60637, County of Los Angeles, State of California, signed by Judge Michael D. Abzug, September 29, 2010, investigation page ID no. 00262–00264.

39. Ibid.

CHAPTER SEVEN

1. "CDC Releases Report on Foods and Foodborne Agents Associated with Outbreaks in the United States: More than 1,000 Foodborne Outbreaks Reported in 2008," U.S. Centers for Disease Control and Prevention, September 8, 2011, http://www.cdc.gov/media/releases/2011/a0908_foodborne_agents.html; U.S. Centers for Disease Control and Prevention, "Surveillance for Foodborne Disease Outbreaks: United States, 2006," *Morbidity and Mortality Weekly Report* 58, no. 22 (2009): 609–15, http://www.cdc.gov/mmwr/preview/mmwrhtml/mm5822a1.htm.

2. U.S. Centers for Disease Control and Prevention; "Surveillance for Foodborne Disease Outbreaks — United States, 2009–2010," *Morbidity and Mortality Weekly Report* 62, no. 3 (2013): 41–47, http://www.cdc.gov/mmwr/preview/mmwrhtml/mm6203a1.htm?s_cid=mm6203a1_w.

3. "Listeria Detected in Morningland Raw Milk Cheese," California Department of Food and Agriculture press release, August 26, 2010, http://www.cdfa.ca.gov/egov/Press_Releases/Press_Release.asp?PRnum=10-046.

4. "Morningland Dairy Conducting Nationwide Voluntary Recall of All Cheese Labeled as Morningland Dairy & Ozark Hills Farm Because of Possible Health Risk," U.S. Food and Drug Administration press release, August 30, 2010, http://www.fda.gov/Safety/Recalls/ucm224494.htm.

5. Property Receipt and Inventory, June 30, 2010, investigation page ID no. 0042–0043, attached to Los Angeles County District Attorney, Bureau of Investigation, Supplemental Report, Case 2010-G-1523, August 19, 2010, investigation page ID no. 0038–0040.

6. Plant Inspection Narrative, California Department of Food and Agriculture, Milk and Dairy Foods Branch, Ontario, June 30, 2010, investigation page ID no. 0060.

7. U.S. Food and Drug Administration, Receipt for Samples Collected at Rawesome, June 30, 2010.

8. U.S. Food and Drug Administration, *Regulatory Procedures Manual* (2011), http://www.fda.gov/ICECI/ComplianceManuals/RegulatoryProceduresManual/default.htm.

9. "Del Bueno Recalls Cheese Because of Possible Health Risk," U.S. Food and Drug Administration press release, November 17, 2010, http://www.fda.gov/Safety/Recalls/ArchiveRecalls/2010/ucm234212.htm.

10. "Dole Fresh Vegetables Announces Precautionary Recall of Limited Number of Italian Blend Salads," U.S. Food and Drug Administration press release, June 22, 2011, http://www.fda.gov/Safety/Recalls/ucm260501.htm.

11. "Wisconsin Business Recalls Smoked Fish Spread; May Be Contaminated with Listeria," U.S. Food and Drug Administration press release, November 30, 2010, http://www.fda.gov/Safety/Recalls/ArchiveRecalls/2010/ucm235924.htm.

12. "Morningland Dairy Conducting Nationwide Voluntary Recall," U.S. Food and Drug Administration press release.

13. Ibid.

14. David Gumpert, "The FDA's Crackdown on Small Cheesemakers Fails to Turn Up Many Bugs," Grist, December 8, 2010, http://grist.org/article/2010-12-07-has-the-fda-come-up-short-in-its-crackdown-on-small-cheesemakers/.

15. "United States Public Health Commissioned Corps," *Wikipedia*, http://en.wikipedia.org/wiki/United_States_Public_Health_Service_Commissioned_Corps (accessed November 5, 2012).

16. "U.S. Public Health Service Commissioned Corps Overview FAQs," U.S. Public Health Service Commissioned Corps, November 8, 2011, http://www.usphs.gov/QuestionsAnswers/overview.aspx.

17. "U.S. Public Health Service Commissioned Corps Opportunities," U.S. Public Health Service Commissioned Corps, 3–5, http://www.usphs.gov/docs/pdfs/bks/USPHS_Physician_111111.pdf (accessed November 5, 2012).

18. "Proper Uniform Wear," U.S. Public Health Service Commissioned Corps, Junior Officer Advisory Group, Communications and Publications Committee, Uniform Sub-Committee, October 26, 2011, http://www.usphs.gov/corpslinks/JOAG/documents/JOAG_Proper_Uniform_Wear_Revised_102611.pdf.

19. Paul Ebner, "CAFOs and Public Health: Pathogens and Manure," Purdue University Extension, August 2007, http://www.ces.purdue.edu/extmedia/ID/cafo/ID-356.pdf.

20. Gregory L. Armstrong et al., "Emerging Foodborne Pathogens: Escherichia coli O157:H7 as a Model of Entry of a New Pathogen into the Food Supply of the Developed World," *Epidemiologic Reviews* 18, no. 1 (1996): 46, http://epirev.oxfordjournals.org/content/18/1/29.full.pdf.

21. "Michael Beverly: The 1996 Odwalla E. Coli Outbreak," Bill Marler website, http://www.billmarler.com/key_case/odwalla-e-coli-outbreak/ (accessed November 6, 2012).

22. Ibid.

23. Bill Marler, "Put a Trial Lawyer out of Business: Pass Meaningful Food Safety Legislation by Thanksgiving," Marler Clark press release, October 6, 2009, http://www.marlerclark.com/press_releases/view/put-a-trial-lawyer-out-of-business-pass-meaningful-food-safety-legislation-/.

24. "Food Safety and Raw Milk," U.S. Centers for Disease Control and Prevention, March 22, 2012, http://www.cdc.gov/foodsafety/rawmilk/raw-milk-index.html.

25. Jeff Benedict, *Poisoned: The True Story of the Deadly E. Coli Outbreak That Changed the Way Americans Eat* (Buena Vista, Virginia: Inspire Books, 2011), 300.

26. "Print/Blog Interviews," Marler Clark, http://www.marlerclark.com/media_relations/archive/C127 (accessed November 6, 2012).

27. Patricia Cohen, "For Personal-Injury Lawyer, Michael Pollan's Book Is Worth Fighting For," *New York Times*, May 28, 2009, http://www.nytimes.com/2009/05/29/books/29poll.html.

28. "CDC 2011 Estimates: Methods," U.S. Centers for Disease Control and Prevention, April 19, 2011, http://www.cdc.gov/foodborneburden/2011-methods.html.

29. "CDC Releases Report on Foods and Foodborne Agents Associated with Outbreaks in the United States," U.S. Centers for Disease Control and Prevention press release, September 8, 2011, http://www.cdc.gov/media/releases/2011/a0908_foodborne_agents.html.

30. Matt McMillen, "CDC: 1,000 Food-Borne Disease Outbreaks in a Year," WebMD Health News, September 8, 2011, http://www.webmd.com/food-recipes/food-poisoning/news/20110908/cdc-1000-foodborne-disease-outbreaks-in-a-year.

31. Bill Marler, "Raw Milk Outbreaks Do Happen Despite What the Weston A. Price Foundation and The Complete Patient (a.k.a. David Gumpert) Say," *Marler Blog*, October 18, 2009, http://www

.marlerblog.com/legal-cases/raw-milk-outbreaks-do-happen-despite-what-the-weston-a-price
-foundation-and-the-complete-patient-aka/.

32. Benedict, *Poisoned*, 299.

33. "Marler vs. Gumpert: A Raw Debate About Milk," *Simple, Good, and Tasty* blog, July 1, 2010,
http://simplegoodandtasty.com/2010/06/30/marler-vs-gumpert-a-raw-debate-about-milk.

34. Colin Caywood, "Missouri Dairy's Raw Milk Cheese Production Stopped Due to Listeria and
Staph," *Food Poison Journal*, August 26, 2010, http://www.foodpoisonjournal.com/food-poisoning
-watch/missouri-dairys-raw-milk-cheese-production-stopped-due-to-listeria-and-staph/.

35. "Raw Milk Cheese from Morningland Dairy Has Been Ordered to Halt Production and
Distribution," *Listeria Blog*, August 27, 2010, http://www.listeriablog.com/listeria-recalls/raw
-milk-cheese-from-morningland-dairy-has-been-ordered-to-halt-production-and-distribution/.

36. Bill Marler, "Missouri Attorney General Seeks Destruction of Morningland Dairy Cheese," *Marler
Blog*, October 30, 2010, http://www.marlerblog.com/case-news/missouri-attorney-general-seeks
-destruction-of-morningland-dairy-cheese/.

37. "Food at the 2009 Food Conference," program guide presented at the 2009 Hazon Food Conference, Asilomar Conference and Retreat Center, Pacific Grove, CA.

38. Ibid.

CHAPTER EIGHT

1. "Chicago Seven," *Wikipedia*, http://en.wikipedia.org/wiki/Chicago_Seven (accessed November 6, 2012).

2. Adam Liptak, "U.S. Prison Population Dwarfs That of Other Nations," *New York Times*, April 23,
2008, http://www.nytimes.com/2008/04/23/world/americas/23iht23prison.12253738.html
?pagewanted%3Dall.

3. Ibid.

4. "Intelligent Sentences," *The Economist*, October 6, 2012, 19, http://www.economist.com/node/21563948.

5. Mike Riggs, "Rand Paul Introduces Amendment to End the FDA's Insane Police Powers: 'I See No
Reason to Have the FDA Carrying Weapons,'" Reason Foundation, *Hit & Run* blog, May 24, 2012,
http://reason.com/blog/2012/05/24/rand-paul-calls-for-an-end-to-the-fdas-i.

6. United States of America v. Daniel Allgyer d/b/a Rainbow Acres Farm, Case 5:11-CV-02651,
United States District Court, Eastern District of Pennsylvania, Complaint for Permanent Injunction, April 19, 2011, 3.

7. Stephen Denan, "Mothers Crying over Raw Milk," *Washington Times*, May 16, 2011, http://www
.washingtontimes.com/news/2011/may/16/mothers-crying-over-raw-milk/?page=all.

8. Jonathan W. Emord, "About," Emord & Associates, http://www.emord.com/Jonathan-Emord
.html (accessed November 7, 2012).

9. Stephen Colbert, "Rawesome Foods Raid," *Colbert Report*, October 6, 2010, http://www.colbert
nation.com/the-colbert-report-videos/361307/october-06-2010/rawesome-foods-raid.

10. Ibid.

11. Ken Ward, Los Angeles County Bureau of Investigation, Supplemental Report, Case 2010-G-
1523, August 12, 2010, investigation page ID no. 00115.

12. Ibid., investigation page ID no. 00117.

13. ProAdvocate Group, home page, http://www.proadvocate.org (accessed November 7, 2012).

14. United States of America v. Daniel Allgyer, Memorandum and Order by Judge Lawrence Stengel,
July 28, 2011, 3, http://www.thecompletepatient.com/sites/default/files/Allgyer-Vonderplanitz
JudgeDenial.pdf.

15. Ibid., 6–7.

16. Richard Ballou, Los Angeles County Bureau of Investigation, Supplemental Report, Case 2010-G-
1523, June 23, 2011, investigation page ID no. 002.

17. "Today's Raid on Rawesome Foods," YouTube video posted August 3, 2011, https://www.youtube .com/watch?v=tgrnVrYZ9x0.

18. "Rawesome Farm Buying Club Raided Again," Farm-to-Consumer Legal Defense Fund press release, August 3, 2011, http://www.farmtoconsumer.org/press/press-03aug2011-rawesome.htm.

19. Ibid.

20. Ibid.

21. The People of California v. Healthy Family Farms, Sharon Ann Palmer, James Cecil Stewart and Eugenie Victoria Bloch, Case BA385253, Superior Court for the State of California, County of Los Angeles, Felony Complaint for Arrest Warrant, June 30, 2011, http://www.thecompletepatient .com/sites/default/files/RawesomeCriminalCompl08-11.pdf.

22. Ibid., 17.

23. Michelle LeCavalier, State of California, County of Los Angeles, Search Warrant and Affidavit, description of Rawesome property to be searched, August 1, 2011, 10–11.

24. "Raw Milk Dispute Spills into Courtroom," NBC Los Angeles, August 4, 2011, http://www.nb closangeles.com/video/#!/on-air/as-seen-on/Raw-Milk-Dispute-Spills-into-Courtroom/126810558.

25. Ron Garthwaite, comment on "Before We Go Judging Accused in Rawesome Case, Let's Make Sure We Don't Get Distracted from Rights Issues," *The Complete Patient* blog, August 4, 2011, http://www.thecompletepatient.com/article/2011/august/4/we-go-judging-accused-rawesome -case-lets-make-sure-we-dont-get-distracted.

26. Mark McAfee, comment on "Holding Open the Gate at Rawesome, and Cutting through the Confusion on Private Food Groups," *The Complete Patient* blog, August 5, 2011, http://www .thecompletepatient.com/article/2011/august/5/holding-open-gate-rawesome-and-cutting -through-confusion-private-food-groups.

27. Maurice Kaehler, comment on "Holding Open the Gate at Rawesome, and Cutting through the Confusion on Private Food Groups," *The Complete Patient* blog, August 6, 2011, http://www .thecompletepatient.com/article/2011/august/5/holding-open-gate-rawesome-and-cutting -through-confusion-private-food-groups.

28. Rachel McGrath, "Santa Paula Woman Arrested on Multiple Felony Counts," *Ventura County Star*, March 2, 2012, http://m.vcstar.com/news/2012/mar/02/santa-paula-woman-arrested-on-multiple-felony/.

29. The People of the State of California v. Sharon Palmer, Larry Otting and James Cecil Stewart, VCIJIS Case: 2011013198, Felony Complaint, February 27, 2012.

30. Sean Newell, "Judge Who Set Unsecured Bail for Jerry Sandusky Is a Second Mile Volunteer," Deadspin, November 13, 2011, http://deadspin.com/5859075/judge-who-set-unsecured-bail-for -jerry-sandusky-is-a-second-mile-volunteer.

31. United States District Court for the Eastern District of Michigan, Subpoena to Testify Before a Grand Jury, Grand Jury No. 11-3-230-2, dated October 13, 2011, addressed to David Hochstetler/ Forest Grove Dairy and Richard Hebron/Family Farms Cooperative.

32. Ibid.

33. Ross Goldstein, e-mail message to Aajonus Vonderplanitz, Right to Choose Healthy Foods organizer, November 13, 2011, subject: Your communication with Mr. Weier.

34. Aajonus Vonderplanitz, e-mail message to Ross Goldstein, November 13, 2011, subject: U.S. Department of Justice - attack on farmers and people who only want to eat healthy food.

35. County Sheriff Project, "About" page, http://www.countysheriffproject.org/ (accessed November 8, 2012).

36. Brad Rogers, e-mail message to Ross Goldstein, U.S. Department of Justice attorney, December 2, 2011, subject: Mr. David J. Hochstetler/Forest Grove Dairy.

37. Ross Goldstein, reply to e-mail message from Brad Rogers, December 2, 2011.

38. Ibid.

39. State of Wisconsin v. Vernon D. Hershberger, Case No. 2011-CM-696, Criminal Complaint, October 28, 2011, http://www.doj.state.wi.us/news/files/criminal-complaint-hershberger-vernon-20111207.pdf.
40. State of Wisconsin, Sauk County Circuit Court, Bond and Conditions of Release in Case No. 11CM696, January 11, 2012.
41. "DATCP. Attempted Inspection at Hershbergers,'" YouTube video posted February 11, 2012, http://youtube/Y4uoeR3XuCY.
42. Eric D. Defort, letter to the Honorable Guy D. Reynolds, February 21, 2012.

CHAPTER 9

1. Alexis de Tocqueville, *Democracy in America*, vol. 1, trans. H. Reeve (London: Saunders and Otley, 1835), 88, http://books.google.com/books?id=-b5LAAAAYAAJ&pg=PA88&lpg=PA88&dq=#v=onepage&q&f=false.
2. Ibid., 90
3. "Food Safety and Raw Milk," U.S. Food and Drug Administration, November 1, 2011, http://www.fda.gov/Food/FoodborneIllnessContaminants/BuyStoreServeSafeFood/ucm277854.htm.
4. Hal Prince, letter to milk distributors, November 25, 2009.
5. Donald E. Hoenig, e-mail message to Hal Prince, November 29, 2009, subject: RE: Letter to raw milk dealers.
6. Donald E. Hoenig, e-mail message to Hal Prince and Caldwell Jackson, Director, Division of Agricultural Resource Development, Maine Department of Agriculture, Food, and Rural Resources, March 28, 2011, subject: FW: raw milk.
7. Cathleen Cotton, Laboratory Evaluation Officer, Maine Department of Agriculture, Food, and Rural Resources, e-mail message to All Deering Building personnel, August 3, 2010, subject: Milk license required.
8. "Poultry Processing Needs in Maine," Maine Department of Agriculture Survey, March 17, 2011, http://www.maine.gov/tools/whatsnew/attach.php?id=216851&an=1.
9. de Tocqueville, *Democracy in America*, 65
10. "Parasites: Cryptosporidium (also known as 'Crypto')," U.S. Centers for Disease Control and Prevention, March 10, 2011, http://www.cdc.gov/parasites/crypto/.
11. Jonathan S. Yoder et al., "Cryptosporidiosis Surveillance: United States, 2006–2008," *Morbidity and Mortality Weekly Report* 59, no. SS06 (2010): 1–14, http://www.cdc.gov/mmwr/preview/mmwrhtml/ss5906a1.htm.
12. "Parasites: Cryptosporidium (also known as 'Crypto'): Prevention – Immunocompromised Persons)," U.S. Centers for Disease Control and Prevention, November 2, 2010, http://www.cdc.gov/parasites/crypto/gen_info/prevent_ic.html.
13. Vicki Rea, Field Epidemiologist, Maine Center for Disease Control and Prevention, e-mail message to Amy Robbins, Epidemiologist/Data Manager, Maine Center for Disease Control and Prevention, August 3, 2010, subject: Raw milk exposure in confirmed cryptosporidiosis case.
14. Donald E. Hoenig, e-mail message to Ned Porter, Deputy Commissioner, Maine Department of Agriculture, Food, and Rural Resources, Robert Batteese, Maine Board of Pesticides Control, Amy Robbins, and Hal Prince, August 13, 2010, subject: Quill's End Farm.
15. Ibid.
16. Ibid.
17. Donald E. Hoenig, e-mail message to Hal Prince, Steve Giguere, Program Manager, Division of Quality Assurance and Regulations, Maine Department of Agriculture, Food, and Rural Resources , Amy Robbins, and Stephen Sears, State Epidemiologist, Maine CDC, August 31, 2010, subject: Quill's End Farm, results.
18. Ibid.

19. Donna Guppy, Regional Epidemiologist, Maine CDC, e-mail message to Amy Robbins, August 31, 2010, subject: Re: raw milk and crypto case.

20. Kate Colby, Field Epidemiologist, Maine CDC, e-mail message to Amy Robbins, May 9, 2011, subject: Crypto Case with Raw Milk Exposure.

21. Megan Kelley, Field Epidemiologist, Maine CDC, e-mail message to Amy Robbins, March 9, 2011, subject: Cryptosporidiosis Case from Islesboro.

22. Amy Robbins, e-mail message to Donald Hoenig, March 15, 2011, subject: RE: Cryptosporidiosis Case from Islesboro.

23. Donald E. Hoenig, e-mail message to Amy Robbins, March 10, 2011, subject: RE: Cryptosporidiosis Case from Islesboro.

24. Amy Robbins, e-mail message to Donald Hoenig, March 15, 2011, subject: RE: Cryptosporidiosis Case from Islesboro.

25. Donald E. Hoenig, e-mail message to Amy Robbins, March 21, 2011, subject: RE: Cryptosporidiosis Case from Islesboro.

26. Town of Sedgwick, State of Maine, The Warrant for 2011–2012 (Fiscal Year July 1–June 30), http://www.sedgwickmaine.org/images/stories/warrant-11-12-pdf.pdf.

27. John F. Sheehan, Director, Division of Plant and Dairy Food Safety, Office of Food Safety, Center for Food Safety and Applied Nutrition, U.S. Food and Drug Administration, Testimony before the Joint Standing Committee on Agriculture, Conservation and Forestry, State of Maine Legislature, March 21, 2011 (contained in supporting documents for Maine Department of Agriculture v. Dan Brown d/b/a Gravelwood Farms, State of Maine Docket No. ELLSC-CV-11-70).

28. Paul LePage, Governor of Maine, memorandum to Sheila Pinette, Director, Maine CDC, and Walter Whitcomb, Commissioner, Maine Department of Agriculture, Food, and Rural Resources, September 19, 2011.

29. An Act Regarding the Sale of Raw Milk, HP0292, LD366, Item 1, 125th Maine State Legislature (2011).

30. John O'Donnell, farmer from Monmouth, Maine, Meeting with Governor Paul LePage (transcript of talk), September 17, 2011.

31. Steven Giguere, letter to Heather and Philip Retberg, December 21, 2011.

32. Heather Retberg, e-mail message to Steven Giguere, February 2, 2012, subject: RE: retail license.

33. Steven Giguere, e-mail message to Heather Retberg, January 17, 2012, subject: RE: retail license.

34. Christopher Braden (U.S. Public Health Service), Memorandum ("The Ongoing Public Health Hazard of Consuming Raw Milk") to State and Territorial Epidemiologists and State Public Health Veterinarians, May 3, 2011.

35. Walter Whitcomb, form letter regarding local food sovereignty ordinances in reply to constituent concerns expressed to Maine Department of Agriculture and Maine Governor Paul LePage, no date.

36. Ibid.

37. de Tocqueville, *Democracy in America*, 55.

38. Walter Whitcomb, letter to Blue Hill Municipal Officials, April 6, 2011, https://salsa.democracyinaction.org/o/1221/images/Whitcomb_Letter_Local_Food_Ordinance.pdf .

39. Steven Giguere, e-mail message to Hal Prince, June 14, 2011, subject: RE: Gravelwood Farm.

40. State of Maine and Walter Whitcomb, Commissioner, Department of Agriculture, Food and Rural Resources v. Dan Brown d/b/a Gravelwood Farms, Docket No. CV-11-70, Summons and Complaint for Injunctive Relief and Civil Monetary Penalties, November 3, 2011, https://salsa.democracyinaction.org/o/1221/images/gravelwood%20summons-1.pdf.

41. "We Are All Farmer Brown," Facebook page, http://www.facebook.com/wearefarmerbrown?sk=wall (accessed November 9, 2012).

42. "Farmer Dan Brown Tells His Story," YouTube video posted November 14, 2011, http://www.youtube.com/watch?v=NeS4RZ50uWU&feature=youtube.

43. Ibid.
44. State of Maine and Walter Whitcomb v. Dan Brown, Plaintiffs' Opposition to Defendants' Combined Motion for Summary Judgment and Opposition to Plaintiffs' Motion for Summary Judgment, July 16, 2012, http://www.thecompletepatient.com/sites/default/files/attachments/Maine-SummaryJudg-8-12.pdf.
45. Ibid.
46. Ibid.
47. Amy Robbins, e-mail message to Cookson Beecher, contributing writer, *Food Safety News*, November 29, 2011, subject: RE: raw milk/farmers markets.

CHAPTER TEN

1. Mark Steil, "Family Sues Farmer, Claims Son Sickened from *E. Coli* in Raw Milk," Minnesota Public Radio News, September 7, 2011, http://minnesota.publicradio.org/display/web/2011/09/07/e-coli-raw-milk-lawsuit/.
2. United States of America v. Daniel Allgyer, Memorandum by Judge Lawrence J. Stengel, February 2, 2012, 9, http://www.thecompletepatient.com/sites/default/files/allgyerjudgedecision2.pdf.
3. Ibid., 8.
4. "NMPF Urges Food and Drug Administration to Defend Laws against Raw Milk Sales," National Milk Producers Federation press release, November 1, 2011, http://nmpf.org/latest-news/press-releases/nov-2011/nmpf-urges-food-and-drug-administration-to-defend-laws-against-r.
5. United States of America v. Daniel Allgyer, Order of Permanent Injunction by Judge Lawrence F. Stengel, February 2, 2012, 1, http://www.thecompletepatient.com/sites/default/files/allgyerjudgedecision2.pdf.
6. Farm-to-Consumer Legal Defense Fund, Laurie Donnelly, et al. v. Kathleen Sebelius et al., Case No. C 10-4018-MWB, Iowa Northern District Court, Western Division, Memorandum Opinion and Order Regarding Defendants' Motion to Dismiss, March 30, 2012, http://www.farmtoconsumer.org/docs/order-033012-dismissing-case.pdf.
7. United States of America v. Daniel Allgyer, Memorandum by Judge Lawrence F. Stengel, February 2, 2012, 12, http://www.thecompletepatient.com/sites/default/files/allgyerjudgedecision2.pdf.
8. Tim Wightman, comment on "Maybe Dan Allgyer's Decision to Shut Down His PA Farm Will Help Us See More Clearly the Importance of Vernon Hershberger's Struggle; Debate on Raw Milk," *The Complete Patient* blog, February 14, 2012, http://www.thecompletepatient.com/article/2012/february/14/maybe-dan-allgyers-decision-shut-down-his-pa-farm-will-help-us-see-more.
9. Ibid.
10. Angela Doss, Online Petition in Support of Sharon Palmer and James Stewart, September 26, 2012, http://www.change.org/petitions/free-the-farmer-release-the-milkman-stop-the-wrongful-prosecution-of-sharon-palmer-james-stewart-drop-all-charges-immediately.
11. "Max Kane 'Calls Out' FDA to Enforce Law Against Moms.....WILL THE FDA SHOW UP on November 1st?" YouTube video posted October 22, 2011, http://www.youtube.com/watch?v=F8KfB7005UY.
12. State of Missouri et al. v. Morningland of the Ozarks, LLC, d/b/a Morningland Dairy, Case SD31390, Missouri Court of Appeals, Southern District, Division One, Appeal from the Circuit Court of Howell County, September 27, 2012.
13. "Caught on Tape: MN Dept of Ag Illegally Blockades Hartmann's Vehicle & Families' Food," YouTube video posted December 9, 2010, https://www.youtube.com/watch?v=ASahQ_cvHVE.
14. "MDA Statement on State of Minnesota v. Alvin Schlangen," Minnesota Department of Agriculture press release, September 20, 2012, http://www.mda.state.mn.us/news/releases/2012/nr-2012-09-20-milk.aspx.

INDEX

abbreviations for organizations, xiv
Abzug, Michael D., 119–20
Acheson, David, 152
Adesina, Kunle, 117, 118–19
Ali, Muhammad, 165
allergies, research on raw milk benefits, 55, 56–57
Allgyer, Daniel
    decision to leave farming, 205–6, 231
    FDA investigation, 35–36, 58, 77–79,
        150–51, 181, 203
    formation of Grassfed on the Hill, 14,
        15–16, 17–18
    inspections, 19–21
    judicial proceedings, 157–58, 203–5
    ProAdvocate Group relationship, 157
    rallies for, 150, 202
    RTCHF participation, 36, 99, 107, 157, 203
    Vonderplanitz, Aajonus relationship, 36,
        151, 157–58, 169
Allgyer, Rachel, 205
Alta Dena Dairy, 46–48
American Association of Medical Milk
    Commissions, 44
American Cheese Society, 129, 132
American Public Health Association, 47
Amish farmers. *See also specific people*
    allergy research on families, 56–57
    increasing food club participation, 17–18,
        65, 82, 83–85, 88
    ProAdvocate Group relationship, 155–57
    RTCHF participation, 99–107
    technology use, 81, 82, 83–85, 99, 175
    traditional agricultural practices, 13–14
antibiotics, routine use in meat production, 9
ARAMARK, 145–46
Ashmore, Audra, 133
asthma, research on raw milk benefits, 55, 56–57

bacteria. *See also specific types*
    pathogenic vs. friendly, 10
    research on, 59–60

baker's bills, 33
bake sales, regulatory crackdowns on, 6, 27
Ballou, Richard, 159
Beam, Stephen, 127, 128
Béchamp, Antoine, 42
Belle's Lunchbox, 67. *See also* Kane, Max
Benedict, Jeff, 139
Bernard, Claude, 42
Biblical references to food, 37
Blain, Tony, 116–17
Bledsoe, Laura, 25–27
Bloch, Victoria
    arrest, 161–64
    bail posting, 165, 166
    e-mail account search warrant, 120
    farmer's market work, 112
    judicial proceedings, 166–67, 207, 208
Blome, Jessica, 135–37
Blue Hill, Maine, food sovereignty ordinance,
    192, 195
Boston Tea Party (1773), 164
Bouis-Towe, Karine
    Allgyer, Daniel support, 150, 205–6
    FDA undercover investigation, 79
    food rights activism, 201
    Grassfed on the Hill involvement, 16–18, 229
    search for nutrient-dense foods, 12–16
Brown, Dan, 196–98, 230
Brown, Laura, 135–37
Brucella bacteria, 46, 67–68
Burgess, Warren, 75
Bush, George H. W., 148
Buttery, Lela, 152

CAFOs (concentrated animal feeding operations)
    Alta Dena case, 46
    ban on undercover filming of, 31
    distillery milk production, 39–41
    rise of, 137–38
California. *See also* Rawesome food club
    Alta Dena case, 46–48

Claravale Farm, 48, 50, 51, 87
GMO labeling bill defeat, 31
increase in raw milk sales, 50–54
lack of herdshare provisions, 180
Los Angeles raw milk sales, 50, 51
Organic Pastures Dairy Company, 51–52, 54, 86–87, 205
raw milk standards legislation, 127
San Francisco regulatory crackdowns, 6, 24, 27
Santa Cruz food sovereignty ordinance, 192
California Dairy Research Foundation, 64
California Department of Food and Agriculture (CDFA)
herdshare cease-and-desist notices, 180
Morningland Dairy case, 123–24, 127
Palmer, Sharon case, 95–97, 111–14, 118
Rawesome case, 113–16, 123–24, 158–59, 160, 162
California Franchise Tax Board, 160
Campbell, Karyn, 78
Campylobacter
chicken contamination, 9, 122
food club case, 104
Carter, Jimmy, 28
caseins, 56
CDC. *See* U.S. Centers for Disease Control and Prevention
CDFA. *See* California Department of Food and Agriculture
cell theory of disease, 42
Center for Food Safety and Applied Nutrition (CFSAN), 68
certified raw milk, 44
Chicago Seven trial, 147–48
chicken, pathogenic bacteria in, 9, 122
children, research on raw milk benefits, 55, 56–57
civil disobedience
Kentucky food club action, 209–10
overview, 200–201
Raw Milk Freedom Riders actions, 201, 210–11
civil liberties restrictions, 28
civil rights movement, 200
Claravale Farm, 48, 50, 51, 87
Cohen, Laurie, 201
The Colbert Report (television show), 152
Colby, Kate, 189
Colorado, herdshare legality, 110
commerce clause, 33–34

Commins, Denise B., 102
Community Alliance for Responsible Eco-farming (CARE), 65
Cooper, Anne, 70
Coppola, Eleanor, 90
Corabest, Ronald, 115
cottage food laws, 33
Cotton, Cathleen, 183
County Sheriff Project, 170, 171–72
cowshares. *See* herdshares and cowshares
Coxiella burnetii contamination, 46
Craig, Wayne, 173
criminal justice policy, 147–49
Cryptosporidium-related illnesses, 187–90
Csengeri, Emoke, 116

Dahlstrom, Karl, 155–57
dairy industry. *See* raw milk
DATCP. *See* Wisconsin Department of Agriculture, Trade, and Consumer Protection
deaths, from food-borne illness, 143
Debre, Patrice, 42
Declaration of Food Freedom petition, 186
Declaration of Food Independence, 237
Defort, Eric, 176
Del Bueno, 130
Democracy in America (de Tocqueville), 179, 185
de Tocqueville, Alexis, 179, 180, 181, 185, 186, 195
disease, competing theories of, 41, 42–43
Dixon, Denise
closing of dairy, 230
embargo and recall of cheese, 129, 131, 132
FDA inspection, 133–34
history of Morningland Dairy, 125–27
trial, 134–37
Dixon, Isaac, 133
Dixon, Joseph
closing of dairy, 230
embargo and recall of cheese, 129, 132
FDA inspection, 133–34
history of Morningland Dairy, 125–27
trial, 134–37
Doffing-Baynes, Michelle, 214, 218–19, 220–22, 223
Dole recall, 131
Dominguez, Raymond, 153
Donnalley, Robert, 112–13, 116
Dukakis, Michael, 148
E. coli O157:H7

CAFOs and, 138
Hartmann, Michael case, 71–72, 202
Jack in the Box case, 139
spinach outbreak, 63
sprouts outbreak, 189
The Economist (journal), 60
Ehlenfeldt, Robert, 67–68
Emord, Jonathan, 150–51
Estrella, Kelli, 193–94
Estrella Family Creamery, 34, 193–94
Evans, Deborah, 184–85, 187, 192
expansion of regulatory authority. *See* regulatory
authority expansion

Fallon, Sally, 37, 55, 88
Falls, Don, 128, 129, 130, 135–36
farms. *See also* industrialized food system;
small-scale food producers
difficulties of local agriculture, 87–89
perception of sanitary conditions, 29–31
FarmTek, 97
Farm-to-Consumer Legal Defense Fund (FTCLDF)
Brown, Dan case, 196
guidance on herdshares, 100–101
Hochstetler/Hebron case, 104
interstate raw milk ban case, 34–35, 204–5
Maine raw milk conflict, 182
Manna Storehouse case, 24
Morningland Dairy case, 230
Quail Hollow Farm case, 25, 26
Schlangen, Alvin case, 215
Traditional Foods Minnesota case, 75
Vonderplanitz, Aajonus and, 101
Wagoner, Eric case, 70–71
FDA. *See* U.S. Food and Drug Administration (FDA)
fermented foods, 60–61
Ferris, Phillip, 67, 176
Fiedler, Patrick, 173
Filburn, Wickard v. (1942), 33
Florida
CAFO undercover filming ban legislation, 31
food club delivery confiscation, 1–4
Florida Department of Agriculture and
Consumer Services Food Safety Division, 1
Florida Department of Alcohol, Tobacco, and
Firearms, 1
Food, Drug, and Cosmetic Act (1938), 137,
170–71, 204

Food and Drug Administration. *See* U.S. Food
and Drug Administration (FDA)
food-borne illness. *See also specific types*
CDC estimates, 9, 55, 122, 142–43, 187, 197
deaths from, 143
focus on pathogens, 31–32, 61–62
food clubs. *See* private food arrangements;
specific groups
Food for Maine's Future, 88
"foodie" trends, 29
food safety. *See also* food-borne illness
crisis atmosphere, 141–42
increasing focus on pathogens, 10, 31–32, 137–44
terrorism concerns, 27–29
Food Safety Modernization Act (2011), 32,
62–63, 140
food security, 28–29
food shortages, 7–8
food sovereignty
conflict with state laws, 194–98
growing number of state initiatives, 199
Maine initiatives, 183, 185–87, 191–98
Forage SF, 6, 24
Forbes, 22–23
Forest Grove Dairy. *See* Hochstetler, David
Freedom Farms Co-op. *See* Schlangen, Alvin
FTCLDF. *See* Farm-to-Consumer Legal Defense Fund

GABRIELA study, 56
Garthwaite, Ron, 50, 51, 163–64
genetically-modified organisms (GMOs), 31
Georgia Department of Agriculture, 69, 70
Georgia food club case, 68–71
Gerard, Chris, 113
germ theory of disease, 41, 42–43
Giguere, Steven, 194
Glassburner, Mary, 144
Goldstein, Ross, 169, 170–71
*Government Bullies: How Everyday Americans Are
Being Harassed, Abused, and Imprisoned by the
Feds* (Paul and Paul), 149
Grade A milk, 45
Grassfed on the Hill food club. *See also* Allgyer, Daniel
FDA lack of action against members, 150
FDA warning letter, 58
formation of, 16–18
loss of Daniel Allgyer, 205–6
resurrection of, 229

RTCHF participation, 36, 99, 107, 203
undercover investigation of, 77–79
Grazin' Acres farm. *See* Hershberger, Vernon
Greenberg, Blue, 146
Green Oaks Creek Farm, 145
Guidry, Diana, 133

halacha (Jewish law), 146
Haney, Deborah, 19
Hansen, Nathan, 215, 216–18, 219, 223
Hardin, Jesse, 78
Harman, Chris, 167
Hartley, Robert, 39–41
Hartmann, Michael, 71–74, 202, 208–9
hazard analysis critical control points
(HACCP) plans, 146
Hazon, 144–46
Healthy Family Farms. *See* Palmer, Sharon
Healthy People 2020 initiative, 62
Hebron, Richard, 61, 102–5, 110, 168
Hemingway, Eric, 225–26
herdshares and cowshares
judge mistaken view of, 203–4
lease agreements vs., 99–101
Maryland ban, 16, 204
Michigan case, 110
Ohio case, 109–10
Schlangen, Alvin jury question, 223
varying interpretations of regulations, 101,
105, 110, 180
Wisconsin case, 35
Hershberger, Andrew, 176
Hershberger, Vernon
judicial proceedings, 172–77, 231
raid and searches by DATCP, 105–6, 172, 176
rallies for, 202
RTCHF participation, 106
Vonderplanitz, Aajonus relationship, 174, 175
Hetherington, Eric, 167, 208
Hetherington, Mary, 94–95, 167, 208
Hochstetler, David, 102–5, 110, 168–72, 202
Hoenig, Donald, 182–83, 188–89, 190
Hoffman, Abbie, 147
Holst, Ted, 112–13, 115–16
homeschooling movement, 200
homogenization implementation, 45
Horton, Willie, 148
Human Microbiome Project, 59

Ike's Pump & Drilling Inc., 97
Illinois
CAFO undercover filming ban legislation, 31
Hochstetler/Hebron case, 102, 104, 168
Kane, Max case, 68
Raw Milk Freedom Riders actions, 211
immune system, 42–43, 61–62
Indiana
Hochstetler, David case, 102–5, 110, 168–72, 202
Kane, Max case, 68
industrialized food system
consolidation of, 22–23, 138
distillery milk production, 39–41
evolution of, 22–23
food safety fears, 144–46
unintended consequences of, 8–10
unsanitary milk production, 39–41, 43–45
International Milk Genomics Consortium, 57
Internet use. *See also* YouTube videos
Brown, Dan, 196
Marler, Bill, 139–40, 141–42, 143–44
interstate commerce
confusing food safety oversight, 180
raw dairy ban, 6, 17, 47–48, 181, 204–5
investigational new drug (IND) applications, 64
Iowa
CAFO undercover filming ban, 31
food sovereignty proposal, 199
interstate raw milk ban case, 34–35, 204–5

Jack in the Box *E. coli* case, 139
Johnson, Kathryn Niflis, 74–75, 216–19, 225
Jones, Cathy, 116–17
Joseph, Inge, 7

Kaehler, Maurice, 159, 164
Kane, Max, 66–68, 121–22, 173, 210–11
Kansas, CAFO undercover filming ban, 31
Kelley, Megan, 189–90
Kennedy, Pete, 75, 174
Kentucky
food club civil disobedience, 209–10
Oaks, Gary case, 61
Kentucky Department for Public Health, 209

labeling
Allgyer, Daniel inspection, 20–21
defeat of GMO labeling bill, 31

medical claims on food, 64
lease agreement model, 99–101, 104–5
LeCavalier, Michele, 116
Lemonade Freedom Day, 27
lemonade stand shutdowns/protests, 27, 211
LePage, Paul, 192–95
licensing issues. *See also* food sovereignty;
   herdshares and cowshares
     Hershberger, Vernon case, 105, 173, 174
     lemonade stands, 27
     Maine two-tier raw milk regulation, 181–83,
       184, 187, 189, 193, 197, 230
     Manna Storehouse case, 24
     Palmer, Sharon case, 95–96, 97, 207
     Sandvig, Rae Lynn case, 73–74
     Schlangen, Alvin case, 76, 211, 212, 216,
       219, 220, 222, 225, 226
     Schmitmeyer, Carol case, 109
Listeria bacteria
     FDA recall cases, 130–31
     Morningland Dairy case, 123–24, 127, 134,
       135, 136, 146
Liu, Anita, 116
Lorain County Health Department, 23–24
Los Angeles, California. *See also* Rawesome food club
     private raw milk distribution, 52
     raw milk retail sales, 50, 51
Los Angeles County Department of Public
   Health, 115, 116, 160
Los Angeles County District Attorney
     Bloch, Victoria case, 161, 163
     Palmer, Sharon case, 152–54, 161, 163
     Rawesome food club case, 115–16, 117, 119,
       120, 124, 160
     Stewart, James case, 161, 163
Los Angeles Department of Building and Safety, 160
Los Angeles Police Department, 160
Los Angeles Times, 117
Louisville Metro Department of Health and
   Wellness, 209

Mack, Richard, 170
Maine
     Brown, Dan case, 196–98, 230
     chicken slaughter regulations, 184
     cryptosporidium-related illnesses, 187–90
     food sovereignty initiatives, 183, 185–87,
       191–92, 194–98, 199

home rule provisions, 197
     private raw milk sales proposed legislation,
       56, 192, 193
     two-tier raw milk regulation, 181–83, 184,
       187, 189, 193, 197, 230
Maine Center for Disease Control and
   Prevention, 188, 190
Maine Department of Agriculture, Food, and
   Rural Resources
     Brown, Dan case, 196
     chicken slaughter regulations, 184
     cryptosporidium-related illnesses, 187, 190
     efforts to defeat private raw milk sales
       legislation, 192
     raw milk regulation crackdown, 182, 183, 192–95
Maine Freedom of Access Act, 182
Malcolm X, 164–65
Manfredi, Joe, 108
Manna Storehouse food club, 23–24
Markel, Wayne, 93–94, 167
Marler, Bill, 138–42, 143–44
Maryland. *See also* Grassfed on the Hill food club
     formation of food clubs, 16–17
     intolerance of raw dairy, 16, 204
     loss of revenues to neighboring states, 88
     pasteurization requirements, 45
     Raw Milk Freedom Riders actions, 210–11
Massachusetts
     herdshare cease-and-desist notice, 180
     raw milk permit limitations, 45
Mayo Foundation, 43
McAfee, Mark
     FDA open-ended inspections request, 205
     Kane, Max support, 67
     protest for Rawesome Three, 163
     raw milk sales, 51–52, 54, 86–87
     Stewart, James bail posting, 168, 207
     Vonderplanitz, Aajonus relationship, 51, 86, 87
MDA. *See* Minnesota Department of Agriculture
Meadowsweet Dairy, 30–31, 34, 111
Metchnikoff, Élie, 42–43
Michigan
     cherry health benefits labeling, 64
     feral pig ban, 63–64
     Hebron, Richard case, 61, 102–5, 110, 168
     herdshare legality, 110
     Kane, Max case, 68
     pasteurization requirements, 45

Michigan Department of Agriculture and Rural Development, 103
Michigan Department of Natural Resources, 63–64
microbiome research, 59–60
Miles, Danny, 97
milieu theory of disease, 42
milk, raw. *See* raw milk
Miller, Amos
    farming operations, 81–87
    FDA search and inspection, 154
    ProAdvocate Group relationship, 155–57
    RTCHF participation, 101–2
Miller, Becky, 81, 84
Miller, Ben, 84
Minneapolis Star Tribune, 74, 76, 225
Minnesota. *See also* Schlangen, Alvin
    CAFO undercover filming ban legislation, 31
    Hartmann, Michael case, 71–74, 76–77, 208–9
    Traditional Foods Minnesota case, 74–77
Minnesota Department of Agriculture (MDA)
    Hartmann, Michael case, 72
    relationship with FDA, 76–77
    Sandvig, Rae Lynn case, 72, 73–74, 208–9
    Schlangen, Alvin case, 212–13, 214–16, 225, 227, 230–31
    Traditional Foods Minnesota case, 74–77
Miranda rights, 148
Missouri, Morningland Dairy case. *See* Morningland Dairy
Missouri Milk Board, 126, 129, 130, 131, 134, 135
Mitterholzer, John, 74, 75
Montana, CAFO undercover filming ban, 31
Moody, John, 199, 209–10
Morningland Dairy
    CDFA and FDA press releases, 123–24
    closing, 230
    embargo and recall of cheese, 127–32
    FDA inspection, 132–34
    history of, 124–27
    Marler, Bill blog posts, 143–44
    order to destroy cheese, 134
    previous voluntary recall, 136–37
    Rawesome food club relationship, 54, 123–24, 126
    trial, 134–37, 146
Muhl, Levi J., 215, 216

Nader, Ralph, 47

National Institutes of Health, 59
National Milk Producers Federation, 204
Nevada, Quail Hollow Farm dinner inspection, 25–27
New York City, pasteurization implementation, 43–44
New York Department of Agriculture and Markets, 111
New York State
    Meadowsweet Dairy case, 30–31, 34, 111
    raw milk permit limitations, 45
Ngo, Celene, 116
Nguyen, Terrance, 117
Nolt, Mark, 36, 61
nutrient-dense foods. *See also* raw milk
    research on microbes and, 60–61
    types of, 57–58

Oaks, Gary, 61
Obama, Barack, 32
O'Donnell, John, 193, 194, 195
Odwalla apple juice case, 139
Ohio
    food sovereignty proposal, 199
    herdshare legality, 110
    Manna Storehouse raid, 23–24
    pasteurization requirements, 45
    Schmitmeyer, Carol case, 109–10
Ohio Department of Agriculture, 23–24, 109–10
The Omnivore's Dilemma (Pollan), 141
Ontario, Canada, herdshare case, 110
Organic Pastures Dairy Company, 51–52, 54, 86–87, 205
Organic Valley Family of Farms, 66
Otting, Larry
    bail posting, 167
    Organic Pastures Dairy Company support, 51
    Palmer, Sharon relationship, 91, 92, 95, 153–54, 231
Owens, Jackie, 176

Palmer, Sharon
    arrests of, 114, 161–64, 167–68
    bail postings, 166, 167–68
    e-mail account search warrant, 120
    farmer's market visits by investigators, 111–14
    financing for Healthy Family Farms, 91–95
    judicial proceedings, 166–67, 206–8, 230
    Otting, Larry relationship, 91, 92, 95, 153–54, 231
    outsourcing allegations, 152–54

raids of farm, 95–98, 114, 117–18

Rawesome food club supplier relationship, 89, 92–95, 151, 152–54

real estate financial troubles, 89–91

Stewart, James relationship, 89, 91, 92, 95, 153–54

Vonderplanitz, Aajonus relationship, 93, 151, 153–54, 231

PARSIFAL (Prevention of Allergy-Risk Factors for Sensitization in Children Related to Farming and Anthroposophic Lifestyle) study, 55–56

Pasteur, Louis, 41–43

pasteurization

effects on whey proteins, 56

history of, 41, 43–45

pathogens. *See also specific types*

increasing focus on, 10, 31–32, 137–44

in industrial food, 9

Paul, Rand, 149

Paul, Ron, 149, 152, 205

Pearce, David, 20

Pennsylvania. *See also* Grassfed on the Hill food club

Florida food club confiscation incident, 1–4

increasing popularity of food clubs, 65

Miller, Amos case, 81–87, 101–2

Nolt, Mark case, 36

Rawesome food club suppliers, 86–87

Raw Milk Freedom Riders actions, 210–11

raw milk market, 45, 88

Penobscot, Maine, food sovereignty ordinance, 192

PFGE (pulsed-field gel electrophoresis), 71–72

Poisoned: The True Story of the Deadly E. Coli Outbreak That Changed the Way Americans Eat (Benedict), 139

Pollan, Michael, 141

Powell, Terrance, 117

Prince, Hal, 182, 183, 188

prison population increases, 148, 149

Pritzker, Fred, 141

private food arrangements. *See also* herdshares and cowshares; *specific groups; specific people*

food sovereignty initiatives, 183, 185–87, 191–92

history of, 21–22, 199–200

labeling issues, 20–21

lack of constitutional coverage, 33

lease agreement model, 99–101, 104–5

regulatory authority expansion into, 4–7

varying interpretations of regulations, 179–81, 212

ProAdvocate Group, 155–57

probiotics research, 64

Public Citizen, 47

Public Health Security and Bioterrorism Preparedness and Response Act (2002), 28

pulsed-field gel electrophoresis (PFGE), 71–72

Pure Food and Drug Act (1906), 137

Quackwatch, 47

Quail Hollow Farm, 25–27

Quill's End Farm. *See* Retberg, Heather

Rabins, Iso, 24

Rainbow Acres Farm. *See* Allgyer, Daniel

Rawesome food club

Amish suppliers, 86–87, 102, 154

formation and growth of, 52–54

judicial proceedings, 116–17, 166–67, 206–8

member responses to raids, 118, 159–60, 162–63, 164

Morningland Dairy relationship, 54, 123–24, 126, 128, 129

Palmer, Sharon involvement, 89, 92–95, 151, 152–54, 206–8

raids and regulator visits, 52–54, 113–16, 123, 160, 162

reopening after raid, 118–19

sealing of search warrant supporting documents, 119–20

splintering into new groups, 229

success in standing up to regulators, 53–54, 99

testing of confiscated foods, 123–24, 128

undercover purchases from, 158–59

raw milk. *See also* herdshares and cowshares

attempted cryptosporidium link, 187–90

CDC memo, 37–38, 194

CDC survey, 55, 64

certified, 44

criticism of, 37–38, 56

difficulty acquiring, 12–13

distillery milk production, 39–41

fermented products, 61

FTCLDF case, 34–35, 204–5

Georgia black dye proposal, 69

health benefits of, 43, 55–57, 103

history of pasteurization, 41

increasing popularity of, 54–55

industrialized production of, 38–41, 43–45

interstate commerce ban, 6, 17, 47–48, 181, 204–5

lease agreements, 99–101

Maine two-tier regulatory approach, 181–83, 184, 187, 189, 193, 197, 230

production quality standards, 100

traditional consumption of, 38

varying state and federal regulation, 180–81

Raw Milk Association of Colorado, 110

Raw Milk Freedom Riders, 201, 210–11, 237

Reader's Digest Canada, 60

Reagan, Ronald, 47

Reardon, Joseph, 77

regulatory authority expansion. *See also specific agencies; specific cases*

economic impact of, 88

Food Safety Modernization Act powers, 32

overview of, 4–7

varying interpretations of, 179–81

Regulatory Procedures Manual (FDA), 130

Reiners, Jim, 125, 126

Reiners, Marge, 125, 126

Reitzig, Liz

Allgyer, Daniel support, 150, 205

FDA undercover investigation, 79

food rights activism, 201–2, 210–11

Grassfed on the Hill involvement, 16–18, 229

Retberg, Heather

food sovereignty activism, 183–86, 187, 192

regulator interactions, 187–89, 193–94

Reynolds, Guy, 176–77

The Rights of the People: How Our Search for Safety Invades Our Liberties (Shipler), 28

Right to Choose Healthy Food (RTCHF)

Allgyer, Daniel participation, 36, 99, 107, 157, 203

formation of, 34

Hershberger, Vernon participation, 106

Hochstetler, David participation, 102–5, 168–72

lease agreement model, 99–101, 104–5

Miller, Amos participation, 101–2

quality standards, 100

Rawesome food club relationship, 53, 93

Robbins, Amy, 190

Roettger, James, 214–15, 216

Rogers, Brad, 170–72

Rosborough, Michael, 68

Rosen, Tommy, 118

Rostami, Edward, 89–91

RTCHF. *See* Right to Choose Healthy Food

Rubin, Jerry, 147

Rushing Waters Fisheries, 131

Sakir, Kelly, 165

Salatin, Joel, 88, 121

Salmonella bacteria

Alta Dena alleged contamination, 46–47

chicken contamination, 9, 122

Sanders, Mary Ellen, 64

Sandvig, Greg, 72, 76, 209

Sandvig, Rae Lynn, 72–74, 76, 208–9

San Francisco, California, regulatory crack-downs, 6, 24, 27

Santa Cruz, California, food sovereignty ordinance, 192

Schafer, Joshua, 19, 20

Schlangen, Alice, 212–13, 214

Schlangen, Alvin

administrative case against, 230–31

defense arguments, 216–19, 223

delay in trial, 211–12

e-mail to supporters, 224

jury deliberations and decision, 223–27

prosecution arguments, 214–16, 222, 223

searches of property and van, 76, 212–13

testimony at trial, 219–22

Schmid, Ron, 46

Schmidt, Michael, 110, 201–2

Schmitmeyer, Carol, 109–10

Schuler, Irene, 90

Schwarzenegger, Arnold, 127

Scott, Fred, 113

Sedgwick, Maine, food sovereignty ordinance, 191–92

September 11, 2001 terrorist attacks, 27–28

Shapley, Stephanie L., 78, 79

Sharma-Wilson, Ajna, 230

Sheehan, John

Grassfed on the Hill case, 77

lack of response to Raw Milk Freedom Riders, 211

raw milk criticism, 37, 56

testimony on Maine legislation, 56, 192

Sheen, Martin, 51

Shipler, David K., 28

Small, Robert, 214

small-scale food producers. *See also specific people*

Food Safety Modernization Act partial exemption, 32, 62–63

lack of help from state legislatures, 185, 193

low prices for dairy, 65

Smith, Barb, 111

Smith, Steve, 111

Smithfield Foods, 22
Solorio, Marco, 116
South Carolina, raw milk suppliers for food clubs, 69
spinach *E. coli* outbreak (2006), 63
Staphylococcus aureus
    Alta Dena alleged contamination, 46
    Morningland Dairy case, 127
Stengel, Lawrence J., 157–58, 169, 203–5
Stewart, James
    arrests of, 160–64, 167–68
    bail postings, 165–66, 167–68
    The Colbert Report appearance, 152
    hearing, 116–17
    judicial proceedings, 166–67, 207–8, 229–30
    McAfee, Mark relationship, 51–52, 87
    Morningland Dairy relationship, 126
    Palmer, Sharon relationship, 89, 91, 92, 95, 153–54
    private raw milk distribution, 52
    ProAdvocate Group relationship, 155
    Rawesome food club involvement, 52–54, 86–87, 114, 116–17, 118, 120, 229–30
    retail distribution of raw milk, 50, 51–52
    Vonderplanitz, Aajonus relationship, 48, 49–54, 151–52, 154, 201, 231
Stowers, Jacqueline, 23–24
Stowers, John, 23–24
St. Peter, Bob, 88, 192
Straus, Nathan, 43
Stringer, Larry, 68
Strong, Mia, 192
Swigart, John Richard. *See* Vonderplanitz, Aajonus

terrorism, food safety concerns and, 27–29
Tester-Hagan amendment, 32
Thompson, Michele, 130, 131
Traditional Foods Minnesota, 74–77, 218–19
Trenton, Maine, food sovereignty ordinance, 192
Treviso, Scarlett, 96–97, 111–16, 159, 231
Tyson Foods, 22–23

Underground Market (San Francisco), 24
unpasteurized milk. *See* raw milk
U.S. Centers for Disease Control and Prevention (CDC)
    Alta Dena case, 46–47
    food-borne illness estimates, 9, 55, 122, 142–43, 187, 197
    food-borne illness website, 140

Healthy People 2020 initiative, 62
historical summary of pasteurization, 44–45
Maine case supporting material, 197
memo on raw milk, 37–38, 194
survey on raw milk consumption, 55, 64
U.S. Constitution
    commerce clause, 33
    County Sheriff Project and, 170
    fugitive slave clause, 164
    privacy protections, 108–9
    right to jury trial, 227
    supremacy clause, 170–71
U.S. Department of Agriculture (USDA), 1, 2, 57, 58
U.S. Food and Drug Administration (FDA)
    Allgyer, Daniel case, 19–21, 35–36, 77–79, 150–51, 181, 203
    cheese producer inspections, 132–33
    claimed lack of action against individuals, 181, 204
    Estrella Creamery case, 34, 193–94
    Florida case possible involvement, 2, 3
    Food Safety Modernization Act powers, 32, 62–63
    food security actions, 28–29
    Georgia case possible involvement, 69–71
    Grassfed on the Hill case, 77–79
    Hershberger, Vernon case, 173
    Hochstetler/Hebron case, 103, 104–5, 168–72
    Maine raw milk legislation defeat, 192, 193
    medical claims on food, 64
    Miller, Amos search and inspection, 154
    Minnesota cases possible involvement, 76–77
    Morningland Dairy case, 123–24, 130, 131–37
    proposed amendment to decrease powers, 149
    raw dairy crackdowns, 64, 66, 69–71
    raw dairy interstate commerce ban, 6, 35, 47–48
    Rawesome food club case, 115, 116, 117, 123–24, 160, 162
    Raw Milk Freedom Riders response, 210–11
    recalls, 130–31
    state-level relationships, 77
U.S. Justice Department
    Allgyer, Daniel case, 150, 157, 203
    Chicago Seven trial, 147
    Hochstetler/Hebron case, 169, 170, 171, 172
    Wagoner, Eric case, 70
U.S. Public Health Service Commissioned Corps, 132–34
U.S. Supreme Court, 33–34, 109, 148, 156, 157, 200
Utah, CAFO undercover filming ban, 31

vaccination, history of, 42
Ventura County, California
    Palmer, Sharon investigation, 97, 118,
        152–54, 161, 166, 167–68, 207, 230
    Stewart, James investigation, 167–68,
        207, 229–30
Villasenor, Teresa, 116
Virginia
    food sovereignty proposal, 199
    formation of food clubs, 16–17
    pasteurization requirements, 45
Vonderplanitz, Aajonus. *See also* Right to Choose
Healthy Food
    Allgyer, Daniel relationship, 36, 151,
        157–58, 169
    cross complaint filing, 157–58
    e-mail account search warrant, 120
    FTCLDF and, 101
    Hershberger, Vernon relationship, 174, 175
    Hochstetler/Hebron case, 168, 169
    McAfee, Mark relationship, 51, 86, 87
    nutrition interests, 48–49, 50, 107–8,
        116, 121
    Palmer, Sharon relationship, 93, 151,
        153–54, 231
    Rawesome food club involvement, 52–54,
        86–87, 118, 119, 165
    Stewart, James relationship, 48, 49–54,
        151–52, 154, 201, 231
    success in standing up to regulators,
        53–54, 99–107

Wagoner, Eric, 68–71
Wallace, Mike, 198
Walters, Ann, 215–16
Ward, Ken, 112–14, 117, 119, 153
Washington, DC
    formation of food clubs, 16, 17, 18
    Raw Milk Freedom Riders actions, 211
Washington State, Estrella Family Creamery
    case, 34, 193–94

Washington State University, 141
Weber, Susan, 30–31
Weston A. Price Foundation
    national conferences, 81, 82, 94, 95
    support for nutrient-dense foods, 37, 57, 143
whey proteins, 56
Whitcomb, Walter, 193, 194, 196
Whole Foods, 143
Wickard v. Filburn (1942), 33
Wightman, Tim, 206
Willis, Marybeth, 70
Winterhawk, Jerel, 116
Wisconsin
    failed raw milk sales legislation, 143
    Hershberger, Vernon case, 105–6, 172–73,
        176, 202, 231
    judge on right to own and use cow, 6, 35, 111
    Kane, Max case, 66–68
    Raw Milk Freedom Riders actions, 211
Wisconsin Department of Agriculture, Trade,
    and Consumer Protection (DATCP)
    contaminated fish case, 131
    FDA funding, 173
    herdshare case, 35
    Hershberger, Vernon case, 105–6, 172–73, 176
    Kane, Max case, 67–68
Wiseman, Gene, 126, 127–29, 135
World War II (1939-1945), food shortages,
    5–6, 7–8
Wyoming, food sovereignty proposal, 199

Yao, John, 116
York, Jedadiah, 129, 130, 131, 133
YouTube videos
    Brown, Dan, 196
    Hershberger, Vernon, 175, 176
    Kane, Max, 67, 211
    Rawesome food club raid, 115
    Wagoner, Eric, 69, 71

Zinniker, Mark, 173

ABOUT THE AUTHOR

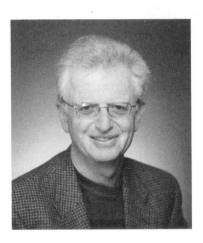

DAVID E. GUMPERT has become a nationally recognized writer and authority on the intersection of food, health, and business by virtue of his widely acclaimed book *The Raw Milk Revolution: Behind America's Emerging Battle Over Food Rights*, as well as his provocative and popular blog, *The Complete Patient* (www.thecompletepatient. com), and his many articles about food rights on Grist.org and The Huffington Post. He gained behind-the-scenes access to the key participants and vast government documentation necessary to write *Life, Liberty, and the Pursuit of Food Rights*. A former reporter with *The Wall Street Journal* and editor at *Inc.* and *Harvard Business Review*, Gumpert has brought his considerable investigative and journalistic experience and business expertise (author or coauthor of seven books about small business and entrepreneurship) to bear in articulating the corporate, legal, and political forces driving *Life, Liberty, and the Pursuit of Food Rights*.